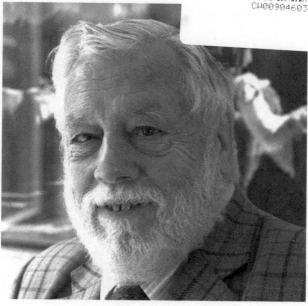

Roger Windsor studied at the Royal (Dick) Veterinary College, part of the University of Edinburgh. After spending some time in veterinary practice in the UK, he went to work in Kenya and soon became head of the Veterinary Diagnosis Laboratory there. Back in the UK a spell at Norwich Veterinary Investigation Centre made Roger realise that he had found his niche as a 'vet detective', a career he went on to pursue with great success in Kenya, Argentina and Botswana. This book is his story up to that point, although he later also worked in Peru, and was awarded an MBE for his work there. Now retired, he runs an art gallery in Scotland.

MORE SHERLOCK HOLMES THAN JAMES HERRIOT

The Veterinary Detectives

Roger S. Windsor

The Book Guild Ltd

Published in Great Britain in 2016 by
The Book Guild Ltd
9 Priory Business Park
Wistow Road, Kibworth
Leics, LE8 0RX

Typeset in Times

Printed and bound in Great Britain by
CPI Group (UK) Ltd, Croydon, CR0 4YY

A catalogue record for this book is available from
The British Library.

ISBN 978 1 911320 11 1

Dedication

This book is dedicated to my former boss, mentor and friend,
Sherwin A. Hall,
with thanks and affection.

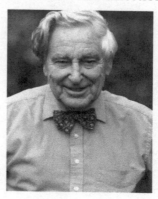

Sadly Sherwin died on Wednesday 20 August and so never saw the published book; however he lives on in these pages.

It is also dedicated to the memory of three other teachers and friends who had a great influence on my work and career:

Professor	Maurycy	Professor Walter
Ian S. Beattie	**(Maryk) Gitter**	**Plowright**
		CMG FRS.

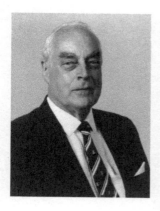 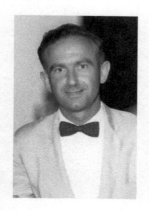 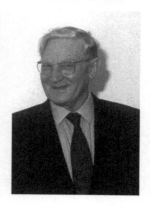

Contents

Foreword
by Sir Ketumile Masire,
former President of the Republic of
Botswana

I am delighted that Dr Windsor has decided to write a memoir of his life and work; he arrived in Botswana at a time when we were experiencing a dramatic increase in our exports of beef. To achieve our European quotas we needed to build up our services to the live-stock industry. We were lucky that the Food and Agriculture Organisation of the United Nations had sent a team under Dr Nick Buck to assist with the animal husbandry aspects of livestock production, and that Dr Jack Falconer and his team in the Department of Veterinary Services, thanks to the excellent vaccine produced by the Botswana Vaccine Institute, had finally brought foot and mouth disease under control. What was needed was a good veterinary diagnostic labora-tory to provide our farmers with the services they required. Dr Windsor set about this task with knowledge and enthusiasm and soon he built, in his own words, 'a rainbow coalition' of scientists both male and female: Batswana, British, Dutch, Indian, Kenyan, Lesothan, Norwegian, Sri Lankan and Tanzanian, all dedicated to providing my people with these services. Once his team was complete Dr Windsor set about field investigations to determine what were the diseases limiting animal production, and teams from the laboratory visited farms and 'cattle posts' throughout the country, including my own farm in Ghanzi, where they identified our problems.

When he arrived the laboratory was housed in temporary build-ings that were erected when the capital of Botswana was moved from Mafeking to Gaborone. These premises were shared with the medical laboratory and were totally inadequate for the tasks that were

ix

required. With financial assistance from the African Development Bank, Dr Windsor and his team were able to design, build and equip what is now the National Veterinary Laboratory at Sebele, a building that is as beautiful as it is useful and must rank as one of the most elegant buildings in Botswana.

What he does not say in his book is that within a few weeks of arrival in the country he was invited to become President of the Botswana Veterinary Association and he converted what had been a political talking shop into a fully fledged scientific association, which took up membership of the Commonwealth and World Veterinary Associations, and held an annual scientific meeting. I was guest of honour at the last annual dinner over which Dr Windsor presided and I noticed that there were visiting scientists from outside my country giving talks to the meeting.

Roger's services to Botswana were not only in the field of veterinary medicine but he and his wife, Maxine, were very active in the cultural life of the capital. My wife and I attended many concerts at which Maxine either gave a solo piano performance or accompanied choirs, individual singers or solo instrumentalists. Roger was responsible for staging *Cry the Beloved Country* – the play that tells of the travails of our neighbour South Africa during the apartheid regime, and bringing schoolchildren from the whole country to see it. Dr Alan Paton, the author, and his wife graced the premiere of the production, which was staged on my birthday, and it gave me great pleasure to entertain Dr Paton at State House during his visit. My wife Gladys was able to use Roger's talents when she was involved with the design and construction of our National Youth Centre.

Having previously worked in Kenya and Argentina, Roger went on to use his knowledge and experience to develop veterinary services in southern Peru, but returned to Botswana to assist us when we experienced a devastating outbreak of contagious bovine pleuropneumonia in the north of my country. On the occasion of his last visit to Botswana with his wife we were able to have lunch together in Lobatse.

I am delighted that he has written a memoir of his stay in my country and it is obvious from what he has written that he, like many other visitors to Botswana, fell in love with the land and its people. I wish Roger and his family all happiness and I hope that many people will read and enjoy this delightful book and then decide that they must come to Botswana.

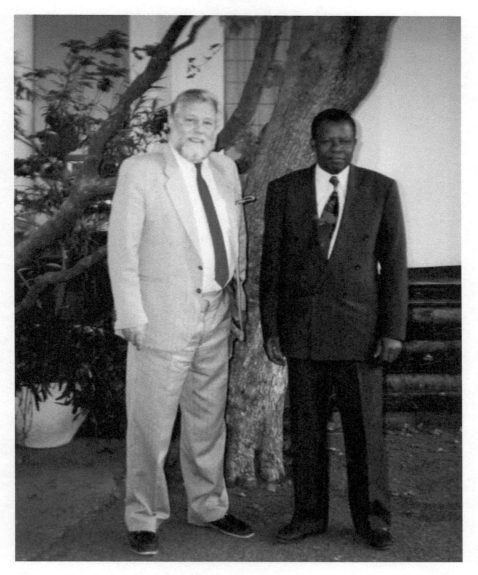

The author with the then President of Botswana, HE Sir Ketumile Masire, in the garden of State House, Gaborone.

Acknowledgements

I thank my wife, Maxine, for her encouragement and help: she corrected the spelling and the grammar and removed the bits she did not like. Frank and Mary Barrie were of great assistance to me and their boundless enthusiasm kept me at the keyboard; they were responsible for a change in the format of the book and advised me either to increase or reduce the amount of explanation of the technical terms! Their help was invaluable. The surgeon Iain McLaren and his physician wife Fiona read the manuscript and gave me very good advice. I sent pertinent sections of the book to many colleagues who are mentioned in the book for their assistance in checking that I had my facts right and I am indebted to Varshika Manji, Monyi Gadek (Brenda Mtui in the early chapters), Ken Digby and Eddie and Jean Bradley for their comments: I made the necessary corrections. That said, all the errors are mine alone. Sherwin gave me his photograph and I am grateful to Elliot Beattie and David Gitter for the photographs of their respective fathers and to Dorothy Plowright for the photograph of her husband. Jean Sanger provided some of the photographs of Ashmore, Brian Ranson gave me the photographs of my days at Bancroft's School, and Ken Digby provided photographs of working in the field in Botswana.

The author is grateful to the Director of the Veterinary Research Institute, Onderstepoort, South Africa for permission to publish the photograph of the great rinderpest outbreak of 1896.

Finally I thank my son Richard for his work in cleaning photographs, which in some cases were more than fifty years old.

And last, but not least, my thanks to Shirley Newall, my former secretary, for all her hard work with the index.

PART 1
What it's all About

1

How it All Began

'I am inclined to think –' said I.
'I should do so,' Sherlock Holmes remarked impatiently.
Sir Arthur Conan Doyle, *The Valley of Fear*

'Roger, I think that you had better come to reception, there is a farmer here who suspects that his pheasants are dying from Venezuelan equine encephalitis.' That was Joan the receptionist in the Cambridge Veterinary Investigation Centre.

'I'll be right there,' I said, and put down the phone. As its name implies, Venezuelan equine encephalitis is a disease of horses restricted to the Americas. The disease is unpleasant, usually fatal and manifests itself with various nervous signs. It is spread by migrating birds flying from South America to Mexico and the United States. The infected birds are not usually ill, but species that are not normally involved can become diseased and die showing the same type of nervous signs as horses: incoordination, fits and violent tremors.

Mr Smithers the farmer was a perky little man sporting a large moustache and wearing a loud, checked cloth cap. Before I could introduce myself he burst out with this tirade:

'I've been reading this book, which tells you all the symptoms of this Venezuelan equine encephalitis, and, bang to rights, that is what my pheasants have got: there's no doubt about it: they're havin' fits, droppin' down, kickin' their little legs in the air and then they snuff it.' In his enthusiasm he was dropping his gs.

'I only started keeping pheasants last year and it was a huge success, I bought a thousand day-old chicks, and reared almost all of them and made a bomb when I sold 'em to a shoot down the road, to put out, and so this year I bought ten thousand, and for the first four weeks they was goin' great and then they started to die and they have not stopped dyin' and I just don't know what to do.'

3

'Have you talked to your vet?' I said, as their local man should be the first line of defence.

'Oh no,' he replied, 'this is much too serious for 'im. I read in this book how it was such an important disease that the Government Vets should be told and if my pheasants 'as this disease then they will come and kill 'em all and pay me compensation.'

The penny was beginning to drop – he was more interested in getting his money back than in the welfare of his birds.

'First of all we have to decide what the problem is and then see what we can do to help. Have you brought any birds with you?'

'An 'undred,' came the prompt reply.

And so Mr Smithers filled in the forms under Joan's benevolent care, giving all the details of his farm and what had happened to the birds since they arrived, and he left, having been assured that we would phone him the moment we had finished our examinations. The laboratory practised a system of 'duty vet', in which we took it in turns to be responsible for the samples that came in that day and carry out post mortem examinations on the corpses. That day it was my turn.

They were a sorry lot of birds that I examined, skinny and bedraggled, and I noticed that they had been savagely debeaked, a process that I deplore but which is widely practised in the poultry industries where large numbers of birds are held in a confined space. Because they do not have adequate room to move, feed and preen they get irritable and peck at each other, causing serious damage to their neighbours, which can result in infection and death. In order to maximise the number of birds in a confined space the farmer snips off what should be a small piece of the upper beak, so preventing them from 'eating' each other. While this might be a justifiable practice for birds raised for human food, in my view it can never be justified in birds raised for sport. Mr Smithers had been rather generous in his removal so the birds had been unable to pick up the food from the troughs and had starved to death, probably in the midst of plenty!

However, when farmers 'know' why their animals have died you have to be careful. Our Mr Smithers was looking to the tax-payer to make good his error. I rang through to my boss, Sherwin Hall, the Veterinary Investigation Officer, and asked him to come to the post mortem room and take a look. Or rather 'Crockie' did, because she was in the PM room taking down notes of the examination. She was the duty laboratory technician and the 'clean pair of hands in the PM room'. You must have a clean pair of hands in the PM room to ensure that you don't get blood on the report sheet, to open the bottles, to stick the sterile swab into the abscess or the uterus and to hold the bag while you fill it with faeces.

'What's up squire?' was Sherwin's breezy entry to the PM room. Dapper, with spotted bow tie to the fore and as always quick in movement, clear in thought and precise in speech, he was a great boss to have – with his view that all vets were equal and that he was only *primus inter pares*. We were left to make our own decisions, write and sign our own reports (rare for those days when the head of the laboratory liked to sign all reports leaving 'his laboratory'). 'You sign the reports with your MRCVS [Member of the Royal College of Veterinary Surgeons, the governing body of the profession]; you get the credit for the successes and the kicks up the arse for the cock ups.' However, should advice or help be needed he was there.

Sherwin and I were both from east London, and although he was ten years my senior we soon became firm friends and have remained so to this day. Sherwin was a great believer in method and order and ensuring that all aspects of the history, clinical and pathological findings and laboratory tests were taken into account in the final diagnosis, if there was a diagnosis. 'Remember Roger, we are in the business of solving problems and sometimes to solve the problem you need to make a diagnosis, but solving the problem for the farmer is the key.'

Another of his methods to ensure we were a team was the regular morning meeting in the General Laboratory, where each of the cases was discussed. Woe betide any sloppy thinking or careless work, for Sherwin could cut you down to size with a simple phrase: 'Tell me Tom, do pigs normally ruminate?' When undertaking a disease investigation on a farm his view was, 'It is best you have an ordered approach to investigation, saves trouble in the long run, particularly when dealing with farmers who have lost a great deal of money, often through their own pig-headedness.' When writing a report it is essential that you tell the vet or farmer what he needs to know, in clear simple language, free from jargon even if not devoid of technical words, because there is no way you can say 'staphylococcal mastitis' in any other meaningful way. How well Sherwin's advice and guidance were to serve me over the years to come.

'Let's have a butchers.'

I gave him the story, showed him my findings and said I thought that the birds had starved to death because they were unable to pick up the food.

'Right on,' was the reply. 'But we will need to play this canny: no farmer likes to be told that he has killed his own animals, and we have the welfare of the remaining birds to think about. We have to get Smithers on our side. We have to persuade him to do what he is told without making him feel he is a murderer. Phone him and tell him that we think he has a nutritional problem and that we will visit his farm tomorrow. We can drive up there tomorrow morning and sort him out.'

While he was not sure that we had got the diagnosis correct, Mr Smithers was more than happy to see us the following day. Before setting off the next morning we checked the bacterial cultures that had been set up from the organs of the dead birds, to ensure that, in addition to the debeaking, there was no underlying infectious cause for them failing to eat. The culture plates were all clear and so we set off for the Glenby Pheasant Farm. It came as no surprise that this enterprise was a bungalow with several sheds in its large garden, on the outskirts of Grantham.

'If you don't mind, I think that it might be better if I handled this one: bad news comes better out of an old mouth, and we could be in trouble with Smithers.'

'Go ahead,' I said. 'The important thing is to get the remainder of the pheasants eating before they all die.'

Before we arrived at the door Mr Smithers had it opened, still wearing the cloth cap of the previous day – I idly wondered if he ever took it off. He did. Later that morning off it came to enable him to scratch his bald head in puzzlement.

'I'm glad you're 'ere,' he said, before even saying hello. 'There's another two 'undred of 'em dead this morning.' The death of a single animal often causes concern, but deaths on an industrial scale seem to deprive people of all feelings.

'Well the sooner we get started the sooner we can stop the deaths,' replied Sherwin and we trouped out to the sheds. The place was clean and tidy and the pens were well constructed: Mr Smithers had obviously spent money when he set up the business. The food was kept in a neat store and there was no sign of vermin. Those young pheasants that had not been debeaked were plump and healthy and tucking into food laid out in shallow troughs for them. The pens

6

containing the debeaked birds were a different matter, with some birds obviously trying to pick up the food but, as their beaks could not close properly, they could not get a grip on the food which slipped from their mouths as they lifted their heads to swallow. Without saying a word, Sherwin picked up one of the trays and emptied its contents into another. Immediately one bird was able get its lower jaw under the food, scoop it up, and commence eating: others followed suit: it was not a very economical way of feeding but it would ensure that most birds would be able to get something in the way of nutrition.

It was at this juncture that Mr Smithers scratched his head. It was now obvious to him that the birds wanted to eat and that they were not sick in themselves. Without saying a word or casting any blame we had convinced the farmer that our diagnosis was accurate. Now all that remained was to sort out the mess. We suggested that he put a teaspoonful of glucose in the drinking water to immediately give them an energy source, and get from his vet some multi-vitamin mix which he could also add to the drinking water. The food being fed was a meal and so we suggested that if the farmer purchased some pelleted feed (the meal is steam heated and put through a nozzle to produce pellets of various sizes) the birds would find it easier to pick up these small pellets. In the short term the food had to be offered in deep trays so that the young birds could scoop it up. We recommended that he reduce the numbers of birds in each pen to discourage the cannibalism. We tactfully suggested that only the extreme tip of the beak should be removed, and not half the total: a visit to a neighbouring chicken hatchery would allow him to see how the professionals do it, but perhaps he should consider not debeaking the birds at all? It has never ceased to amaze me that people think that they can learn practical skills by reading a book! Practice and experience are the best teachers.

We left Mr Smithers a much happier man than we had found him but he would not be 'making a bomb' this year. His losses would continue for a few days more as the weakest would not have the strength to pull back from the brink, but with a bit of luck not many more would die. Luck plays a massive part in disease investigation; knowledge and experience are important but good luck is vital. We had had a bit of luck during the visit; had that pheasant chick not scooped up the food on cue, we might never have convinced Mr Smithers.

7

First stop was the pub, for a pint of Greene King bitter and a sandwich, before I drove us back to the laboratory to write the report and start on the next case. This was not a normal problem as seen in the laboratory: the standard practice was for a vet to refer his client to us and he would send us the details of the case: the history, his findings, and treatments. Exceptions had been made in the case of birds; because their economic value was so low, owners were permitted to submit samples without involving their vet. However, it was our normal practice to send all reports to the vets concerned because it was they who had to prescribe any treatment required. We discussed the details of the farm and farmer during the journey back – both of us failed to understand why people went into keeping large numbers of animals when they had no experience and training, and we wondered if perhaps they should not be allowed to do so.

The laboratory of which Sherwin was the boss, was the Cambridge Veterinary Investigation Centre, one of a chain of laboratories throughout England and Wales (Scotland and Northern Ireland had their own services), run by the Ministry of Agriculture, Fisheries and Food, which provided farmers and veterinary surgeons with a complete laboratory and consultancy service, which, until the arrival of Margaret Thatcher, was free of charge: the idea was to boost food supplies and to reduce imports, so that the perilous position in which we found ourselves during the Second World War, should never happen again.

But I am jumping the gun. I have not introduced myself. My name is Roger Windsor, and at the time of the visit to Mr Smithers I was in my early thirties and a vet, trained at the Royal (Dick) School of Veterinary Studies in Edinburgh. Once qualified, I had a year in general veterinary practice, putting some practical experience onto the university theory and learning about farmers and how farms worked. Then I went off to Kenya for a couple of years, which completely changed the course of my life, and ensured that I would end up as a detective working for the Veterinary Investigation Service.

But I must put some flesh on the bones: I was born in London and seven days later Mr Hitler invaded Poland. So before I was many weeks old my mother, two sisters and I were sent off, away from the bombs: we were evacuated to Dorset and billeted in the home of Ray and Gladys Bealing and their daughter Jean. Ray was a head

8

cowman on a dairy farm in Fontmell Magna, but I have no recollection of my time there. We spent much of the next six years with Ray and Glad and they remained firm friends of the senior Windsors to the ends of all their lives.

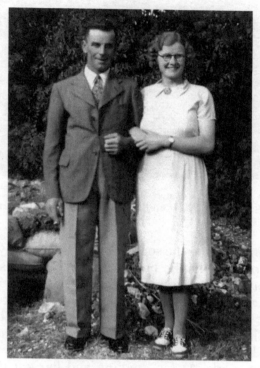

Ray and Gladys Bealing, the wonderful hosts to the Windsor evacuees.

Ray and the rest of his extended family moved to Compton Abass and then to Ashmore, which is where my earliest memories begin. The village of Ashmore is high, on the top of the chalk downs, and is splendid cattle country. The road down to Shaftesbury was a mass of bends known by all as Zig-Zag Hill and was a splendid road for training tank crews for the invasion of France, so there were tanks driving into the village daily and then descending the hill at top speed. At the first sound of the tanks the children of the village all rushed off to greet them, to be showered by the GIs with sweets, a rare treat in a Britain fighting for its life, with massive food shortages and strict rationing of everything.

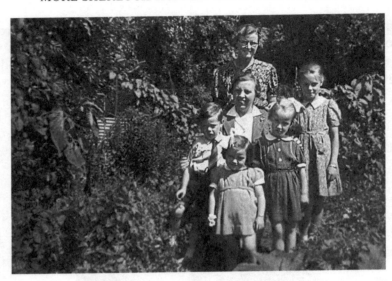

In the garden at Masons Cottage, Ashmore; Gladys Bealing, Cissie (Amelia) and Mary Windsor, Roger and Margaret Windsor and Jean Bealing.

Life on a dairy farm in the south of England was idyllic for a small boy; there were nests in the hedges and sticklebacks in the village pond and streams. There were copses and woods to play in and hide and there was always an unrationed cup of milk in the dairy. Summers were always hot in those far-off days and life so pleasant that my sister has returned to live there in her retirement. But it was not all play. There were times of the year when even the smallest of children had to work. At hay making and harvest there were jobs that even little children could do. The hayrick was made by laying the dried grass on a base prepared by the men: then the horse and cart would arrive and the men would toss the grass onto the developing rick. The children, equipped with small wooden rakes, would keep the surface level: it was not hard work and there were frequent breaks waiting for the next load to arrive during which there would be fun and games. As the stack increased in height falling off could have become a hazard (luckily there was no 'elf and safety' in them days!), but to my knowledge no one ever did. The carts were left in the field as the big old Shire horse was removed from the shafts and then it was the children's time to have fun, as we returned to the farmyard aboard Dobbin – yes he was really called 'Dobbin'. Six or more children would travel in style on that broad strong back but again I do not remember anyone falling off, or if they did, being hurt. Perhaps the children of yesteryear were more intelligent, or perhaps not having a nanny state telling you what could and, more importantly, what could not be done, they acted in a more responsible fashion. In those far off days, common sense was not legislated.

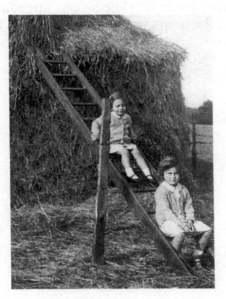

Haymaking in Ashmore before the Second World War.
Photo © Charles Sturge.

Horses were the main source of transport in Dorset: the farmer had a big car in the garage but because of petrol rationing it was rarely used. From time to time we returned to our London home to see my father, who had been invalided out of the army not long after the start of the war and now ran his shop by day and drove an ambulance in the East End of London by night. We travelled to the station at Shaftesbury by pony and trap. I have glorious memories of clip trotting down Zig-Zag Hill to Shaftesbury station. It was always sunny in my memory!

The only man who regularly used a car was the vet. He was a frequent visitor to the farm. In those far-off days when the relative value of an animal was far greater than it is today, a sick animal had to be seen and treated by the vet: there was no do-it-yourself in those days. Farm animals also received more respect; the cowman knew

11

them all by name, with their likes and foibles, and he knew when one was off colour. Ray was a wonderful cowman with an uncommon empathy with his animals and so the vet was called at the first sign of trouble. When he arrived on the farm all work stopped; this very important man was too busy to be kept waiting and the children were banished from the byre while he was attending the animal, but we peeped round the doors until we were spotted and shooed away. Was this the reason I decided to become a vet? Probably!

2

TB . . .

'It is quite a three-pipe problem.'
Sir Arthur Conan Doyle, *The Red-Headed League*

Alex Scott, the highly respected vet from Bedford, sounded worried. 'Roger, we have a strange problem in the abattoir. Good, healthy pigs are coming in from a farm owned by a local supermarket and when we get them on the line they are showing a great number of tiny lesions in the liver but nothing elsewhere.'

Such lesions are called miliary because they resemble a grain of millet seed. The liver drains all the organs in the abdomen and chest and acts as a huge filter cleaning up the blood before it is returned to the lungs to be re-oxygenated. It is therefore not uncommon for bacteria to be filtered out and to develop into an abscess, sometimes obtaining a huge size; if large numbers of bacteria are spread round the liver, many tiny abscesses can develop (this is also a common way of spreading cancer cells.) but it is rare to find more than a single animal in a herd or flock with the problem.

'What percentage of the animals going through are affected?' I asked.

'This is the strange thing, in some batches there are none and in others almost every pig slaughtered shows a healthy number of these tiny abscesses, and every one with the lesions is being condemned. It is costing the supermarket a bomb and they are getting very touchy.'

'The first thing to do is to get the abattoir to let us have three or four of the affected animals and we need all the organs and they must be those of the carcases: can you organise that?'

'No problem! Recently I have been going to the abattoir each time they slaughter a batch to see what is happening. The next time we see any I will try to stop them removing the organs so you can have a complete animal.'

'Good man,' I said. What a delight it was to work with a colleague

13

so positive, friendly and helpful. Sometimes people in trouble become very belligerent, but not Alec, always cool, always the gentleman.

'I do hope you can get to the bottom of this one because it is one of the best managed farms in my practice and the manager is a personal friend.'

'We will do our best.'

It was a few days before we heard from Alex again and work in the centre went on its usual way with the regular batch of students from the vet school coming for training.

'It's the school's job to teach the students what a problem could be, and our job to teach them what it is likely to be,' was one of Sherwin's favourite sayings. He was right: it was possible that a dog showing nervous signs had rabies, but in Britain it was far more likely to be distemper.

I loved having the students about me as they kept me on my toes and made sure I read up on my cases and kept abreast of the literature. Sherwin and the other young vet, John Simmons, felt the same: John loved to pontificate and could talk for hours on almost any topic, but his knowledge was soundly based as he read extensively. He was slightly older than me and unmarried, but had just bought a sports car with which he hoped to attract a wife; the speed of the car making up for the slowness of the deliberation. He was a reasonable spin bowler and at matches he went on and on about how he had been at school with Derek Underwood, the England spinner.

Jock Dawson did not enjoy the students; to him they were 'just a bloody nuisance'. Jock had not wanted to be part of the investigation centre and had joined the Ministry of Agriculture Fisheries and Food's Cattle Fertility Service many years before. One of his two passions was cattle breeding and the other the Boy Scout Movement. He always kept a well-thumbed leather-bound copy of Rudyard Kipling's *Kim* in his back pocket and would pull it out when there was not much going on; he considered it to be the best book ever written, and I agree with him. Jock had been born and brought up in India, and I think he resented the British having to leave at independence. His surrogate was the Scouts and he ran the only mounted troop of boy scouts in Britain, providing all the horses out of his own pocket. For many years he had run a sub-centre of the Veterinary Laboratory Service from his large house in north Essex, where Crockie was employed by the Ministry to assist him with the samples and the paper work. When a team was sent to decide whether the sub-centre should be closed and moved to Cambridge, Jock had not helped his case when they asked to speak to Crockie and were informed that she was 'in the house making the beds'. Jock came to Cambridge with a bad grace, but he had an encyclopaedic knowledge of cattle breeding and was always prepared to share that knowledge.

The fifth member of the veterinary team was also a specialist: Blackie was a poultry man who had worked at the Central Veterinary Laboratory in Weybridge for years. He was coming to the end of his career when the unit he worked in was closed down and he was moved to Cambridge as his home was in north Essex, to replace a colleague who had been seconded to the Kenya Veterinary Department. He tried hard to fit in with the routine work, because Sherwin had informed Head Office that in a staff of five he could not afford to have two specialists not doing the general work. Whereas Jock was small and scruffy, with the inevitable aroma of cow dung, Blackie was tall and elegant and always immaculately turned out.

The technical team was excellent, with Peter Edwards in charge although he never gave that impression. He seemed to be permanently in a state of disarray bordering on panic and yet he always managed to get the job done: he was a considerate manager, and a quiet, careful, meticulous and neat worker, perhaps the result of his artistic talents. Despite having a young family, Peter, to the despair of his wife, was often the last to leave the laboratory in the evening. By contrast Denis was balding and ebullient, a very able biochemist, willing to turn his hand to anything but keen to ensure that the work was out of the way by 5 pm so that he could get off.

Then there was Cyril, the final member of the senior technical team: Cyril the sublime, or Cyril the unequalled as he was known. Quiet, small and dark, with a disabled wife, Cyril was our histopathologist – there was no one within a hundred miles of Cambridge who could cut histological sections like Cyril. When scientists wanted sections to be photographed for publication in scientific journals they beat a path to his door and begged him to cut and stain them for the journal. He never refused. The man had such amazing pride in his work, a true expert.

These senior members of the technical team were assisted by a variety of juniors of both sexes and all ages. Crockie you have met, a helter-skelter of a technician, always rushing about and looking for the next job before the first was finished and so there were some mix-ups. I think that she would have been happier working in a pony club or riding school but, then as now, such jobs were in short supply. She was not in her first youth, small and wiry with unkempt black curly hair. She had worked with Jock for many years and was devoted to him and his family.

Every lab has to have a comedian, to keep everyone sane, and ours was Stephen. Perhaps his masterpiece was during Ted Heath's 'three day week' when everything was in short supply. Stephen was the lab store-keeper and kept it neat, very tidy and well documented. When Joan asked for toilet paper for the ladies' loo, Stephen handed her two rolls with the admonition, 'Make sure you use both sides!'

Joan was the receptionist and more importantly the backstage organiser of the lab, making sure that everything ran smoothly, things were in their place and the files kept up to date. Silver-haired but still an attractive woman, Joan knew everybody and everything: phone numbers, addresses, where you could buy anything, who could get you what you wanted. She was a tower of strength and worth her weight in gold, and she ran her administration team with a light touch. Poor old Flossie was tiny, with short, curly, dark but greying hair and was the butt of all the jokes, but dearly loved by all: nearing retirement she cycled to work on her mini-bike. She coped well with all the ribbing and was an excellent shorthand typist (we did not truly realise their value until the dreaded computer robbed us of their services). I believe that everyone looked on Flossie as a much loved, slightly eccentric granny and treated her as such. Winifred arrived soon after me and she also came to work on two wheels much to the merriment of the male members of staff. She sat bolt upright on her small motorbike with her helmet barely concealing her prematurely white hair. Why she never married remains a mystery because she was such a kind caring person and, then in her late forties, she had not given up looking. She was a wonderful aunt to her nieces and nephews (surrogate children perhaps) and she liked to mother us poor vets. She was an excellent shorthand typist even if she never quite mastered the spelling of the technical words: in an attempt to remedy this defect she kept a notebook for spelling – the problem was the notebook kept getting lost or she could not find the word in it and it ended up being quicker to ask Flossie or the vet concerned.

Then there was Mrs Parker, the self-appointed shop-steward and complainer: nothing was ever right with her terms of service. She knew every rule in the book and used them whenever she could. She was away more than she was in the lab and was always 'sick'. She knew how many days off you could have per year without a note from a doctor and made sure she took them in full. Sherwin ran an easy ship but all the work had to go out on time. 'Animal lives depend upon it and possibly human ones as well,' was his view, and so if reports were not finished then people had to stay until they were. The other side of this was that when we were not busy the staff could get away early: it was a system that worked well for everyone but Mrs Parker. She antagonised her workmates to such an extent that they started to ostracise her; eventually it was made plain by the administrative and technical staff that she was not wanted and she resigned.

Ron and Ray kept the place clean and tidy, washed down the post mortem room after each examination had taken place, disposed of the carcases and other bits of bodies, fed the animals that we kept and were general handymen round the building. (The incinerator was a great bone of contention with the neighbours. The lab had been operating some fifteen years when the farmer across the road obtained planning permission to build a small estate of houses. People purchased their houses in full knowledge of the incinerator across the road but the complaints rolled in. The Ministry had to spend a large fortune extending the chimney and putting in scrubbers.) Although similar in age and size Ron and Ray could not have been more different in appearance: Ray was always immaculately turned out and spruce; dear old Ron was scruffy; but they both had a love of cricket and encyclopaedic knowledge of the game. Ron organised his local cricket team and arranged fixtures for a combined Vet School and lab team. We played on a Wednesday evening, the original twenty–twenty overs match and a good way to spend a summer's evening, before adjourning to the pub to replace the lost liquid. I cannot say that I ever distinguished myself in any of these games other than by dropping vital catches.

The founding fathers of the veterinary investigation service were men of vision who realised that a veterinary school and investigation centre could complement each other and strengthen the services offered by both, feeding off each other. We exposed their students to a much wider variety of material than was seen in the school, as it was sent in by the vets in practice in several counties and the vet

17

school offered us the services of specialists in limited fields. And so, when the vet school was built in Cambridge, money was found to build a veterinary investigation centre in its grounds. This continued for more than forty years until the accountants and money men took over the Ministry, the Cambridge and Norwich centres were closed and their services merged into a new centre at Bury-St-Edmunds. It is called progress.

The call came. 'Alex here. I will bring four affected carcases in to you later this morning.'

'Great,' I replied, we did not waste words: John was on duty that day but had no qualms about relinquishing the case to me and offered to help with the necropsies: I did not refuse. The carcases arrived and Alex joined us in the post mortem room as we started work.

As he had promised, although the carcases had been opened, the organs were all intact. This was slow demanding work, meticulously dissecting the carcase and examining every organ and more import- antly every lymph node, those strange glands in the body that swell up when there is an infection: I do not know how many there are in the pig body, but it runs into several hundred. The animals were in splendid condition – good, big, bacon pigs ready to produce hams and cuts of bacon. Alex watched for a while and then had to return to his clients. John and I worked our way doggedly through the bodies but the only things that we could find that were abnormal were the livers – they teemed with tiny abscesses. Tissues were selected and samples taken. Smears of these tiny lesions were put onto glass microscope slides and they were stained by various methods, the two most important in regular use being Gram's and the Ziehl-Nielsen's Stains. Bacteria are either Gram Positive or Gram Negative depending upon whether they appear either blue/ black or red down the microscope. With one test it is possible to reduce the possible causes of disease by half, a very useful tool. The Z-N stain is a specific stain for the organisms that cause tuberculosis and allied disease.

There was great excitement in the lab when all the Z-N smears were positive for 'acid fast bacteria'. Clumps of fine red bacteria were seen when we looked down the microscope. We had a preliminary diagnosis of tuberculosis at least. But this gave us a bigger headache: most people only know of human TB, some will know of bovine TB;

however, in addition there is avian TB affecting birds, including the domestic hen, and most confusing of all, the so-called cold-blooded strains of TB that infect reptiles and insects.

Trying to understand this disease is like walking in a minefield but let me try and explain a little to the reader. Human tuberculosis is normally caused by the human strain called *Mycobacterium tuberculosis*; readers aged over about fifty will remember seeing people with scars under one or both ears, this was a manifestation of the bovine strain, *M. bovis*, in humans and the scars resulted from the surgery to remove the infected gland (lymph nodes). This condition no longer occurs because of the pasteurisation of milk and the formerly successful campaign to eradicate the infection from cattle.

Sadly the disease is making a massive return to our herds thanks to a campaign by so-called 'animal lovers' who have opposed the killing of badgers, little realising that the badger that transmits the disease to cattle dies a dreadful death from TB. It makes much more sense to eradicate the disease from cattle and badgers so that both species can live a healthy TB-free existence. Cattle can be infected with *M. tuberculosis* but this is not commonly seen and usually it results when a stockman is suffering from TB and has a close association with his animals. Normally this disease in cattle is 'self-limiting' – that is to say the animal throws off the infection, having shown little or no signs of the disease: however, it can interfere with the test used to identify bovine TB in the animals. *M. avium* strains have been known to cause disease in humans but it is very rare; unfortunately the same is not true of animals and avian TB regularly causes the liver abscesses in pigs that we had found, but not on the scale we were seeing. The cold-blooded strains keep themselves to their cold-blooded hosts, or that was what the books said and what I thought.

John, Peter and I worked late that night putting up cultures for the TB organism, putting tissues into formalin so that when they were fixed Cyril could cut sections; they normally take several days to become hard enough to be cut with the micro-knife. There were tissues to be sent to the Central Veterinary Laboratory in Weybridge, where they had a specialist TB Unit with the expertise required to isolate and identify the more exotic types of mycobacterium, which is a slow and tedious job. All mycobacteria grow slowly and so the preliminary cultures can take in excess of four months. We knew we were in for the long haul and every day's delay could result in more animals becoming infected and more losses to the farmer in the slaughterhouse.

Meat inspection and food safety is in some ways a balancing act, where you have to weigh up public safety against economic reality. If, for example, every sheep that had a small subcutaneous abscess was totally condemned, then there would be no mutton to eat. A compromise was reached in the legislation and it is permissible to remove small lesions. Similarly a bullock which shows an infestation of flukes (a small heart-shaped liver parasite) in its liver is not totally condemned: the liver is destroyed but the meat is allowed to go for human consumption. When it comes to TB the regulations are quite specific – if only one organ is infected then that organ is condemned but the rest of the carcase may be eaten. If, however, there is more than one organ affected or there are lesions in the lung or liver then the whole carcase is condemned. These regulations had been drawn up for bovine TB in cattle but were applied indiscriminately to pigs with TB where the cause was different. It seemed to me that a great deal of human food was being wasted because the regulations did not really apply. I decided I would have to discuss this with Sherwin.

I thought it strange how two East End boys had ended up together in a Cambridge laboratory. The war had ended and in 1946 we returned to take up permanent residence in London. I had a sickly childhood involving several stays in Ward 8 of the Royal Northern Hospital. The first was in the bad winter of 1947: it started with getting soaking wet in a great snowball fight, I developed a chill which became a severe fever, and I was sent off to hospital. I was attended by Dr Coward, who was at a complete loss and so the great child doctor Dr Bruce Williamson was sent for (unknown to me at the time of course, he was a great friend of my future father-in-law). Such symptoms had not been seen in a child before; at one point in the day my temperature would be 95°F and a few hours later it had risen to 105°F. I ate nothing and the flesh fell off me. I was fed dried liver extract and milk and was filled with vitamins and minerals. Although they failed to diagnose the problem, I slowly recovered and made a paragraph in Williamson's book on childhood diseases!

In later years I suspected that I had suffered from brucellosis, a common disease of cattle in Britain until it was eradicated in the 1970s. I probably picked up the infection while living on the farm. Tonsillitis and then glandular fever sent me back to the hospital. This took its toll on my education, and my parents were desperately keen on education, particularly as my grandfather had not allowed my father to take up a scholarship at London University. Special tutors were employed to bring me back up to standard and I duly obliged by winning a scholarship to Bancroft's, a local public school. The most stupid thing that any Labour government has done was to close down the 'Direct Grant' which enabled boys and girls from poorer homes to attend those public schools that accepted this grant. The school excelled at producing senior civil servants, insurance brokers, bankers, lawyers, accountants and classicists, together with a few doctors and actors, but the last vet produced by the school was in the early 1930s.

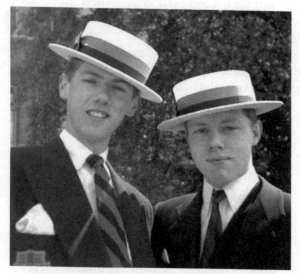

Tom Barker and Roger Windsor in their smart Bancroft's School boaters.

Our headmaster, Sidney Adams, was an inspirational man for me, with his regularly aired view that 'You boys have had a privileged education and it is your duty to put something back into society'. I have tried to live by this maxim. Even Sidney had difficulty in pronouncing the word. 'So, Windsor, you want to be a *veterererererinany* surgeon, why should you want to do that?'

'Well Sir, I spent several years on a farm and I have maintained an interest by regular summer trips back to that farm and although we have no pets at home I take a great interest in dogs and horses.'

21

'Do you think that you are clever enough to be a *vetererererer-inany* surgeon?'

Today only those just short of genius are guaranteed entry to a veterinary school. It was much easier then, but there was still considerable competition for places.

'I passed all my GCEs with flying colours Sir, and I have a great interest in the biology and chemistry classes. I think that, with luck, I might get a place.'

'Worth a try then I would say. We will have to see what we can do to assist.'

A few days passed, then I had a message from the school secretary telling me to contact Goddard and Allen in Wanstead, a local veterinary practice. I arranged to go and see Arthur Goddard and he was charming.

'I have arranged with your headmaster that you are to come here for two hours on Wednesday and Friday mornings as that fits with your timetable. I hope that that is all right with you.'

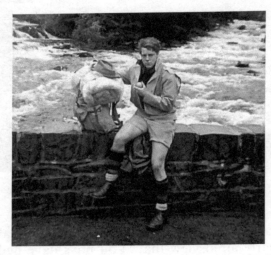

The holiday in Scotland that decided Roger to study in Edinburgh.

'Thank you Sir,' I blurted out, as this was too good to be true. Today, unless you have experience in every imaginable type of practice no vet school will look at you. And so I assisted in surgeries, helped at operations, treated and dressed wounds and obtained some idea of what my future work was going to be.

22

Not one but two vets were produced from my year at school. Fred (Christopher) Chesney and I went up for interview to the Royal Veterinary College in London. Fred was offered a place but I, knowing almost nothing of Thomas Hardy (because I was reared in Dorset they thought that I should know all about that county's greatest author), was rejected. Then it was the turn of Edinburgh and the interview there was much more amenable. The only interviewer that I remember was Tommy Graham, the Professor of Anatomy, president of the college rugby club and an ardent fan.

'So Windsor, you hooked for the first fifteen at school and had a trial for the Eastern Counties Schools?'

'Yes Sir.'

'Do you intend to play rugby at College as we will need a new hooker for the first fifteen the year after next?'

'Definitely Sir, if I am good enough.'

'Excellent, no more questions from me, Chairman.'

I was offered a place at the Royal (Dick) School of Veterinary Studies. By a quirk of fate, Fred was turned down! Before I knew it my trunk was packed and I was on the midnight sleeper to Edinburgh and a new phase of my life.

3

... or Not TB, That is the Question

'I am afraid,' said Holmes, smiling, 'that all the Queen's horses
and all the Queen's men cannot avail in this matter.'
Sir Arthur Conan Doyle, *The Bruce–Partington Plans*

Problems never come singly. No sooner had we started investigating
Alec' s problem in Bedford than what seemed to be a similar
problem was reported in the Haverhill abattoir, even if it was on a
smaller scale. The first link was that the abattoir was owned by the
same supermarket whose herd in Bedford was affected. The second
was it was another herd in the supermarket ownership that presented
with the disease. Not only did Keith Harrison carry out the veterinary inspections in the abattoir, he was the vet to the farm: as with
Bedford so with Essex, there was no overt disease on the farm. We
took the same action with Keith as we had with Alex and within a
few days we had three carcases in the necropsy room for examination. Again the pigs were in excellent condition but were being
condemned because of the lesions in the liver. Again John and I
carried out the detailed examinations of all body organs and a large
number of glands and again the problems were confined to the liver –
but here there was a big difference from Bedford; whereas there were
a massive number of miliary abscesses in the Bedford livers, there
were far fewer in the Essex ones.

The same operation as before was put into play and again it was
obvious that we were dealing with the same problem, namely avian
TB in pigs. It was time for a serious discussion. A meeting in my
office was arranged with Alex and Keith, the regional manager of the
supermarket chain, Paul Carwardine the consultant vet to the
supermarket for the interested parties, and Sherwin, John and myself
for the laboratory. We had to assume that we were dealing with avian
TB in the pigs because that was the likeliest diagnosis. This put me in
mind of my old pathology teacher Morton Gellately, who preceded

almost every lecture with the statement, 'Gentlemen, [in those days almost the whole class was male; a different story today where 80% of the students are female] you must remember that common diseases commonly occur.' Another quotation flashed through my mind, this time from Sherlock Holmes: 'It has long been an axiom of mine that the little things are infinitely the most important.'

We decided that the first thing to do was to determine the source of the infection; however, until we knew what the infection was, we might be chasing our tails. It was agreed that I should visit all the farms that had produced affected pigs and make a list of the possible sources of the infection. These would be investigated one by one and eliminated. There were three farms in this group that were basically managed together. However, one of the farms had produced no diseased pigs, one only produced a small percentage of diseased pigs, and one farm had a large number of infected animals. It was like a quadratic equation and so it should be easy to solve the calculation by sound detective work, and identify the source of the problem.

The boss of the supermarket indicated that the real problem for his company was not a few dead pigs which could be claimed for on their insurance; no, the real trouble was in the Haverhill abattoir. The company owned the abattoir, and he pointed out that if the pigs came from a private supplier they would refuse to accept more pigs until the problem was resolved, because each time the disease was seen, the line was stopped while the affected pigs were moved to the 'Examination Line'. If that filled up then the production line was stopped until that line was emptied to take more. Each time the line stopped, the slaughtermen lost money: they were paid a flat salary and a bonus for every pig above seventy per hour slaughtered. When the line stopped the slaughtermen got very stroppy.

It was decided that for the foreseeable future all pigs from the three farms would be slaughtered at Haverhill. There were about 600 sows on the three farms which would produce an average of 20 piglets per year, and so the throughput would be about 12,000 fat pigs for slaughter each year, or 250 a week, or 50 per day. Deliveries to the abattoir would be such that there were always fifty on any one day for slaughter (what you can do if you are a big rich organisation). These fifty would be slipped in at the end of the day and the Examination Line would be expanded to accommodate thirty carcases awaiting examination. This meant that the routine slaughter work would not be disrupted.

At the end of a very productive meeting I slipped in my suggestion that we should undertake a detailed investigation of the problem in the pigs to see whether or not the infection was confined to the liver, or whether we could demonstrate the presence of bacteria in seemingly healthy tissues. The supermarket agreed to supply us with one infected carcase a week for twelve weeks. We would dissect out the glands and make cultures, and undertake animal inoculations on pooled samples of these glands in an attempt to detect the presence of living bacteria in them. It was a laborious task for John and me, and I suspect even more so for the technical staff, mincing up the glands and producing thirty or more cultures and a guinea pig to be infected from each of these pigs.

I have never had any problems with properly conducted animal experimentation which is carried out for the benefit of animals or human health (only the opponents call it vivisection – we do not cut up live animals). As animals have no obligations they can have no rights. However, as civilised human beings it is our duty to look after animals, and the animals in the laboratory were cared for by the staff who looked upon them as pets and made sure they were clean, comfortable and well fed. I always visited my animals each day to see how they were faring. During the 'experiment' the guinea pigs were subjected to a single injection and a daily rectal temperature examination. Not even the guinea pigs injected with liver abscesses developed TB and we isolated organisms only from the liver: these we had to send to Weybridge for further examination, as we did not have the expertise or the facilities for identifying mycobacteria, a seriously difficult task and one for the specialist.

I drew up a plan for visiting the farms with their vet and Paul Carwardine. It would be tedious to recount the visits because all three farms were almost identical. Similar houses, similar management practices, similar levels of staffing, identical farrowing houses and similar food provided for all three by the same mill. However, there was a significant difference in the provision of the bedding – in all cases they used sawdust/wood shavings. The clean farm received its wood shavings from a local sawmill. The farm with moderate infection also received bedding from the same source. The severely affected farm only occasionally received supplies from this source, when they had much more than usual. The deficiency was made good by a sawmill in Thetford Forest.

Together with staff from the supermarket I visited the sawmill, where there was a veritable mountain of sawdust at least thirty feet high. It was certain that this mountain was alive with every type of wildlife. The sawmill obviously could not be bothered looking for customers for its by-product and so the mountain grew and grew. Farmers were free to come and collect but only the supermarket farms did so.

We now had to involve the local pest control people, because we needed to know what species of animals were around and we needed to examine some of them for TB. John Malcolm was a real Norfolk boy and I could barely understand a word he said. Despite being a pest control officer he had a real 'feel' for animals and I think he did his job because it meant he could spend most of his time in the country. He set big traps and small traps and over a month he trapped two deer (I could never make out what species they were), three feral cats, five badgers, twenty hedgehogs and many mice of various species. We killed and examined at least one of each species, in the case of hedgehogs we examined five, and about a dozen mice. We also cultured the sawdust in the pile, collecting from more than twenty randomly selected sites. How on earth did bacteria in the bedding get into the pig? Simple, little pigs will eat anything – they love picking at the grot on the floor, food gets spilled on the floor, and so bits of sawdust and shavings are eaten. I remember a fascinating case where a wood yard started working with an obscure type of mahogany and produced a dark brown sawdust. The little pigs just loved this sawdust and ate it instead of their food: unfortunately it contained a kidney poison and the little pigs died one by one: they were taken off that sawdust.

The incubators in the laboratory were beginning to fill up with cultures as more and more samples were collected and examined: the bill for the culture media was getting larger and larger and there seemed to be no end in sight. People looking for quick results should not work with mycobacteria as each culture has to be incubated for up to six months before a definite negative can be given. As an interim precautionary measure the farms had stopped collecting sawdust from the forest and had found an alternative source of the bedding. Since this was the only difference between the three farms there was a strong possibility that it was the source of the problem. Because the sows and boars were moved between the farms on a regular basis it was possible to rule out the breeding stock as the source of the infection.

We now had to sit and wait for the results to come in. Once the first ones were in, it developed into a regular torrent and we had the whole problem sorted out. The first surprise was that the organism was not *M. avium* but two cold-blooded types, *M. intacellulare* and *M. xenopi*. The natural habitat of the latter was on and in the bark of pine trees. It had first been identified in the pine forests of Eastern Europe and is a parasite of a small mite that also lives on the bark. The mycobacteria had been isolated from all sawdust samples examined and even more interesting was the fact that the mite was seen in all the samples. The mycobacteria were not isolated from the deer or cat but from some of all the other species – badger, hedgehog and mice. However it had only been isolated from the intestinal tracts and not from any of the organs, and so we deduced that it was just passing through and was not causing any problems. None of the wildlife species was infected and none was involved in the outbreak of disease that we had seen.

We never found out why the organism had invaded the piglets' bodies, nor why such huge numbers of lesions resulted. The lesions took their time to disappear from the pigs – a bacon pig takes six months to reach slaughter and the lesions only completely disappeared after all those pigs reared on the infected bedding were slaughtered. Another case successfully resolved, another happy customer and two relieved vets. But the story is not completely finished.

John and I had carried out dissections on twelve carcases provided by the Bedford abattoir, together with several other carcases from other farms that the two abattoirs had submitted, and the culture results were beginning to trickle out. *M. creatophagus* was the only organism isolated from the livers of the pigs from the supermarket farms – it was not isolated from any other tissue or glands in the pigs and inoculation of material from the glands did not cause disease in any of the guinea pigs inoculated. *M. avium* was isolated from some of the livers from other farms but by no means all. We also failed to isolate the organism from the other tissues and glands. We had shown that there was no danger from eating the meat of those pigs that had miliary lesions confined to the liver, as the organism was not lurking in the tissues to infect some unsuspecting human who ate the meat.

We wrote a letter to the Meat Inspection Section of the Ministry suggesting that a change in the Meat Inspection Regulations was required. We described all the work that we had done and tabulated all the results. The reply came: 'Nobody has ever complained about these regulations and so we will be taking no action.' Well, we had complained about them! All our hours of work, all the materials and the time of the staff at the Central Veterinary Laboratory had been dismissed in a single sentence. Such are the ways of the Ministry and truth to tell, it has become worse under subsequent anti-agriculture governments.

There had been some interesting staff benefits from this study: we decided to practise what we were going to preach. We had considered that these carcases were no risk to human health and, with the agreement of Sherwin, after we had finished work with a carcase it was carefully butchered into joints and distributed among the staff. The meat was excellent; my wife and I cured the hind and forelegs by the York Ham method and the unwanted meat we minced and turned into sausages. A friend in the village where we lived lent us a war-time Ministry of Food booklet on preserving and using meat, and the local butcher gave us his old machine for making sausages, sold us the skins and taught us the art of linking the sausage into a string. It was all very time consuming but we had no television and so most evenings of the week were taken up in the preparation of hams and sausages. These came in handy because times were hard: inflation was soaring, mortgage rates were going up almost daily and Ministry salaries were fixed. Those carcases helped to keep us afloat. When there were visitors to the Windsor house my wife invariably offered them some product of the pig for dinner.

I had met my wife when in my second year at the Dick Vet. While not a virgin when going off to Edinburgh, I knew little about sex and the opposite sex. On that first Friday I went to a dance at the Men's Union which in those days was known as the 'Cattle Market'. I was dancing with a young lady from Leith and, for want of anything better to say, asked, 'What's a nice young lady like you doing in a place like this?' She dropped my hand, turned on her heel and walked away. Lesson number one, do not be facetious. I then met a young Irish nurse, working in the Royal Infirmary to complete her training before returning to Dublin, and we spent the rest of the evening together. At the end of the dance I was invited back to her flat, which she shared with another Dubliner nurse, for coffee. I was taken into the sitting room while Bernadette went to make coffee.

29

After a few minutes of idle chat the flat mate made her excuses and left (they had obviously trodden this path before). Bernadette returned wearing a dressing gown and bearing coffee. As we drank our coffee it became apparent to me that Bernadette had nothing on underneath that dressing gown. I was too flummoxed to take advantage of the situation; I drank up my coffee and fled. I never saw Bernadette again: should she read this, all I can say is sorry.

The Saturday night dances in the Dick Vet College were much more genteel. The admission charge was half a crown (12½p), we had a live band, and the dances resulted in a great number of permanent unions and raised a great deal of money for the Veterinary Students Committee, the student body that was responsible for all student affairs. It used this income for subsidising trips to the British and International Veterinary Student Unions Meetings and Conferences, and underwriting the college One-Day Equine Event, and the dramatic society productions. No alcohol was sold on college premises but during the interval coffee and soft drinks were sold in the college refectory; however, there were two pubs within a hundred yards and here many a young man raised his courage for the second half of the proceedings.

I have to admit that I was not the most studious of students and I scraped though my first year by explosive episodes of studying at the last minute and a great deal of good luck in the questions. The second year was worse. Brian Ranson, an old friend from Bancroft's, and I took a flat in the prestigious Castle Street, just off Princes Street in the heart of the city. The rent was not excessive, the address was central and we became the centre of night life for vet students and arts students alike. There was a twenty-first birthday party that started on Friday evening in Castle Street and ended on Monday lunchtime at the same address having moved venue several times over the weekend. Nobody survived the whole party without sleep but that was usually taken between 10 am and 6 pm, and from Saturday morning onwards there was always somebody asleep somewhere in the house or flat, often not alone. But it was mostly very innocent fun, with much alcohol consumed but little drunkenness, no smashing up of furniture and only a smattering of sex as far as I know.

It was in Castle Street that I first met Maxine, a small, shapely brunette with a great dress sense and a very smart ladies' college accent. She had studied music at the Reid School but became bored

30

by the theory and history and the lack of playing and had left at the end of the first year. She had decided that music was not to be her career (how wrong she was) and so she returned to London to train as a secretary. She had come up to meet old classmates and was brought to the flat by a mutual friend. We enjoyed some light banter, supper was organised and we all went off to the Dick Vet Dance. I liked her well enough to get her London phone number but thought no more of the matter (how wrong I was).

Mark Allen was a contemporary of Fred's at the Royal Vet College in London but lived in the same suburb as me. His father was a pharmacologist at the local hospital who brewed his own beer and mead in the days before such activity was made legal, and they lived in a huge house which was just right for parties, when his parents always made themselves scarce. Mark was throwing a party for New Year's Eve and there was a shortage of women. I thought of Maxine. I was already going to the party with a 'steady' but I thought she might enjoy meeting the London gang. I phoned and explained the situation to Maxine, who had nothing planned and so I arranged to meet her at Tottenham Court Road tube station and escort her to the party. I explained that my girlfriend would be coming along later, having been to the theatre with her father; however, Maxine was having none of that and stuck to me like a leech all evening. It was a good party and the start of a lifelong friendship which five years later became a wedding, and then a life. Since then Maxine has been my wife, my lifelong companion, my adviser, my editor, and my closest friend. We have lived in many places and done many things together and we have had three children and a great deal of fun. She chose well.

PART 2

Apprentice, 1958–1973

4

A Little Learning and Much Playing, 1958–1964

'We are moving in exalted circles.'
Sir Arthur Conan Doyle *The Singular Experience of Mr John Scott Eccles*

Edinburgh was a great city in which to be a student, with its myriad artistic venues, great cafés and a dazzling array of pubs, and in the late fifties the Dick Vet was in its heyday as a veterinary school. Without a doubt it was the best in Britain then, although London students would question that claim. It did not set out to train academics, that was why the Cambridge school was set up; no, it set out to produce solid well-grounded practitioners who could look after the health and welfare of animals. In those far-off days students wore a jacket and tie to attend college and indeed on farm visits. Veterinary medicine was a profession to which you dedicated your working life: alternate nights 'on call' and a full weekend off just once a month. Today almost the first question asked by vets attending a job interview is 'What are the time-off arrangements?' and woe betide any practice that requires their services for more than one night a week and one weekend a month.

Where have all the characters gone? Men, and indeed a few women, who were listened to when they stood up and spoke. When I started college the Principal of the Dick Vet, Willie Mitchell, had just retired and had been replaced by Alexander Robertson, later knighted for his services to veterinary education, both in their different ways immense characters. Glasgow had Willie Weipers (also knighted); Liverpool had the great John George Wright of anaesthesia fame; London had the West Indian physiologist Professor Amoroso (a Fellow of the Royal Society); they also had Professor Jimmy McCunn, the anatomist, and Professor C. Formston, the surgeon. Even the new boys in Cambridge had their characters, with

35

Col Hickman, one of the leading horse vets in the country, and Peter Storie Pugh who ended up in the Colditz prisoner of war camp, after numerous escape attempts from other camps. The other new college, Bristol, had Professor Messervey to put it on the map. Now bean counters, bureaucrats, biologists and grant holders have taken over. They do not want to put their head above the parapet lest it be shot off. How many vet students today could name one member of staff from each of the other colleges? We knew many.

Outside the colleges there were men and women of huge character and reputation – the Steele-Bodger brothers, Nigel Snodgrass, Joan Joshua, Mary Branckner the first woman president of the BVA, and Dame Olga Uvarov the first woman President of the RCVS.

Edinburgh had a plethora of characters. Perhaps the finest was Tommy Graham (why is it the greats were all known to students by their Christian name?), professor of veterinary anatomy who probably owned more suits than the remainder of the college staff put together. We were well into our second year before we recognised a suit previously worn. He was never seen without a rose in his buttonhole – he grew roses in a heated greenhouse to ensure a regular supply. He might not have been the greatest anatomist in veterinary history but no student who passed through his hands left without a sound grasp of animal anatomy, and none will ever forget him. He was also president of the Dick Vet rugby club and fiercely proud of his teams: they could hold comparison with the best that the whole university could offer.

We actually beat the University First XV once during my student days. No one in my year will ever forget the morning after the Rugby Club Dinner: we had an anatomy lecture from 9 to 10 every morning: followed by anatomy practicals from 10 to 12. Most of the year had assembled for the nine o'clock lecture in the old Victorian lecture theatre: steeply rising tiers of wooden benches in a semi-circle looked down on the teaching cockpit, which consisted of a large wall-mounted blackboard, a good solid mahogany desk and the complete, assembled skeleton of a horse. We waited and waited: quarter past nine came and the stickler for punctuality still had not arrived. We were thinking of leaving when Tommy walked in, still wearing his dinner jacket, with the bow tie untied. The year sat frozen. Not a word was said. Tommy walked unsteadily up to the blackboard and picked up the blackboard duster. Still without a word, he walked to the skeleton and with a great flourish, draped the duster over the skull of the horse. Then he looked up and said, 'Ladies and Gentlemen, that concludes the lecture.' With that he left, to a huge cheer of acclamation and a stamping of feet. Today he would be reported to the university authorities because the students were not getting value for their money.

The man who taught us biochemistry was a dour Scot called Dr Ramsay who paced up and down with his hands clasped behind his back, while he lectured to us in a monotone; he was the son of the famous admiral who masterminded the evacuation from Dunkirk. The rudiments of biochemistry had been taught by Dr Croft, who made the building blocks of the subject totally fascinating, and we had taken to the subject with a will, and so when Dr Ramsay wrote on the board the formula of one major component of the Krebbs Cycle, and made a mistake in one of the side chains, we stamped our feet, pointing out his error. Dr Ramsay mistook the reason for our stamping, thinking it was that we did not know to what he was referring, and proceeded to give the class a lecture on: the idleness of modern youth; how Dr Croft had tried to teach our useless class about how biochemistry worked; how the youth of today were idle, indolent and lazy; how we were wasting the tax-payers' money; and what a useless bunch of students he was forced to teach. He went on and on, and the more he ranted the more we laughed and stamped our feet, until he realised that something was wrong. Students on the receiving end of a bollocking just did not behave in such a fashion. In mid tirade he stopped, turned and looked at the board. With the cuff of his sleeve he rubbed out the offending item and replaced it with the correct radical. A huge cheer went up from the class and he turned again, looked at us and said, 'Gentlemen, I grovel.'

The cheering doubled until we fell silent and the lecture was resumed. From then on we had no further trouble with Dr Ramsay and he was able to teach us a great deal of biochemistry, and eventually was held in high esteem.

Then there was Johnny Burgess one of the great horse surgeons of his day: his one problem was that he could not operate when sober, as his hands shook too much. It is not generally known that Johnny B operated on that great steeplechaser Merryman the Second, six weeks before he won his first Grand National. He certainly had his problem but it did not interfere with his work.

Professor James Spreull Andrew Spreull was another great character, almost a caricature Scot with his coarse grey three-piece tweed suit with watch chain and fob. He had been the boss of the family practice in Dundee and came to the Dick as a hands-on surgeon. His great remark was, 'I dinnae want to go down to posterity as a mender of ear 'oles and airse 'oles.' He was an avid collector of old Rolls Royce cars and he often gave me a lift to college in his tourer – a two-door model from the thirties. When you opened the door there was no need to put the front seat forward to get in and it was almost a route march to the seat. A generous man, belying the Scottish reputation, he gave one of his great cars to a group of students who wanted to drive round Spain, and no one was more pleased than he when it returned with a picture of the route taken painted on the side of the car. He was a hopeless lecturer, constantly getting muddled up and losing his place, but a wonderful demonstrator in the operating theatre and never afraid to let the student wield the knife. He was a great defender of his profession and a splendid advertisement for it.

George Frederick Boddie was an objectionable little man, who stood there twiddling his thumbs across his dark blue waistcoat while he lectured. He always called me 'the Toon Clairk' because on my first day at college I had arrived wearing my old school uniform. He did not take kindly to students questioning his diagnoses and he never forgave us on a major case when we were right. He might not have been held in high esteem by Edinburgh students but he was known throughout the colleges for his books, and he was one of the few Edinburgh professors to become President of the Royal College of Veterinary Surgeons. Alexander Robertson was another.

Without his 'Wee Free' mentality, Alexander Robertson might well have been one of the truly great members of the profession. He modernised the Dick Vet, capitalised on the college's reputation as the world leader in tropical veterinary medicine, and built and staffed the Centre for Tropical Veterinary Medicine (now called the Sir Alexander Robertson Building, but no longer a tropical centre) out at the Veterinary Field Station at Easter Bush (which will soon encompass the whole vet school, as the old Summerhall building is being closed down and sold to developers). It was his small-town mentality that prevented him from turning the CTVM into a huge international centre, which would have prevented the vandals from closing it down. Sadly it is no more, as molecular biologists and mathematical modellers took over the senior posts, and teaching students from Africa, Asia and South America was swiftly phased out. Those students from poor countries who in the past had been trained in epidemiology, disease investigation and control of epidemics, went on to become directors in their countries, with inestimable benefits for Britain; they were driven out because their countries were unable to pay the huge fees required to fund the running of this institute. They were replaced by people who were not interested in the big picture but only in the sub-microscopic particles which could garner them large research grants and might gain them admission to the Royal Society. There was great talk about how molecular biology was going to revolutionise animal disease control, but little practical benefit has accrued to animal health in almost 30 years. Sadly high-quality teachers are no longer valued and yet that is what a university should be about.

Our year was one of the beneficiaries of Alexander Robertson's rule, as we were the first year of the course that he introduced to modernise the teaching of clinical subjects by the use of small groups. There was a downside to this new system as we started with more than fifty students and they only wanted thirty-two students in final year (eight groups of four), which meant failing a few along the way and they rather overdid it. Only sixteen of our year of fifty survived unscathed and we were joined by eight people from the years above, which meant that there were only twenty-four in the final year (the following year they had more than seventy, which must have played havoc with their groups). This in turn had another unexpected result, as we became a very close-knit group that has met up annually for more than fifty years.

First year is where you find your feet and get the feel of the place: we were all allocated 'digs' and I shared a room with Brian Ranson, an old school friend who was studying anthropology. Mrs Mac 'looked after' us and six more students, and gave us bed and breakfast all week and an evening meal Sunday to Friday for the sum of £4 a week. She put a couple of spoonfuls of tea in the huge enamel tea pot on Sunday morning and added a couple more spoonfuls at each meal until the end of the week, when the grouts were finally removed and the process was repeated. The food was not haute cuisine but we did not go hungry.

There was rugby, football and hockey in the autumn and spring terms, and cricket for some in the summer. Scottish country dancing was a must of a Wednesday night because that was where all the American girls went. There were the college dances on a Saturday evening, held to raise money for student activities, where many met their future partners and much harmless fun was to be had.

The annual gathering of vet students from all over Britain (and Ireland as we were never allowed to forget) in one of the veterinary schools was an opportunity to meet friends from other vet schools and to do battle with them on the rugby field. The night before the rugby match in Dublin we were liberally entertained by the Dublin College team: you can imagine our surprise when a different fifteen turned out the next morning to play us – but we still won!

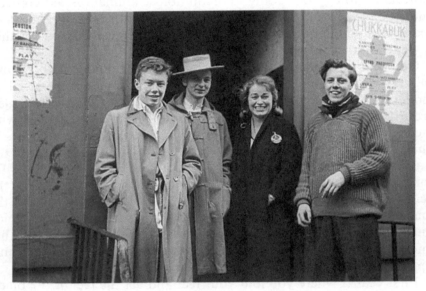

Kidnapping the Aberdeen Charities Queen: outside the Charities Office
(*l to r*) Alan Wilson, John Trethewey, Marlene Luebe and Roger Windsor.

There was the charities fund-raising week in which the students let down their hair, supposedly in the name of raising money for good causes. Our greatest exploit came in our first year when we set out in two vehicles to 'kidnap' the Aberdeen Charities Queen, Marlene Luebe, an American. She was captured and brought back to Edinburgh and displayed in a cage in the Charities Procession. She actually had a wonderful time and was a constant guest of the rector of the university, James Robertson Justice, so attended all the social functions. On the College stand we produced the perfect farm animal – the henhorcoo, which could be ridden, produced milk and laid eggs. The downside was that immediately after the procession we had to return Marlene to Aberdeen as she was returning home to the States on the Sunday and had not packed nor done of any of the many things required to do when leaving a country. She did not mind, but her boyfriend was livid.

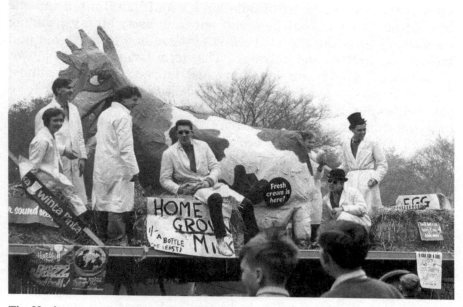

The Henhorcoo – the all-purpose farm animal, producing bottled milk and super large eggs – on the College float. (*l to r*) Pat Yelland, Dick LePage, Roger Windsor, Paul Brown, Anthony Gill, Dick Alexander and Don Eden.

There were balls and parties and clubs and politics. There were ponies to be ridden: Jimmy Speed, an anatomy lecturer, had the finest herd of Exmoor ponies in Scotland which he lent each summer to the Youth Hostels Association for their trekking. He was one of the original self-sufficiency exponents and lived the good life, long before TV's 'The Good Life': his wife collected wool off the fences which she spun, dyed and then wove before making Jimmy his suits. When you took the ponies back to their smallholding in Fife, which meant taking them on the Queensferry ferry, you ate regally off plates made by Jimmy, with knives and forks of similar origin, and the food was mostly home grown. Sheep wandered in and out of the house while you ate; the only house-trained sheep I have ever met.

He was a wonderful man with a delightful wife. They had married late in life and there were no children; I guess we students were their family and he was very generous to the Students' Association in his will.

The second year was the time in which you could feel free, as there were no examinations at the end. For the first term I shared a flat in Queens Street in the centre of Edinburgh with Brian Ranson and one of his friends, which was huge fun but took away all my spending money and so at the end of the first term we had to move out and look to 'old clothes and porridge'. That term I came bottom in two of the three class exams (anatomy and biochemistry) and almost bottom in physiology. Tommy Graham called me into his office for a real bollocking. It did not help that I had overslept for his anatomy practical exam that started at 2 pm.

'Well, Windsor, you have been having a high old time this term and you have done precious little work in any of the subjects and especially anatomy. I have a good mind to kick your airse, because you're no' stupid. Instead I am telling you now, you got twenty percent in this class exam and you need an average of forty percent to take the degree examination. If you don't get sixty percent in the next class exam, then you'll no' be taking the degree examination, which means you will have to resit the whole of third year. Think about it.'

I thought about it. Having no money was a great incentive to study. I moved into a cheap bed sitter and started to remedy the defects in my anatomical, biochemical and physiological knowledge. I must have overdone it a bit because I scored eighty percent in the anatomy class exam and came top, making me the only student in the year to come bottom and top in the same subject – and it was in consecutive exams.

The third year was when the work started to get serious, and fourth was the worst of all. I remained in the bed sitter for third year. Brian my anthropological school friend took the one adjacent and we took turns in cooking. It was during third year that the idea of founding a Bath Club came to the fore. To join, one had to take an unofficial bath in one of the Ladies' Halls of Residence. The founder members were Anthony Gill (who had the transport), Alan Wilson, Brian Ranson, John Shevill (a South African vet student a year or two below us who sadly never completed the course), and myself. St Leonard's Hall (formerly the St Trinian's School of Ronald Searle fame) was selected because Brian had a girlfriend resident therein, and it had a large ground floor common room where the young ladies were allowed to entertain their gentlemen friends. A far cry from today.

On the night in question Brian was duly entertained and while the young lady was preparing the coffee, Brian ensured that the one of the windows was unlocked which would allow us entry. St Leonard's Hall had a long drive down to the main road and so at about 3 am we parked Anthony's van under some trees near the top of the drive. Brian opened the window and climbed in, came to the front door which he unlocked and let us in. The door was left ajar in case a rapid exit was needed. We knew where the first floor bathrooms were situated and we soon had the baths filled. One by one we had our baths; decently we had brought our own towels. We dried ourselves and hung the Mickey Mouse masks, our chosen badge, over the taps and crept down the stairs. At the foot of the stairs there was a splendid Indian gong about three feet in diameter. Anthony, ever the buffoon, picked up the stick and gave the gong several thunderous bangs. We fled into the night, piled into the van and sped down the drive: by the time we got to the end the hall was a blaze of lights. We heard later that a couple of girls, thinking that they had overslept, had leapt out of bed, dressed hastily and rushed down to breakfast … at 4 am!

The Second Preclinical Examination commenced the slaughter of the innocents and our numbers were greatly reduced. There were two sets of Professional Examinations in third year – anatomy, bio-chemistry and physiology at Christmas, and pharmacology and animal husbandry in the summer, when we lost more. And the really tough year was still to come. Pharmacology was overseen by Pro-fessor Frank Alexander, a real gentleman and a stickler for propriety and good behaviour. He was also an honourable man: he told the story of being the external examiner in Bristol, when what he regarded as a 'tarty' girl in a micro mini skirt walked in for her oral examination. As she walked through the door he decided that she had to fail, and so he set about demolishing her knowledge, but on every topic she was able to give him chapter and verse. 'And much as it went against the grain, I perforce had to give her a distinction.' Which was honourable in its way, I suppose.

Professor Alexander introduced a new method of teaching

43

pharmacology as well as a novel method of selling a book. At his first lecture he informed us that he had written a small book on veterinary pharmacology and if we knew everything in that book then we would have no difficulty in passing the examination. Consequently he was not going to lecture to the syllabus: at each lecture he would tell us which chapter we should read and he then proceeded to lecture us on topics that he found interesting. As a result the lectures were a real stimulus to us to want to know more; they were great fun and enjoyed by both the professor and the students. Most of us found that the system worked, but Tony Stewart had problems and had not done well enough in the class exams to sit the professional examination in pharmacology and so he went to Frank Alexander to plead his case.

'There is no point Stewart: you stand no chance whatever of passing the exam and so I will not let you take it.'

'Please sir, I have been working at the subject; do let me have a go.'

'Very well, Stewart; you will be wasting your time and mine, not to mention that of the external examiner. You may take the examination, but YOU WILL NOT PASS.'

Tony took the examination and did pass. Alexander could have worked the marking for him to fail – but that was not the man. Many years later when I was standing for election to Council of the Royal College of Veterinary Surgeons I wrote to him asking for his support. He replied that he would willingly vote for me but he could not understand why on earth I wanted to involve myself with that gang of reprobates who sit and talk and do nothing. 'We in Edinburgh do not associate ourselves with that useless London talking shop.'

It was only a few years later that I realised how accurate was his observation. During the 2001 outbreak of foot and mouth disease the government of Blair, determined to have its election, took the control of the outbreak from the hands of vets and put it into the control of the Chief Scientist and the mathematical modellers, with the result that there was massive slaughter and many animals were killed that could and should have survived. I was still an RCVS councillor and furious that, despite the request of myself and several like-minded colleagues, the college refused to act to stop the carnage; it also took no action against those vets who had behaved so unprofessionally. I resigned from both the council and the college. I was greatly dismayed that the professional body of the profession that I loved could behave so badly. However, that was in the future – at this point I still had to qualify.

Fourth year involved courses in pathology, parasitology and bacteriology together with the start of clinical medicine and surgery. It was a tough year and so I decided to go back into digs to be looked after and fed. I teamed up with John Trethewey who had palatial digs in Joppa, where he was waited on hand and foot by Mrs Menzies, a banker's widow with two teenage daughters; a small room was found for me. It was during this year that the feeling was growing in me that I wanted a job which would offer me greater intellectual stimulation than would be found in veterinary practice, and I found myself increasingly drawn to the world of pathology and microbiology. Ian Beattie and his team of pathologists, particularly Ken Head and Alan Rowland, made the whole subject come alive. I was amazed by the different ways that bodies and tissues responded to injuries as they tried to defend themselves. It seemed to me that pathology was the hub around which the whole wheel of veterinary medicine revolved – this was what I wanted to do. 'Bean' Phillips and Gordon Fraser who taught most of the microbiology had a similar effect on waking my interest in the part that microbes play in disease processes.

I was also growing more politically aware of what was going on round the globe: with more colonials than Scots in our year, I became keenly interested in the problems of the emerging countries. Countries that were shrugging off colonial rule were going to lose many of their trained, skilled and experienced staff who would not work under black rule. There was going to be a massive skills shortage as training of indigenous people was only just starting, and it was slowly dawning upon me that I wanted to be part of this new venture. I was a great idealist at the time (thanks to Sidney Adams) and I suspect that, all these years later, I still am. I would have the training and knowledge to really make a difference. But first I had to qualify and so I worked harder in the fourth year than I ever had before, or have subsequently. It did the trick and I sailed through the First Professional Examination. Then it was downhill all the way as, by comparison with what had gone before, the final Professional Examination was a walkover. It was time to enjoy myself again, and so it was out of digs and back into a flat.

Most of our year had had settled living companions throughout their stay and so I was in need of someone to share with. Brian

Ranson had graduated and was working in Turkey. Clifford Harding and Don Eden had shared accommodation since first year but both were to be married before final year and both to girls from home: Don's wife Joyce was to come from Wales and live in Edinburgh but Edith, Cliff's wife to be, had a very good job in her home town in County Durham and decided to continue with it until Cliff qualified. Cliff was at a loose end and so we decided to team up.

We found an attic flat above the Gillespie Boys Preparatory School based in a large house in Morningside. The flat occupied the attic as three sides of a square running round the glass roof (single-glazed in those days) that allowed light into the stairwell in the centre of this Georgian house. On one side there were doors to the bathroom and kitchen. On the adjacent wall there was a door into the bedroom; moving round there was the door into the living room that was about thirty feet long with a tiny fireplace at the far end. There was no central heating but there was a gas geyser in the bathroom and a gas cooker and water heater in the kitchen. It was a cold flat and we were to experience the coldest winter in twenty years. Cliff and I soon established a cosy modus vivendi until one evening there was a ring at the door. A bedraggled Colin Sutherland stood there; he had been thrown out of his digs and wanted to know if we could put him up. Colin and I had gone through four years of armed neutrality, neither caring much for the other. There was a spare bed at the far end of the sitting room which I was going to move into when Edith chose to visit Cliff. We took him in on the understanding that if things did not work out he would have to go. Things worked out; Colin remains a close friend to this day.

There was a definite routine. Cooking was a communal task and we washed up while listening to 'The Archers'; what a great programme it was, dispensing advice and information under the guise of entertainment. From 7 pm we worked until a quarter to ten, when we downed books and nipped round the corner to the pub for a pint before closing time. We were not angels and there were not always three of us in the flat of an evening, although Cliff went out less frequently than either Colin or I. I had purchased an ancient Hillman for £10 which was very useful since we had to travel out to the Bush (the college field station) each morning. The main problem with the car was that it did not like starting in the cold weather and had to be pushed. Luckily there was no shortage of young boys about who were only too pleased to push the car across the icy playground, so we would all pile in, the boys pushed us out of the grounds and down the hill, and we were off. However, some of the parents complained to the headmistress that they did not pay fees for their boys to push-start cars, so we stopped the practice and had to take it in turns to push it ourselves.

The main social event of the year was the organising in January of the Annual Conference of the Association of Veterinary Students of Great Britain and Ireland. As President of the Veterinary Students Committee it fell to me to make the arrangements for the conference, and I wanted to make it a big one and a very successful one, I also wanted it to have a scientific core. The hallmark of a Windsor production, then and ever thereafter, was that everything was done by committees. Giving people 'ownership' of an activity ensures that they do the job to the best of their ability. We had an Accommodation Committee headed by Anne Horne (soon to be Schermbrucker as she married a man a couple of years ahead of us) which was responsible for booking the hotels. It had been past Association policy to put the Irish contingent into the grottiest hotel to be found because they invariably smashed up the joint. Anne decided that if we put them in a smart hotel they would behave, and they did. We were lucky that our regular Saturday night dance profits enabled us to subsidise the accommodation costs so we were able to use decent hotels throughout.

John Trethewey was in charge of the Entertainment Committee and he put on a wow – 'Pulse Beat' in the Eldorado Ballroom in Leith. The principal band was Acker Bilk's Paramount Jazz Band, but the university West Indian Steel Band (in those days there were many West Indian students in the university who supplemented their grants by their musical activity) played and so did Don Lambert's Dance Band (Don was a perennial vet student who financed his way through college by running a huge musical empire. At any weekend Don would have half a dozen bands playing in different venues round the city, including the Dick Vet.) The dance was a sell-out and a huge financial success.

Angus Gordon and Keith Dobson were in charge of the sporting fixtures. Lunches were organised by Dick Alexander's committee and they too were a sell-out because of the quality of the after lunch speakers: Arthur Smith, then Captain of Scotland and the British Lions Rugby teams talked about their recent visit to South Africa.

47

The distinguished comic author Sir Compton Mackenzie spoke of his love of cats, and Jo Grimond, who was Rector of the university as well as being leader of the Liberal Party, spoke on the delights of politics.

On the Sunday morning Dick le Page's committee organised a wonderful series of lectures. 'Physiology and Physique' by Alan Croft started the proceedings. 'How to Influence Genes and Make Profits' delivered by Donald Michie, the famous geneticist, came next. The best was saved till the end when Magnus Pyke, soon to be a regular TV science presenter, thrilled the hall with an electrifying talk on 'The Concept of Biochemical Unity' which showed how all of life was linked.

The success of this conference together with the absence of any complaints from the public helped to restore the reputation of the Association and put it back into the good books of the various schools. Involving so many people in the organisation had reduced the load on us all, which meant that we did not have to take off too much time from our studies.

During this year we spent much of the time visiting farms, attending clinics, going to the abattoir for meat inspection practice. We all enjoyed going out with Ben Mitchell, or 'Crash' Mitchell as he was known, as he allowed us to do all the work and there was always the chance of a prang in the car which was how he earned his nickname. He was a lovely man, a generous and good teacher, and we learned only later that the problems in the car were a prelude to his terminal illness – within a couple of years he was dead from motor neuron disease. This was my first experience of the living hell of a death as the body ceases to function while the inner person continues to remain intellectually competent to the end.

The head of the Large Animal Clinic, Walter McClennan, prided himself on his clinical ability and he was responsible for the teaching of infertility and breeding diseases. There was nothing Walter liked better than getting his shirt off and shoving his arm up the backside of a horse or better still, a cow. Sadly he believed that if he could not solve the problem then no one at the Dick could. This failure to use all the facilities available to him was a further stimulus to me to look for a career outside general practice. The college had a commercial general practice but it provided the laboratories with almost no material. This seemed most short-sighted to me, it being the duty of the vet to use all available tools to ensure that the right diagnosis is made and hence the correct treatment provided. This was an example of George Boddie's failure of leadership: all the disciplines in the college should have been working as a team to provide the clinicians with the best back up; but you cannot provide back up if you are not asked. Some of the finest facilities and staff were not being used.

In Gorgie abattoir John Norval was king. He ran that abattoir with a rod of iron and the place was always spick and span as he would not tolerate dirt in an establishment working with food. No small feat in an abattoir. When making his rounds of the suspect carcases he would hold out his hand and a knife would be slapped into it. Work completed, the knife would be taken away and washed and sterilised. His incisions were always bold and precise and he would bark out his clear instructions concerning the fate of the carcase: 'Condemn liver, pass carcase,' or 'Condemn pluck, and right stifle, split carcase and we will examine again.'

I only saw him perplexed on one occasion and that was when two groups of students were both examining the same line, one group on either side of the organs – in this case the plucks (tongue, trachea, lungs and heart removed as a unit) from cattle. Anthracosis was a regular problem in those days when the coal mines on the outskirts of Edinburgh were in full production. The animals, mostly cattle and sheep, inhaled the coal dust, which was filtered out of the blood and became trapped in the lymph nodes that over time became a solid black colour. These lymph nodes were removed and condemned, and the rest of the carcase was treated on its merits.

'Here is a classic case of anthracosis,' said Norval and he stretched out his hand into which was slapped a sharp clean knife. The lymph node was sliced open. There came a loud shriek from the other side of the line. The lymph node was Mike Buadu's thumb. Mike was in our year; he was a Ghanaian, a small rolypoly man with a great sense of humour and a very good hockey player. He had been examining the pluck from the other side and had the misfortune to be holding the pluck when the 'King' was in full flow – and a thumb through the pleura did look like a lymph node full of coal dust. There was a copious flow of blood, which, given the environment, was probably as well. However, Norval rushed off with Mike to the First Aid Post, all was well and there were no hard feelings. Today there would be a court case.

49

By the start of the summer term I had decided that I wanted to be involved in confirming diagnoses rather than working on hunches, and so I applied to the university to study for an honours degree in pathology. On the strength of Ian Beattie's recommendation and my unhindered progress through the vet college, I was accepted by the medical faculty for the BSc (Honours) (Pathology) course: the veterinary faculty did not run honours BSc courses. Before I started the course it was found that one of the statutes governing the degree course only permitted medical students to study for the pathology degree (there was some requirement to examine dead human bodies) so I had to settle to study for the bacteriology degree, as it required an Act of Parliament to change the statutes. In those days the Horse Race Levy Board was giving good grants for postgraduate studies even if they were not directly related to horses. I flew down to London for an interview, the day before our final examinations began, and came back on the midnight flight. Because of fog the flight was diverted to Glasgow and I arrived back at the flat at 4 am with a 9 am examination in medicine to be sat. A couple of hours' sleep was enough in those far-off days. The written examinations went well and I was buoyed by the news that I had been awarded a Horse Race Levy Board Scholarship.

The written exams were over: we had had the Final Year Dinner and now only the practicals and oral examinations stood between us and a job. Being a 'W' I was always one of the last to be examined and so all my practicals took place on the Saturday morning. It was common knowledge that you only needed to worry in medicine if, when you went into your practical, the examiner said to you, 'Now Mr Windsor, how would you go about examining this cow?'

I could have dropped dead when I walked into the stall where there was a tethered cow and the examiner said, 'Now Mr Windsor, how would you go about examining this cow?'

I was certain that I had passed the written examination and to be confronted with this completely threw me. I do not think that I recovered throughout the whole interview. I tried to pull myself together and I believe that I made a reasonable job of the oral without doing myself justice. I do not remember much of the rest of the sessions, save the one with Johnny Burgess, who twice left the interview to restore his whisky level.

Lunch was taken at Bush House in the knowledge that the results would be on the college noticeboard at 2.30 pm. Much as I disliked

George Boddie, I will always be grateful to him; as I was standing forlornly in the queue waiting to get lunch, Prof. Boddie came up to me put his arm round my shoulders and said quietly, 'I wouldnae worry if I was you Mr Windsor.' And with that he was gone.

It was a happier man who downed his lunch and then stood expectantly by the main college noticeboard waiting for the secretary to come. When she did, there was my name right down near the bottom. I had gained no medals but I had not failed any professional examination on the way. I rushed to phone my father and give him the good news.

'No more than I expected,' came the reply. My father might have shown some reaction had I failed, but I am not even sure of that: however, I knew that he was delighted that one of his children had succeeded at what had been denied him.

I was now a qualified vet and had set my feet on the path of research and investigation. I had decided to become a 'Sherlock Holmes' rather than a 'James Herriot'. It remained to be seen whether I had made the correct decision.

5

First Steps in Detection, 1965–1967

'You are brought in contact with all that is strange and bizarre.'
Sir Arthur Conan Doyle, *A Case of Identity*

One of Sherwin's great dictums is: 'He who never makes a mistake, never makes anything.' I was lucky to have been able to make most of my mistakes in Kenya, under the benevolent eyes of my boss, Bill Bruce, the Chief Veterinary Research Officer who ran the Veterinary Research Laboratory at Kabete, and Ian Beattie and Maryk Gitter. It was in Kabete that I started what was to become the work for most of my professional career; it was where I learnt that solving problems was fun and that a good veterinary detective could save many animal lives, or make them more comfortable or productive and at the same time make money for the farmer. I have never regretted my decision to follow in the animal footsteps of Sherlock Holmes!

It is amazing how responsibility concentrates the mind. I was in charge of the only diagnostic laboratory in Kenya: qualified for two years, three months in Africa, no experience of laboratory work and little knowledge of African diseases. I could offer a reasonable intellect, a great desire to learn, an unquenchable thirst for knowledge and an ability to work hard. It was not quite 'blood, sweat, toil and tears' but only the tears were missing. Bob Roach, the New Zealander who ran the Diagnosis Section, was a very good pathologist and he knew his African diseases, but he was not interested in administration or making sure that reports went out on time. He was a true dilettante who could be working away at one case when if something new and interesting came his way, the first case would be dropped and left for a week or more. He presided over a team of young vets new to Africa, two European laboratory technicians and a bunch of experienced African technicians. He had a very short temper and could be very rude: he upset Arthur Cole, a large estate owner and brother of Lord Enniskillen and cousin of Lord Delamere, two of Kenya's leading farmers.

When called by the Director, Tony Dorman, to explain his actions, knowing that he was 'irreplaceable' Bob was not in the least contrite and blustered about the incompetence of the new field veterinary officers, finally tendering his resignation as Head of the Diagnosis Section. He had thought that he was indispensable with only three young vets in his department none with any African experience. He was shattered when Dorman accepted his resignation. He never forgave me for agreeing to take over.

First the laboratory had to be put into some sort of order and then there had to be control of samples coming in and reports going out. I had no knowledge of how a laboratory worked as I had only ever been on the receiving end, but I was certain that vets wanted their results the day before yesterday not in three weeks' time. Fiona McCrudden was on her way to Naivasha to marry another young British vet, Pat Dawes. Jürgen Wegener from Germany was the third; his doctoral thesis was on the subject 'The Histology of the Sausage'. Wally Ashford (the Chief Laboratory Technician) and I sat down and planned out a system for running the laboratory, which involved a 'duty vet' with responsibility for all the work that came in on the day, regular case meetings and a daily check on the reports going out. The system creaked a bit at first but we soon made the necessary adjustments and within weeks there was a marked increase in the number of submissions. Wally was a tower of strength in the section and kept the bacteriology under his special supervision. He had worked for many years for Burroughs Wellcome making vaccines, until getting itchy feet; he had seen an advertisement for a bacteriology technician's post in Kenya. He took to Africa like a flea to a dog's back.

Expatriates lived very sheltered lives in those days, protected by our good jobs, our neat little houses with big gardens and a plethora of cheap servants who did all the unpleasant jobs. The Veterinary Research Laboratory at Kabete was going through a transitional phase with many experienced members of staff retiring, for age reasons not because of the political changes, and some had transferred to the East African Veterinary Research Laboratory at Muguga about 10 miles further out of town, where I was later to work. Young people were arriving by the day from Britain, Australia, Germany, the Scandinavian countries, and young Kenyans were returning from their training abroad. It was an exciting place to work: there were enough old heads to keep you on the straight and narrow and enough space to develop.

At the laboratory we had plenty of staff mostly of excellent calibre and we had a band of young African trainees who had been selected for their academic ability and an aptitude for the work. Once they had learnt that they were not God's gift to the farming community, they became solid laboratory staff. I remember walking into the general laboratory one morning and noticing that the jars of stains were almost all empty. I said to young Christopher Muroke, 'Please Christopher, fill the staining jars from the stock bottles.'

Christopher looked at me in horror, his big, round, brown eyes wide open; he put out both hands palms up and said, 'But, Sir, I cannot soil my educated hands.'

I looked him straight in those big brown eyes and replied, 'If you do not, Christopher, I will kick you up your educated backside.'

He filled the jars. There was of course no possibility of my kicking his backside, educated or otherwise, because it would have resulted in instant deportation and anyway violence has never been my style. Christopher became a Member of the Institute of Laboratory Technicians and a valuable member of the Bacteriology Department, which was finally built.

The staff of the Diagnosis Section were the general dogsbodies of the Vet Labs and were called on to perform almost any task that nobody else wanted to do. The lab had its own farm for supplying the experimental animals required and so it was the vets from Diagnosis who provided all the clinical services. It was in that capacity that I was called upon to attend a bullock that was developing bloat. The bovine animal produces a great deal of gas from its large fermentation tank which we call the rumen: this is released by regular belching. However, should the passage to the exterior become blocked then the animal blows up like a balloon and if not treated then the pressure of the rumen on the heart and lungs rapidly results in death. The animals were being fed on surplus potatoes – a notorious villain in the cause of bloat, as the passage from mouth to rumen is not a nice straight tube but curves to pass over the heart and it is here that lumps can get stuck. If the animal is not too large then it is not too difficult to put your hand in and pull out the offending object. Consequently I had put a gag into the mouth of the bullock to prevent him closing his mouth and biting off my arm. I stripped off my shirt, put my hand into the mouth of the beast and found the opening of the oesophagus and was working my hand down trying to find the potato when Bill Bruce passed and said to me in his quiet west of Scotland accent, 'Roger, do you know that one of the first signs of rabies in cattle is the inability to belch?'

I think that I blanched, but at that moment my fingers touched a solid object and I was able to grasp and remove a small potato. I felt a great deal better, but I had learnt a salient lesson: 'different countries, different problems'. We never give a thought to rabies in Britain because it does not occur: it is a different story in Africa and much of the rest of the developing world.

Kenya was newly independent, there was massive activity in all spheres of industry and commerce, and agriculture was undergoing a real boom. Farmers were importing stock from various parts of the world to improve their herds and flocks and as a result there were constant batches of animals to be examined at the airport and at the docks in Mombasa. Already the problems of apartheid South Africa were affecting the rest of Africa. A farmer had imported a batch of pedigree Suffolk sheep from Britain: when the plane arrived in Nairobi they were not taken off, and it was not until the plane landed in Johannesburg that the mistake was discovered. It was decided to leave the sheep on the plane and return them to Kenya on the plane's return home. They were taken off this time, but the customs officials decided that since they had come from South Africa they had to be slaughtered immediately, as such contaminated sheep could not be allowed in the country. Of course this happened on a Sunday.

Luckily the farmer was a friend of Bruce Mackenzie, the Minister of Agriculture. A message was brought to the house by Bill Bruce's houseboy (we had no telephone!) informing me that I had to report to the Minister, at Embakazi Airport, *immediately*. I went. Mackenzie had persuaded the customs officials that they did not need to slaughter the animals because, not having been taken off the plane, they had never been in South Africa. That was agreed, but then it was suggested that they might have been infected by some nasty South African apartheid virus by breathing their contaminated air. It was my job to check each one and assure the customs that they were all healthy. They seemed fine to me but they had perforce to be put into quarantine where they languished for two weeks until I examined them again and found them to have remained healthy, when they were released.

At the time in Kenya there were many small abattoirs for local consumption scattered round the country but there was an export abattoir for pigs at Uplands near Limuru, and two export abattoirs for ruminant animals (cattle plus a few sheep and goats), one at Athi River, about twenty-five miles from Nairobi, and one at Mombasa. Animals were trekked to these abattoirs or sent in lorries. A lorry overloaded with cattle was stopped by the police as it was passing through Kabete; they were horrified by what they saw and instructed the lorry to come into the laboratory. As usual the staff of the Diagnosis Section were asked to see what was going on: the police were right to be horrified. Many of the animals had fallen and four had been trampled to death. I instructed the staff to unload the lorry into a field and we set about examining them. They had come from Archer's Post, 350 miles away in the Northern Frontier District and the first half of the journey had been along dirt roads. To make matters worse this was not a proper cattle truck but just a truck used for this and that, with projections for the animals to bump into and injure themselves. Five animals with broken legs were shot and we tended the wounds on the others – many of whom were too weak to stand. Hay and water was brought to them. While this was going on a messenger came up to me and told me that the Director, Tony Dorman, wished to see me in his office, *immediately*. I washed up and tidied myself as best as possible and presented myself, almost for the first time, to the great man.

'Windsor, what is going on? What are all these animals doing in the field? This is a quarantine station and we cannot accept animals here.' From his office at the top of the Administrative Building he had an almost complete view of the estate.

I did my best to explain; I stressed the horrors of the situation and stated that there were four dead and that we had shot another five which would be disposed of in the same way as all our post mortem material.

'Windsor, there is nothing for it, you must load the animals back onto the lorry and send them to Athi River.'

I was incensed, but in my best diplomatic language explained that first and foremost I was a veterinary surgeon and bound by my Royal College oath to do the best for the animals under my care: that this was the worst animal welfare case I had seen in my short career and there was no way I was going to load those animals back onto the lorry.

'Windsor, this is an order: you will load the animals back onto the lorry.'

'Sir, my first duty is to the animals and although I respect your authority as my Director, in the Kenya Civil Service you are not entitled to give me such an instruction. If you insist that the animals be loaded onto the lorry then you must supervise it yourself.'

New boys rarely speak to directors in such terms and with remarkably good grace Mr Dorman decided that he had to see for himself. We walked to the field in silence, each preoccupied with his own thoughts. I had visions of being on the plane home in a few days. However, one look at the animals and the director agreed that they should and could stay. They remained with us for a week until they were fit enough to continue their journey to the abattoir.

An interesting result of this confrontation was that thereafter I was on very good terms with Mr Dorman, who regularly asked me for an opinion when there many more senior people to whom he could have turned. It confirmed in me the belief that I should always stick to my professional principles because in the long run people respect those who behave honourably.

Running the laboratory had its difficult, as well as exciting, times. Such as when Benson Ochido, on my first Christmas in charge, stole a Winchester bottle (about five litres) of methyl alcohol for his Christmas party and died of poisoning in the Kenyatta Hospital. I had a further battle with the director so that Benson's widow could get a pension: Benson had given twenty or more years of service in the laboratory, rising from cleaner to senior laboratory technician, and was a lovely man, a wonderful worker who taught me well about the technical work of a laboratory. Luckily I was well supported by Wally who considered him his deputy. The widow received a pension. Benson just had a weakness for alcohol; if only he had taken the ethyl alcohol he would still have been alive.

The Vet Lab possessed a mobile laboratory that had been donated by USAID (United States Agency for International Development) which had been designed for use in the States, to run on well-surfaced American roads not African bush roads. The first time we took it off the tarmac the air-conditioning unit fell from its bracket, and the second time the centrifuge broke out of its moorings. We also found out that it would only travel about 100 miles on a full tank of petrol. It went into our vehicle workshop and extra tanks were fitted, the suspension and all the fixings were reinforced and we scrapped the air-conditioning unit.

The first time I got to use the mobile lab for real was when Bill Bruce asked me to accompany him on a field investigation of infertility and breeding diseases in cattle in Nakuru District. We parked the lab in the grounds of the District Veterinary Office and the DVO, David Shannon, took us off to the different farms, where I was just an extra pair of hands. Bill asked the questions and then David and I took the samples: these included taking sheath washings from bulls. This is a fairly exciting job – you need your wits about you to avoid being kicked, or worse, by the bull. Once you get started the real danger is over. The bull has to be reasonably well tethered and you need a good man to hold the tail in the vertical position (this reduces the chances of the animal kicking) while a looped rope is put round the hind leg on the side you are working from and this is held by another good man. You then have to crouch down and trim the hair from the end of the prepuce and generally clean the area, while at the same time keeping an eye on that back leg – you can usually sense when the animal is going to take action and surprisingly beef bulls were usually quiet under these strange conditions: it was the dairy bulls that were most fractious. A soft plastic tube is inserted into the prepuce and about 100 ml of warm saline is poured through a funnel, down the tube and into the prepuce, which is then massaged briskly a hundred times (you can now understand why the bull does not object once you get started!). The funnel is then lowered and the saline runs back. With luck, it contains the pathogens that you are looking for. This is back-breaking work. Some ranches have a hundred or more bulls.

In those far-off days we did not have 'Vacutainers' (sealed tubes from which the air has been expelled) and disposable needles, and so cattle had to be bled from the jugular vein using a good big needle; this required that the head of the beast be held. With 'Vacutainers' you can bleed from the caudal vein – and the tail is easier to hold than the head! Tampons were used to collect vaginal mucus from cows and heifers. The samples were all carefully identified and put into a cold-bag with plenty of ice to keep them cool.

Back in the mobile lab all the samples had to be processed: the serum had to be separated from the blood; the mucus and preputial washings had to be spun in the centrifuge and plates had to be inoculated with the samples. Christine Lund and Phillip Otieno, both

58

laboratory technicians, had come with us. Christine was a locally employed expatriate: her husband had been seconded from the Central Veterinary Laboratory in Weybridge and worked in the Virology Section. Christine was also from the CVL, where she was a trained bacteriology technician, Phillip was a rising star at the Vet Lab, as he was the first Kenyan qualified veterinary laboratory technician; he was a very able man with a delightful, open personality, who was prepared to accept responsibility for his own actions and for the staff who worked under him. They set to with a will, assisted (or otherwise) by the CVRO and me.

We spent three days in Nakuru and it was a very useful exercise as we were able to determine that several of the farms were infected with *Brucella abortus* while others had problems with *Vibrio fetus*: some were infected with both pathogens. That trip showed me the benefits of having a local veterinary laboratory so that samples do not have to be transported over long distances under poor environmental conditions. A lesson I learnt and was able to put to good use in later stages of my career. I also found out later that a poorly equipped laboratory or a laboratory without trained staff is worse than useless and so one has to balance proximity of the service against quality. In many developing countries where there is a shortage of good quality staff it is often better to centralise the services. Yet another factor to be considered is cost: laboratory services do not come cheap and it is therefore essential that costs do not outweigh benefits. And so in developing countries with a thriving meat export industry it pays the country to invest heavily in its veterinary laboratory services, whereas in countries with no such exports it is difficult to justify investment in anything more than basic laboratory services which can provide a good early warning system of new diseases.

Not only was I an inexperienced vet (just two years qualified) but I had little knowledge of those diseases specific to Africa in general and Kenya in particular. Two wonderful lifebuoys were thrown to me in the persons of Ian Beattie (on secondment from the Dick Vet) and Maryk Gitter (on secondment from the Weybridge Veterinary Investigation Centre): these two men saved my professional career, if not my life. Ian was the head of pathology at the Dick Vet and was responsible for running the best teaching department at my time in the college. It was a criminal shame that when a Chair of Veterinary Pathology was endowed at the college he was not given it (an indication of what was to befall the veterinary schools of Britain, as high-powered science took precedence over quality of teaching). He was a wonderful teacher, with all the time in the world, and when asked to come and advise in the post mortem room he was never too busy to come. His analysis was always clear, concise and to the point and he had an inexhaustible store of knowledge of the various manifestations of diseases.

I have been blessed throughout my career with a wealth of excellent teachers and Maryk Gitter was another. Maryk had been a member of the Polish Air Force and was captured by the Russians, he escaped from his Siberian prisoner of war camp and walked across winter Russia to freedom. At the end of the war he became a student at the Edinburgh Vet School and by the early sixties was head of the Weybridge Veterinary Investigation Centre. He had been sent by the British government as part of a team to strengthen the East African Veterinary Research Institute (a place I came to know well in later years) and undertake research in diseases caused by salmonella. Maryk's great strength was his ability to sort out problems on farms, and so at a tender age I was exposed to one of the finest pathologists Britain had to offer, and to its leading field investigator. I could not have received better teaching. I have tried to prove worthy of the training they gave me.

Maryk was my first real contact with the English Veterinary Investigation Service (a branch of the State Veterinary Service which was part of what was then the Ministry of Agriculture, Fisheries and Food). It is fair to say that Maryk's contribution to the control of salmonellosis in Kenya was not great, but his contribution came in teaching people (including me) how to investigate outbreaks of disease in the field. I had the good fortune to spend a week in Kitale in western Kenya investigating a disease of pigs that had recently been introduced into the country, in imported pigs. We spent five days going from farm to farm, sorting out the problems. The new disease had already spread to most of the farms in the area; it was swine dysentery.

There was one Danish pig farmer whose farm was a total shambles. Mr Rasmussen had not the first idea about pig management. The farm was a mess and the pigs were all in very poor condition. Farmers are always hospitable and those in Kenya no less so, and so we sat down in the kitchen with a cup of tea and some of Mrs Rasmussen's excellent cakes when Maryk leant forward to Mr

Rasmussen and said in his strong Polish accent, 'Mr Razzmussen, 'ave you ever zought about keeping ze sheep?' It was his way of saying, 'I do not know where to start or what I can do to assist you'. A few weeks later Mr Rasmussen sold up and returned to Denmark but for many years he kept in touch with Maryk.

During the trip we visited the Kitale Prison Farm and there I saw the largest sows I have ever seen, they must have weighed at least 500 lb each. They were enormous and very fat. The farm had been started by a British inmate; in civvy street he had been a farm manager on a European farm but had embezzled a considerable sum of money from the owner. He had served three years of his five-year sentence and had returned to Britain on his release. During his stay in jail he had set up a very good little farm with a small dairy, a pig unit, a vegetable patch and an orchard which grew bananas, guavas, and avocado pears. The prison was now self-sufficient in milk and vegetables and sold some for prisoner amenities. It had also been an excellent provider of pork but for some reason the sows would no longer produce young ones. They had been fed more and more in an attempt to get them to give birth, to no avail. We did our usual detailed investigation and I can still remember the first line of Maryk's report: 'On a pig farm, in the absence of artificial insemination, it is essential to have a boar!' Problem solved. 'Elementary my dear Windsor.'

By the end of the week in Kitale my knowledge of disease investigation had increased significantly and so I was in good shape to handle swine dysentery, one of the major problems that confronted us when I was working in Cambridge. I had also been given the wherewithal to undertake a disease investigation of any type of disease in the field. While I was still feeling my way I had Maryk to turn to for advice and guidance. The importance of a logical and systematic approach to a problem was well learnt. I was learning to follow in Sherlock's footsteps. Thank you Maryk.

Such skills were not required for the next major investigation that we undertook. A lorry pulled up outside the door of the diagnostic laboratory, but the driver knew nothing other than he had come from Mombasa, a drive of about 300 miles. At the time about 100 miles were asphalt; the remainder a very rough murram – the red soil of Africa which makes good roads when maintained but is likely to deteriorate into rumble strips as the surface takes on the shape of corrugated iron spread across the road. The size of the corrugations varies from road to road, depending upon its construction and the types of vehicle that use it. For the novice driver corrugations are a nightmare, as the faster you go the more the car shakes until you reach the magic speed when the car rides the surface and the car stops shaking. But it requires courage to accelerate while the car is being shaken to pieces: the larger the corrugations, the faster you have to travel to reach the magic speed; and the heavier the vehicles that use the road, the larger the corrugations.

The lorry driver was instructed to take his load to the door of the post mortem room and unload the animals. There were five full grown beasts. It was 4 pm and we finished at 4.30, but something told me that these animals should be examined before we left and not put into the cold store until the morning. We set to work. One of the joys of Africa is that there are plenty of staff to carry out the heavy work such as removing the skin. We always examined the animal before the work commenced and these animals were in reasonable condition but showed signs of diarrhoea and dehydration.

I had never seen rinderpest, but I had heard a great deal about it. The name in German means 'cattle disease or plague' and brings fear to the hearts of anyone who knows about animal disease. In the mid nineteenth century it changed the shape of British farming: Willingham in Cambridgeshire had been a major supplier of milk to London, but when the entire population of cattle were wiped out for the second time in a few years, the farmers decided that they would no long keep cattle and instead they went in for fruit growing. Rinderpest was responsible for the birth of the State Veterinary Service which later developed into the Ministry of Agriculture. In 1864 the Archbishop of Canterbury wrote to the government requesting a 'Day of National Humiliation' be established: later Queen Victoria ordered a special prayer be read in churches throughout the land. Hundreds of thousands of cattle died throughout the whole of Britain.

Despite never having seen the disease, within minutes I felt certain that rinderpest was what it was. There were necrotic lesions in the mouth, on the gums, tongue and hard palate; there were ulcers in the oesophagus – the only diseases that cause ulceration in the oesophagus of cattle are rinderpest and acorn poisoning (there are few oak trees in Kenya). There were ulcers in all parts of the stomach and haemorrhages and necrosis throughout the whole of the intestines. This was rinderpest, a disease way above my pay grade. By now it was after 5 pm but Ian Beattie and Bill Bruce were still there and, like Hilaire Belloc's 'All sorts and condition of famous physicians', came hurrying round at the run.' Ian had never seen the disease before, but Bill with his vast African experience had, and both agreed that I was right. Tony Dorman was sent for and had to come from home. Soon there was more brass in the PM room than there is in a bedstead: the heads of the Virology (Dr Pini, an Italian) and Serology Sections (Dr Ogonowski, a Pole who, like Maryk Gitter, had trained in Edinburgh) were called and for good measure Helmuth Ohder (a German virologist who was pioneering new serological techniques) was asked to join us. Despite having made the diagnosis I felt privileged to be present for this high level policy discussion. Samples were taken for confirmation and the post mortem room was cleaned and disinfected before the staff were allowed to leave at 7.30 pm – they did not mind because they were paid overtime.

The first imperative was to find out where the animals came from and so the Provincial Veterinary Officer for the coast was contacted by phone, and telegrams were sent to alert the veterinary officers along the coast. Although we did not know it, we were witnessing the last great epidemic of rinderpest. The story finally emerged: these cattle had originated in the Northern Frontier District of Kenya, along the border with Somalia. There was much unrest at the time as Somalia was demanding the return of great swathes of Kenya that they considered to be theirs, bands of guerrillas called shifta were being sent into Kenya to terrorise people and so the land was in a state of flux. Civil strife is one of the great contributors to epidemic disease. The animals were being trekked down for slaughter at Mombasa when they started to die.

Sadly, I never got to see this outbreak: my presence was deemed unnecessary. Never having had anything to do with rinderpest control, I considered the decision regrettable but reasonable. The Director, the Assistant Director (Disease Control, the Australian, Marcus Durand), the CVRO, the Head of the Animal Livestock Marketing Organisation (Hector Douglas) and several others flew down to see the situation on the ground. They came back with grisly news that the holding ground was like a charnel house, with dead and dying animals everywhere. I could not help but remember the photograph we were shown as students of the outbreak in South Africa during the great pandemic of the 1890s. It was really too late

63

to start a vaccination campaign because it was obvious that many animals were infected, but that was what happened. The animals were run through a crush: anything that looked ill was shot and if it appeared healthy then it was vaccinated. The animals were examined daily for several days and all sick animals were destroyed. After ten days the outbreak came to a halt but 5000 animals died

One of the major responsibilities of the Diagnosis Section was rabies, and we had the entire national responsibility for rabies diagnosis in both humans and animals. The technique for diagnosis in those far-off days was to use what is called the Sellar's stain. The brain was removed from the skull and split in half longitudinally; half was put in formalin to 'fix' for the Histology Section to cut very thin slices of the tissue to be examined under the microscope. The other half was carefully dissected to remove the Ammons Horn from dogs and most other species; however from cats the cerebellum was used. The reason that specific parts of the brain were chosen is that in some parts of the brain there is a greater concentration of the virus and so it is easier to make a diagnosis.

A small portion of the selected brain tissue was smeared thinly on glass slides and 'fixed' to the slide with alcohol. Once the pre-liminaries had been carried out the smear was stained with Sellar's stain and then examined under the microscope: we looked round the smear until we found an area with many nerve cells and then we focused in and looked into the cells. If they were infected with rabies virus we saw a small round or oval inclusion called a Negri body that stained blue against the red cell. This was conclusive: however, if the disease was not very advanced there would be insufficient virus to show up in the smear – that was the reason that in former times dogs suspected of having rabies were not killed but caged and kept under observation. If they did not die within ten days they were not infected with the virus and they were released. Once a dog shows signs of rabies then it is invariably dead within a week and those extra three days are purely an extra precaution. Even so it was not always possible to be completely sure that the absence of Negri bodies meant the animal was free from the infection, and so a bio-logical test was carried out. A small amount of the brain is ground up with sand and a sterile salt solution, and it is hoped that the virus is released into the liquid, then a minute amount is injected directly into the brains of a litter of mice less than a week old. The sucking mice are anaesthetised and a fine needle is injected through the skull which has not yet become bone. If there is virus then the mice start dying from seven days after the injection and they are then checked for rabies in the way described. After thirty days with no deaths the test is proclaimed negative.

It was rabies that gave me my third major headache: Jürgen was on duty and he was injecting baby mice when the needle blocked. Instead of removing the needle and using a new one, Jürgen held the needle and forced down the plunger. The result was that brain material shot out of the syringe end of the needle and went everywhere, including into Jürgen's face and we thought into his eyes. We had a first aid kit for such emergencies and we washed off his face and squirted sterile saline into his eyes and tried to wash out anything that had gone in. Nevertheless we made a trip to the Medical Laboratories, where Dr Lawrence was undertaking research into rabies vaccines, and Jürgen was given the full treatment of the fourteen daily injections of the Pasteur vaccine – seven each side of his belly – that was produced in rabbits. The eyes are the most dangerous place as a portal of entry to the body – the shorter the distance from the place of entry to the brain, the shorter the incubation period and so the less time the person has to develop immune resistance before clinical disease appears. Jürgen survived; both the course of vaccinations and possible infection from the virus.

However, we learnt another lesson – we had no policy for protecting the staff against rabies. After discussions with Dr Lawrence we decided to vaccinate all staff who worked on rabies diagnosis. There was a new experimental vaccine available to workers made from duck eggs. This vaccine was injected into the skin and we had to have four tiny injections at weekly intervals; they itched a bit but it was nothing compared to Jürgen's Pasteur vaccine. The duck egg vaccine was used commercially for some years until it was superseded by the tissue culture vaccine which today is still the rabies vaccine of choice.

It is amazing how fashions change: years later when I was in charge of the National Veterinary Laboratory in Gaborone, Botswana, the general feeling was that you should not vaccinate staff working with the virus. The tissue culture vaccine is so good that there is no need to vaccinate until the person is exposed. The rationale is that knowing that they are protected makes people careless, not so much in their work as in reporting a potential incident. There was a Peace Corps woman in Kenya who had received the course of tissue culture vaccine and thought herself immune: she was bitten by her puppy but did nothing about it even when her puppy died of rabies. A month later she died. Vaccinated people need to be treated with further doses of vaccine following exposure to boost their resistance. And so the scientific arguments are batted back and forth. I have a sneaking suspicion that although we followed this policy in Botswana, we were wrong. There is always the possibility of an incident in the laboratory going unnoticed and a worker receiving a small dose of the virus from which, had they had prophylactic vaccination, they might have adequate protection.

Helmut Oder had been seconded from Bayer, the important pharmaceutical manufacturer in Germany, and he had with him a supply of reagents for a new diagnostic test for rabies and so when we prepared our slides we made three for him. This experimental tool is now the major technique for the diagnosis of the disease. The test is the fluorescent antibody technique in which serum antibodies to rabies virus are concentrated and then a fluorescent dye is attached (conjugated) to the antibody. The smear is stained with this conjugate, the slide is examined under the microscope and a stream of ultra violet light is shone through the slide. If fluorescence is seen, it means that the antibody has attached itself to the rabies virus. Helmut was able to diagnose positive cases when we were unable to find our bodies. It was uncanny that whenever he said it was positive our mice died from rabies, and so a new super test was born. I like to think that we played our part in this development.

When we made a positive diagnosis of rabies there was a strict protocol for reporting. The Directors of Veterinary and Medical Sevices, Provincial and District Veterinary and Medical Officers all had to be informed by telegram and the local vet or doctor also had to be informed by telephone if possible. The war in the north against the shifta was taking its toll on disease control in that area, and its effects on rabies control were devastating. The Kenyan soldiers were systematically destroying the antelopes for their own food and to sell to the villagers. This meant that there was a shortage of food for hyenas and jackals – and the latter play a major role in the epidemiology of rabies. When wild food was in short supply they moved into the villages – just like the urban fox in Europe today. This had a catastrophic effect on canine and human rabies, which was not resolved until the war with Somalia came to an end.

Less than a year after the rinderpest outbreak, the experience was repeated. Again it was late in the afternoon when a lorry pulled up at the laboratory carrying several dead adult beasts. On this occasion they came from a government holding ground near Archer's Post in the Northern Frontier District and so we thought we knew what to expect. However, the post mortem picture was completely different. It was not rinderpest but another disease that I had never seen before: contagious bovine pleuro-pneumonia. Animals with this disease normally have lesions confined to the lungs and the associated lymph nodes, and what is strange is that in the vast majority of cases only one lung is affected. However the reaction to the infection can be so severe that the whole lung dies. In acute cases there is a massive outpouring of pleural fluid, severe congestion and haemorrhage in the lungs and the animal dies from the poison caused by the breakdown of the tissue: it could be likened to a gangrene of the lung. Not all cases die; unlike rinderpest, the vast majority recover. But in many animals the lung never really recovers; the affected portion dies and then becomes walled off, being surrounded by a thick layer of fibrous tissue. The great Edinburgh teacher, Professor Thomas Whalley, described the chronic lesion of CBPP to be 'like a mummy in its case'. Sometimes the dead tissue becomes completely detached from the case and will rattle if shaken. It was always said, but without any evidence, that it was the breakdown of these sequestra as they are called that set off new outbreaks.

Again we had a similar collection of senior staff in the post mortem room, but with a few changes in personnel, because the Veterinary Department had a section purely for dealing with CBPP, and so the head of that section, Andrew Bygrave, was present. There was not the same degree of urgency that there had been with the rinderpest outbreak for several reasons: first, CBPP does not have a huge mortality; second, the incubation period of CBPP is lengthy (it was later shown to be about six weeks); third, the animals belonged to the Kenya Government as they had been purchased by the Animal Livestock Marketing Organisation and were being held in a quarantine, before being shipped down by truck to the abattoir at Athi River. Despite all this it was 9 pm before we were able to switch out the lights in the post mortem room and go home.

At least I was able to see this outbreak: it was decided to renovate the old abattoir at the holding ground at Archer's Post and to slaughter all the animals there and ship the meat down to Athi River.

Andrew Bygrave was sent up to live on the quarantine and he was lucky that there was a delightful house with a garden already established there, from the time that the abattoir had been used as a source of meat for the people of Nairobi, before the construction of the one at Athi River. Andrew was a great man for big game hunting so he was in his element living in the bush, close to the Samburu Game Park but with a shooting block nearby; buck, guinea fowl and yellow necked francolin were often on the menu in Archer's Post.

The Kenya Government decided, in conjunction with the East African Veterinary Research Organisation, to use this outbreak to obtain epidemiological data about the disease. Despite the international importance of CBPP, because it was a difficult disease to examine experimentally, almost nothing was known about how the disease behaved. A large scale investigation project was set up: all the animals (about 2500) were to be bled and their sera examined for antibodies to the mycoplasm (a very small micro-organism, smaller than a bacterium and without a cell wall) that caused CBPP; they were then slaughtered and a detailed post mortem examination carried out on each. The lesions were all recorded and cultures to isolate the causal organism were made from some. It was the first, and to this day the only, large scale investigation into the nature of the disease that has ever been carried out. The scientific paper produced by Andrew Bygrave and his colleagues Jack Moulton and Moshe Shifrine is still the major source of information into the nature of CBPP, almost 40 years after it was written.

It is possible to drive to Archer's Post in a day but it is a long hard drive despite being less than 300 miles. You can either skirt Mount Kenya to the west or east; we went via the west and spent the night with the DVO for Nyeri, Graham Duncanson. For me it was a working trip but for David and Mary Steel and my wife, Maxine, it was purely social and to see the country and its wildlife. David was a biologist who worked in the Tsetse Control Department and like me was a recent recruit. We had two days with the Bygraves, one for work and one purely for game watching. It was possible to see the abattoir from the veranda of the house and it was fascinating to see the large numbers of vultures sitting in the trees around, all waiting to be fed.

This was not a mechanised slaughter house: there was no production line, the animals were killed one by one and meticulous notes were taken of the findings. This slowed down the slaughtermen, but speed was not of the essence and it was important to get the details down and the samples taken. Some detective work is slow, and meticulous yet cumbersome and boring at the same time. The excitement lay in seeing the picture of the disease emerge.

If the journey up was uneventful, the same could not be said for the return. We were sitting on the veranda eating dinner on the Sunday night when at about eight o'clock we heard two loud explosions: at 8.30 pm we heard two more. We were mildly concerned but no more. We left at 8 am the next morning as we had decided to return in a single day; it is easier to return in a day as the road improves the nearer you get to Nairobi and so it is not a problem to drive in the dark. We said our farewells and set off in tandem with me in the front as I had had more experience of bush driving than David. About halfway between Archer's Post and Isiolo the road crosses the Ewaso Ng'iru river and we found the cause of the explosions of the previous night – the bridge had been blown up. Obviously the shifta had set the first charges which had not done the job and they had waited for half an hour to see if the army would come out to check up – the Kenyan army did not work after dark or on Sundays! And so they put down some more charges which this time were successful.

This called for some investigation since we both had saloon cars: the rains were due to start and so the river was low and the bed looked pretty solid. However before we could decide what to do an army lorry arrived with a platoon of soldiers on the back, accompanied by a Land Rover in which sat the commanding officer looking very pukka, with smartly pressed uniform complete with neatly tied cravat.

'Don't worry Saar, we will take you through the bush to the Garissa road. Follow us.' He drove into the bush on the left and we followed, with the lorry bringing up the rear. We drove along a bush track, which divided and sub-divided. After about half an hour we all stopped.

'We are lost, Saar, but sit tight and we will find the right track.'

And so off went the Land Rover and the lorry, leaving the two saloon cars as sitting ducks. Luckily the army returned before the shifta found us and we were taken without hitch to the Garissa road. But it had taken a while. From there it was a short distance to Isiolo and to the gate through which you pass to leave the NFD. At the gate stood an ashen-faced Andrew: you have to sign in when you enter the NFD and sign out when you leave. We had not signed out, it was more than three hours from the time we left and the twenty-mile journey should have taken no more than half an hour. Poor Andrew was thinking that all sorts of terrible fates had befallen us. When he got to the abattoir he heard that the bridge had been blown: he had to carry out some administrative tasks before he could follow us to see if we required help to cross the river; he had a four wheel drive Land Rover. At the bridge he could not see our tyre tracks leaving the road because they had been obliterated by the lorry and he assumed that we had crossed the river and then got into trouble. He was relieved when we turned up safe and sound after our bush escapade. We thanked him for his concern and set off for Nyeri and the south.

As we were crossing the foothills of Mount Kenya it was getting darker and darker as the clouds gathered and then ... down came the rain and it poured. Although the road was murram which is quite passable in the rain, the land on either side was black cotton soil, a very devil to get stuck in: as we neared the bottom of one hill I noticed that David had slid off the road and was obviously stuck. I continued my way to the top of the next hill so that I would be able to start again with the car going downhill. We locked the car, a sad sign of modern times, and started the walk back in the pouring rain – of course we had no raincoats or wellingtons. The great thing about rain in Kenya is that it is warm and so although we were soon soaked we were not cold.

David had got the car well and truly stuck in the black cotton, but by a process of digging out, and putting down vegetation and whatever stones we could find, we finally got the car out of the mud and back onto the road. Another hour lost and it was getting on for 2.30: however we still had four and half hours of daylight left. By this time the sun had come out and we were rapidly drying out. David gave Maxine and me a lift back to our car and set off in front. The remainder of the journey home was without incident.

After rabies, rinderpest, and pleuro-pneumonia, what else was going to turn up? It had to be either foot and mouth disease or tuberculosis, and it was ... both! But it was not the TB that I knew. A missionary family in Machakos kept a few cows to feed themselves and their parishioners and they suspected that one of their cows was suffering from mastitis, and so they sent us a sample of milk in a medicine bottle. The milk was spun in a centrifuge and the deposit stained and examined. A few 'ghost' forms of bacteria were seen in the routine smears and so we carried out a Ziehl Neelsen stain. Lo and behold acid-fast bacteria were seen which means mycobacteria. No other bacteria were isolated in our routine cultures. Cultures for TB were set up but this would take weeks. To speed up a diagnosis we arranged to visit the farm to carry out a tuberculin test in which you inject a small quantity of TB antigen into the skin and three days later examine the site of injection to see if there is a reaction. At the first visit we drove down and did the injections and came back: we were on the farm for barely half an hour. The second visit was different, we read the tests and carried out a farm investigation, after which we had lunch.

All tests were completely negative and there was nothing about the animals to suggest that they were suffering from TB. I was at a complete loss as to what was going on. And then the penny dropped.

'How did you clean the bottle you sent the sample in?' I asked.

'I washed out an old medicine bottle very carefully and then boiled it in water in a saucepan. When it had cooled down I washed it in rainwater to make sure that it was chemically clean.'

'How do you collect your rainwater?' I asked, knowing the answer because every house had its large rainwater collecting tank made from curved sheets of corrugated iron: this was excellent for irrigating the garden and in some places, where well water contained many chemicals, it was used for drinking water. I have a good memory and my thoughts went back to a day in the bacteriology practical class when we were asked to collect samples from the taps in the laboratory. It was pointed out to us that there are acid fast bacteria that live in an environment where there are metal ions. These are perfectly harmless and indicate that the water is clean. Problem solved. We took a sample of water from the rainwater butt and sure enough it was full of acid fast bacteria. The missionaries were greatly relieved. It was another step in the learning process.

The foot and mouth saga could have been disastrous had good luck not intervened. There are six major strains of foot and mouth virus and many interstrain varieties. The European strains are types 'A', 'O', and 'C' and these were the strains most commonly seen in Kenya. Elsewhere in Africa there are the 'SAT' (South African Type) strains of which two predominate and in Asia the strain is called 'Asia'. Immunity to the virus of foot and mouth disease is not long lasting: a single dose of the tissue culture rinderpest vaccine lasts for

71

a lifetime; at that time no foot and mouth vaccine had been produced which gave protection for more than six months, which necessitates that the cattle are vaccinated twice a year – expensive and time consuming. However, Burroughs Wellcome had produced a new vaccine from tissue culture and it was thought that it would give long lasting protection. A vaccination campaign was started. Not long after vaccination the cattle started dying and dead animals were sent to us for post mortem examination. These were carried out in conjunction with staff from the Embakasi Foot and Mouth Laboratory, who handled all suspect cases of foot and mouth disease as well as carrying out research into diagnostic tests and vaccines.

There were no lesions to be seen in any of the animals: all the tissues appeared to be completely normal, but the animal was dead. It could not have been a reaction to the vaccine because there were no signs of an anaphylactic reaction. We were at a loss to know what to do. We carried out routine cultural examination but there was nothing. One of the vets from Embakasi remembered some old work where foot and mouth virus was injected into the muscles of cattle and the animals had died because of the death of some of the muscle fibres in the heart. We carried out histological examinations of the heart and found the answer to the puzzle. Vaccinations were halted while the company had another look at the vaccine: it was never reintroduced.

It must not be thought that the major epidemic diseases were our prime concern, they were not. The vast majority of samples came from the farmers in and around Nairobi and from the veterinary officers working up country from Isiolo in the north to Narok in the south and from Kisumu in the west to Mombasa in the east. These samples reflected the major concerns of the farmers – tick-borne disease, of which East Coast fever was the most important. It was a killer and once infected the animal invariably died, but there was also anaplasmosis and babesiosis (redwater) in which protozoan parasites invade the red cells and destroy them. These diseases were treatable and if the animal was infected at a really young age it did not become sick then or later, as a long standing immunity was produced. Other tick-borne diseases were heartwater and Ondiri disease (named after the farm on which it was first diagnosed).

There were the usual problems caused by internal parasites, flukes and worms; there was mastitis and infertility and neonatal diarrhoea, the list goes on and on. These problems usually affected individual farms but the losses could be great. And from time to time disease on one farm could spill over into another. The first thing that greeted us in the morning was a line of Kikuyu farmers outside the laboratory each with a straw basket, a kikapu, on their bicycle handlebars. These would contain a variety of organs from an animal that had died the day before or overnight. Eighty percent of all those deaths were from East Coast fever. In those early post-colonial days great moves were being made to persuade farmers to upgrade their breeding animals by buying imported stock. Whilst the principle was sound, the practice was disastrous as local stock did have some immunity to East Coast fever, whereas imported cattle just keeled over and died from the parasite. To prevent this from happening the farmers were supposed to dip their animals every week; where the tick problem was high it might be necessary to dip twice a week. The word 'dip' is used because that is what the big farms did, immersing their stock in a deep bath of the acaricide. Smallholders would use a hand spray, and if they did not do it properly the result was death. The usual chemical used was DDT, but then along came Rachel Carson with her book *Silent Spring* and organo-chlorines were banned. They have been replaced with organo-phosphorus compounds, but these do not work as well and are at least as damaging to the environment; they certainly cause more problems in man. It is my belief that many of the lassitude-causing diseases that are so prevalent today, and possibly even motor neuron disease, are the result of the exposure to this class of compounds, which today are used in every branch of agriculture.

Dipping or spraying did not always work and the result was a visit to the lab with a kikapu on the handlebars. They did not bring us the carcase because that was eaten and they knew if they brought the whole animal we would not let them take the carcase away. We would register the samples and the farmers would sit on the grass outside the laboratory, putting Kenya to rights, while they waited for their results. Making smears from the spleen liver and lungs took but a few minutes and the slides needed to be stained for about 40 minutes so they could expect their results within a couple of hours, and the weather was warm; there were plenty of matters to discuss – if they went home they might have to help their wives with the hand ploughing or weeding. Once the work was completed, a report would be hand written by the vet and typed by the secretary; this would be sent to the local veterinary officer. He in turn might send a livestock officer or veterinary scout (two tiers of semi-trained local staff who were the bedrock of the department) round to the see what was going wrong.

On occasions large outbreaks of the disease were seen: a Danish couple had a large ranch just outside Nairobi on the Mombasa Road; their neighbour was a Mkamba farmer, very enlightened and well trained, and the two farms lived in harmony. The Mkamba man had to go on a long journey and his manager was not of the same calibre: he stopped dipping and he failed to repair fences with the result that the cattle broke through into the Danish farm in large numbers bringing the ticks and the East Coast fever parasite with them: years of work were undone in hours. Within a couple of weeks, the cattle on the Danes' farm became sick and soon started dying and a truck load was brought to us. It was not really necessary to carry out post mortem examinations to determine the cause of death – we could see it in the unopened carcase: the lymph nodes, being swollen, were all very prominent, and the eyes and gums were pale. Nevertheless complete examinations were carried out but East Coast fever was the only problem seen. The farm was visited but we could offer little hope. The fences had to be strengthened and it was recommended that until the losses ceased the farmer should dip his cattle twice a week. The outbreak caused more than 100 deaths.

So often in Africa deaths of livestock occur not in ones and twos but in scores or hundreds: the climate is warm and often moist which means the conditions are ideal for the multiplication of microbes and proliferation of parasites, but it never ceased to amaze me how farmers could survive these catastrophic losses. Joe Jerwood, a farmer near Voi, two thirds of the distance from Nairobi to Mombasa, had purchased 200 young beasts from the Animal Livestock Marketing Organisation, and had trekked them up to Voi. A few days later he noticed one of them was sick and within a few hours it was dead: he thought little of it and gave it to the staff to cut up and distribute the meat. The following morning there were twenty-five animals dead. He put five on the back of his truck and drove them to us. It was a worried man who sat in my office.

'It's a bugger,' he said. 'We've been doing so well of late and we had a bit of spare grazing and I saw that ALMO had brought some young stock down from the NFD and I thought we could fatten them up and sell them for the Eid feast or Christmas but whatever happens now we are shindered even if no more die, the profit's gone and God only knows how many more will die and I do hope that you can do something ...' His delivery was accelerating as he spoke.

'Calm down,' I said, 'and drink your coffee,' which Miriam our cleaner had just brought in for him.

'I am sure we will get to the bottom of the problem,' I said, with more confidence than I felt. 'Just tell me the story.' Which he did.

The animals were eight or nine months old and were fairly scrawny beasts. There was one of the regular droughts going on in the NFD and the government through the ALMO had purchased these young animals to stop them from starving to death (and to give the farmers some cash). Having quarantined them and found them to be free from epidemic diseases such as rinderpest, CBPP and foot and mouth disease, the government were selling them to farmers in the more productive parts of the country who had grazing to spare. As soon as the skin was removed it was obvious that the animals had died acute deaths from septicaemia. Once the chests were open it was clear where the problem lay: there was massive acute pneumonia.

'Not another outbreak of CBPP,' I said to myself. I had not then the experience to know that in CBPP only one lung is affected and all five animals had a bilateral pneumonia. There were a few worms in the stomach and intestines but no other conditions were seen. Even when rabies was not suspected we routinely removed the brains of cattle and sheep to enable us to make smears to check for the organism that causes heartwater and we took our standard tissue samples from spleen, liver and lung to make smears for examination for the common tick-borne parasites and to make cultures to look for bacteria.

Joe Jerwood had been lent boots and a gown and had joined us in the post mortem room; he could not stand still, hopping from one foot to another and walking up and down, he was a bundle of nerves. He had probably overstretched himself to buy the animals and was in danger of losing a pile of money which, I suspected, he had borrowed from the bank. He saw the diseased lungs and wanted to know the cause.

'Just hold fire,' I said. 'With such massive lesions we will be able to get to the bottom of the problem before too long.' This was said with more confidence than I felt.

Benson asked me to come and look at the smears. We had cleaned up and were back in my office. We routinely allowed farmers to come into the post mortem room: it was a form of training, since we

75

could explain to them what we found and show it to them, so that the next time they encountered the problem, they would recognise it for what it was. However, we did not encourage farmers to come into the laboratory since the space was more limited and they were likely to get in the way. I left Joe and went with Benson to look at the smears: they were all interesting but the most exciting was the brain crush smear; they are made as a means of looking at the blood capillaries. The heartwater parasite actually infects the cells that line the blood vessels: in a normal brain the nuclei of these cells look like small lemons and with our stain are coloured dark blue. When infected with the heartwater parasite they look like acorns in their cups: a smooth cell (acorn) with a knobbly end (the parasite). However in this case we were seeing something rather different: the cells were fine, but the capillaries were packed solid with tiny bodies that were intensely blue at either end and pale in the centre, the red and white blood cells were hemmed in by these small bodies. I had no doubt as to what they were – *Pasteurella multocida* – I was seeing my first case of 'shipping fever' or haemorrhagic septicaemia to give it its proper name. We would have to isolate the bacterium and identify it and of course, carry out a sensitivity test but we had enough evidence to suggest a means of treatment.

I went back to my office and said to Joe, 'I think we know what it is, but your problems are by no means solved: the trouble may only just be starting.' I told him that we thought the problem was shipping fever and proceeded to explain that we would not be able to confirm the diagnosis until the next day, and even that would only be a provisional diagnosis until we had carried out the necessary tests to confirm the identity of the organism, which might take a further forty-eight hours. In the meantime we could start taking the necessary action. I explained that pasteurellae were normal inhabitants of the nose and throat of cattle and other animals, and usually lived there quite happily doing no harm. However, from time to time something triggered off the bacteria to start multiplying rapidly: one of the best triggers was to mix together several mobs of cattle and then take them on a long journey either on foot or in trucks. Related problems occurred in barracks of young soldiers or young people going to boarding school.

Once the organism starts to multiply then it becomes self-perpetuating, and it is more able to kill as it spreads from animal to animal. Mr Jerwood had to break this cycle. There was evidence that pasteurellae were particularly susceptible to streptomycin, an antibiotic that had not long been introduced. I suggested to Joe that he should go into Nairobi on his way home and visit Mr Monks, who ran the biggest and best pharmacy and agricultural chemist in Kenya. I suggested that he needed to treat, for three days, *all* the animals that he had bought. A more relaxed Mr Jerwood set off in his truck: he now knew what he was dealing with and what steps he could take to try and resolve the problem. People are always happier when they know the full story, even when that news is bad.

We isolated *Pasteurella multocida* in pure culture from all the animals and all the tissues. We confirmed the identity and the antibiotic sensitivity test showed it to be sensitive to streptomycin. I grew some of the organisms in culture media in small screw-top bottles and sent them off to 'Bean' Phillips in Edinburgh who was an expert on pasteurellae. A few days later we had a phone call from Joe Jerwood to say that there were ten dead animals to greet him on his return. He had got the drug from Mr Monks and they had injected the whole mob that evening and on each of the two following days and there had been no more deaths following that first injection. He would survive.

Between leaving university and setting off for Africa I had worked in a practice in the North Riding of Yorkshire and one of our clients was Flamingo Park Zoo. When Reg Bloom, the manager, learnt that I was going to Kenya he gave me an introduction to his former partner John Seago, a game trapper whose premises were close to the Vet Lab and so regularly after we finished in the laboratory I would visit John to check on the health of his animals; he was delighted to have a vet who was interested in antelopes, rhinos and other game animals and he spread my name round the wildlife community. Early one morning there was a knock at my office door and in came a tall, well-built, bronzed man in his fifties.

'I am looking for Dr Windsor – I have a dying cheetah on the back of my truck.' This was Bobby Cade, the manager of the animal orphanage in Nairobi Game Park. The animal certainly appeared to be at death's door as she lay immobile in the back of an open truck. She did not move as I examined her, took blood from her jugular vein, and faeces from her rectum. Examination of the samples indicated that she was suffering from a severe infestation of hookworms in her intestines, which were drinking her blood through the gut wall. I told Bobby that she was probably too far gone but we gave her pills to treat the hookworms, together with iron and vitamin injections. There were no blood transfusions for wild animals in those days.

The next morning Bobby phoned to say she was sitting up and wanting food. She made a complete recovery. From then on, in Bobby's eyes, I could do no wrong. Even when, one by one, his baby cats – leopard, cheetah and lynx – died from feline enteritis. Next door to the orphanage was the Kenyan Army officers' mess and under the building there was a huge pack of feral cats, which were a constant source of infections for the wild cats in the orphanage. I took the young animals home to nurse, but we had little success.

Using massive doses of vaccine and vaccinating the cubs three times in a month we finally brought the disease under control. Working for Bobby led to more work with the game department and my services were called into play. This work was definitely of the James Herriot variety and involved treating everything from a baby chimpanzee who stole and mangled my sunglasses, and a newborn rhino to young giraffes and adult leopards and antelopes.

The Kenya Government had decided to approve the importation of six white rhinos to try and re-establish them in the country. Because they were a present from South Africa the rhinos could not be established in Nairobi Game Park, the only park free from tsestse fly, which carried the deadly trypanosome that causes sleeping sickness. Once a month I was flown to Meru Park and there examined the rhino, took a blood sample from the ear and checked for the presence of the trypanosome. When we saw this parasite the animal was treated with a very effective drug called Berenil. This was later banned as it can be carcinogenic. The rhinos developed resistance to the parasite and we believed that they were established in the park and they were breeding well until they were slaughtered by poachers.

It was during these visits that I met George and Joy Adamson and got to know their lions (Ugas, Boy, Girl and the cubs) and the cheetah Pippa. Dume was Joy's pride and joy; as he was the only male cub in Pippa's first wild litter and she was distraught when he went lame. A plane was sent for me and when we finally were able to examine him it was obvious that he had broken his leg. Left in the park he would die: going to Nairobi for treatment ran the risk of feline enteritis. I did not enjoy the return flight in the back of a two-seater aeroplane with a semi-sedated cheetah cub on my lap with his head sticking out of a carpet bag. Immediately upon arrival we gave Dume a double dose of feline enteritis vaccine. The following day Professor Donald Lawson did a wonderful job repairing the double fracture and all was going well until he developed feline enteritis …

Kenya belonged to the Kenyans and we were there to teach them how to do things for themselves and to run a bridging operation until they were in a position to take over. The tragedy of Africa was that many of the local people had an inflated idea of their knowledge and ability, and wanted the power and authority without being prepared to take responsibility for their actions. (Years later I was to find a totally different attitude in Peru, where the people did not want to take charge until they felt competent to do so.) Sadly this concept was promulgated by the United Nations Organisation and its agencies, which insisted that all projects were headed by a native Kenyan and that their 'experts' had no executive authority and were only there as advisers. While working for the Kenya Government, I was a civil servant and part of the regular government structure which gave me the authority to take decisions and to carry them out. This is a much better use of skilled labour. Despite my youth and inexperience, I was far better educated than my local colleagues, even those trained in Europe and America. In fact the Americans did Africa a great disservice by ensuring that no African student failed. Veterinarians returned from such distinguished universities as Ohio and Wisconsin with veterinary diplomas which stated 'This degree is only valid outside of the United States of America'. The Russians did exactly the same by setting up the Patrice Lumumba University for training students from Africa.

Throughout my overseas career I have felt that my major role has been to train my counterparts and ensure that they get the benefits of the best training possible. To that end I worked with Mark Anderson an Australian laboratory technician in the veterinary faculty, to set up a laboratory training course for veterinary technicians. Mark had an interesting career in the faculty which had been taken over by the Glasgow Veterinary School. At one time it seemed that there were more Glasgow teachers in Nairobi than there were in Glasgow; it got so bad that the students in Glasgow revolted and a semblance of order was restored. With the aid of Ian McIntyre, the Dean of the Nairobi School and later the Glasgow faculty, Mark, a microbiology laboratory technician, enrolled in the Nairobi Faculty to study veterinary medicine while at the same continuing his work in the

Bacteriology Department (and his wife ran the student hostel): hard work but he made a success of it. He then worked in the Glasgow School while he studied for his Royal College examinations – the Royal College of Veterinary Surgeons did not recognise the Nairobi degree.

Mark had discussed setting up a course of laboratory technology with the head of the Nairobi Technical Training Institute who was in favour. A committee was set up to sort out a syllabus and a time scale. It was decided that the course should aspire to the same status as the British Institute of Medical Laboratory Technicians, membership of which, at the time, was probably the most prestigious qualification that could be obtained and a fellowship of which was only rarely given. Every institute in Nairobi with an interest in animal health sent a representative to the committee and we produced a syllabus based on that of the IMLT but tailored to local conditions. The course commenced amid high expectation as the IMLT had given it its blessing. And a very good course it proved to be: at first the teachers were all expatriates but over the years they were replaced by local people.

At the time I was receiving more training than I was imparting! But we set up a system for teaching the veterinary students from the faculty which was only a short walk away. Had I had the Cambridge experience (which I obtained later) we would have done things differently. The system that we evolved meant phoning the vet faculty when we had animals for examination in the post mortem room. In Cambridge the laboratory was on the regular rota for group teaching and when there were no animals for post mortem examination they spent their time learning laboratory skills. Nevertheless we were able to show the young students how to set about finding out why the animal died. I belonged to the school that believed in the dictum 'To hear, is to forget; To see, is to remember; To do, is to understand.'

And so I have stood there, itching to take the knife from the student's hand and speed up the business, but then I have remembered my own tentative early steps and held back. I cannot say that I produced any pathologists, but it was easy to identify the good students and it was gratifying to note that some of them did make it in the long run. I remember many years later when I was carrying out a consultancy in Kenya and I had an interview with the Director of Veterinary Services. I was sitting in the office where I had had my set-to with Tony Dorman all those years ago, when Dr Richard

Masiga said to me, 'You do not remember me, Dr Windsor, but I remember you.'

I had to confess that I did not remember him.

'I was a student when you were teaching in the Vet Lab PM room.'

Then the penny dropped: the tall gangly student with the big eyes who asked a succession of intelligent questions and was forever keeping me on my toes trying to answer him.

'Oh, yes I do,' I replied. 'But you have filled out since your student days!' Success had filled his figure. He had not forgotten the genial teacher and I was given all the assistance I needed for my consultancy.

The British Ministry of Agriculture, Fisheries and Food was playing its part in the development of its ex-colonies and Ivor Field, the Director of the Central Veterinary Laboratory, was instructed that he could second vets and laboratory technicians from the CVL and the Veterinary Investigation Service to aid in development in Africa. This was not a totally altruistic move, because it was to result in a cadre of vets and technicians well versed in African diseases which would be useful in fighting any future invasions. Ivor Field came to Kenya to find out what was required: did they need bacteriologists, virologists, pathologists, biochemists, or a combination of them all? He was also on recruitment mission, looking out for likely talent to employ in Weybridge, or the Investigation Centres. He came to Kabete and undertook a tour of the whole laboratory and spent more than an hour in the Diagnosis Section looking at what we were doing: he knew Christine Lund, of course, as she had been a member of his staff and like all good bosses he knew all his staff, even the most humble. A few days later he came back to see me. He sat in my office and told me that he was interested in recruiting me for a permanent job in the Veterinary Investigation Service, with a view to sending me back to work in Kenya.

'Bill Bruce tells me that your two year contract is about to come to an end. Do you plan to renew it?' he asked.

'I am certainly enjoying working here,' I said, 'and there is still much work to be done to improve the service that we offer.'

'I was thinking that we might send an experienced member from a veterinary investigation centre to help in this section and you might find it rather embarrassing to have a member of staff with rather more experience than you. Why not come and join us and I will guarantee to send you back to Kenya once you have served your probation?'

This was an offer too good to turn down: to obtain a permanent job in a prestigious service, and the VIS paid considerably more than the Kenya Government, even with the British overseas allowance.

'I would not want to stop working in Kenya, there is so much to do and there are so many problems,' I said. 'Besides we love living here, there is so much to see and do and we have barely scratched the surface.'

'Don't worry, I am looking for people to work at the East African Veterinary Research Organisation, as we are part of a large consortium undertaking research into CBPP, and Bill Bruce tells me that you have had experience in the control of this disease and realise the gaps in our knowledge. You do not have to make a decision now, but do come and see me in Weybridge when you get home.' And on that happy note Ivor Field departed.

A few days later I was called to see the new director, Ishmael Muriithi. Ishmael had been the year below me at the Dick Vet and although we had not been friends we knew each other well enough. He had been selected by Tony Dorman and other senior colleagues for training in Britain. He had undertaken the Vet Diploma at Makerere University in Kampala, Uganda and was definitely the brightest star in the Veterinary Department. Providing he did well in Britain he had been pencilled in as the first African Director. Tragically he was not permitted to demonstrate his skills for very long: after less than ten years as director, he was struck down by a heart attack.

'I understand that you are thinking of leaving us.'

'I have to think of my future career, as you will not offer me a permanent job here.'

'You know, Roger, it is not in my power to keep you here indefinitely because it is the policy of the government that we localise the jobs as quickly as possible. We have to provide jobs for our people.'

'I understand completely,' I said, 'but that does not change my position, I have a wife and we hope to have a family in due course, and I must look to them first.'

'I will be most unhappy if you leave the department, and I would not want you to go to work at Muguga [the East African Veterinary Research Organisation]. You must realise that my laboratory has already lost many of its most able staff to them and it has to stop.' Sadly there was no love lost between these two institutes. 'If you go and work there, you will receive no cooperation from me.' On that veiled threat, the interview was terminated.

On my return to Britain I went to see Ivor Field and told him about Muriithi's threat.

'Think no more about it: he will get over it in a few days.' He did not know the Kikuyu mind. 'I have decided to send you to the Norwich Centre, because Geoffrey Holmes is off to Kabete to take your place and Edward Gibson is very good with young vets.'

I had decided to take up the offer and before leaving Kenya I had written a letter of resignation.

'You can start in Norwich as soon as you wish, and I hope you enjoy it there but before you know where you are, you will be off back to Kenya.'

Little did he know how wrong he was.

6

A Prolonged Norfolk Interlude, 1967–1968

'I find many tragic cases, some comic, a large number merely strange,
but none commonplace.'
Sir Arthur Conan Doyle, *The Speckled Band*

I never did discover the origin of the name Unthank Road, one of the main roads into Norwich from the south, but that is the road in which I lodged for the first weeks of my stay, while I looked for a house. Before we left Kenya we had ordered a new Renault 16: when we were informed that it was ready for delivery, we went to Paris to collect it. We drove to the coast and it was flown across the sea to Southend and given a temporary importation certificate for six months. At the time Renault 16s were virtually unknown in Britain and with its red French licence plates it caused quite a stir. The laboratory was on the east side of the city on the ring road leading to the Yarmouth road in a small industrial estate which we shared with a Remploy factory and several other small factories together with the Driving Test Centre: one of the examiners looked at the car and shook his head.

'It's an interesting looking creature but it will never replace the motor car.'

The Renault 16 was the first of the hatchbacks, which subsequently took over the family car market.

The laboratory was in an old converted factory building and was spacious if not well designed. The staff were warm and welcoming: the boss, Edward Gibson, was from my part of London and was a kindly soul; apart from Edward there were Geoff Holmes, and Roy Gilbert, who were the senior vets. Geoff was to take my place in Kabete. Roy was also destined for Kenya; we ended up living in the house next door to Roy at Muguga. John Simmons who was a new boy like myself was a generous man and very kind, but he was slow of mind and speech and once primed he was unstoppable;

84

irrespective of interruptions he went on like a steamroller in his slow expressionless way until he had finished what he was going to say. A classmate of John's at the Royal Veterinary College once said of John that he could 'bore for England'. With many of my colleagues I develop an intuitive relationship and often know what they are going to say before they complete the sentence and they stop to let me comment. Not John.

The technical staff were friendly and efficient but there were no outstanding characters such as we had later in Cambridge. The chief tech was Stanley Harrison a small wiry man with a balding head. I later felt that with different management he could have been a truly splendid technical staff leader. However, there was a distinct social difference between the grades in Norwich: I might be wrong but I attributed this to Geoff in particular. As a result there was little mixing of professional, technical, cleaning and admin staff.

I shared an office with John, and Geoff and Roy set about instilling in us the way the Veterinary Investigation Service worked. I was interested to note that there was not much difference in the system we had established in Kenya and that practised in the VI Service. The submission form for the samples closely resembled that which we had developed, but there were certain refinements which made control of the movement of specimens in the laboratory much simpler.

The Norwich Lab served the vets in Norfolk and East Suffolk an area of rich arable land which had once been the home of sheep at the time when wool was England's wealth. This could be seen in the magnificent cathedral in the city and the glorious medieval churches that dotted the landscape. It was said that Norwich, a city of 100,000 people, had a church for every week and a pub for every day. (Time has taken its toll, many of the churches now serve other functions and most of the pubs have closed.) Sadly there were very few sheep and even fewer cattle. Most farms now grew wheat and barley, potatoes and sugar beet. Some kept pigs to turn their barley into pork and there were numerous hatcheries, broiler houses and egg producing units. A few dairy herds remained and there were more than fifty practising vets in sixteen or so practices attending to the needs of the farming community. Today there are only two practices working with livestock and they employ just five vets.

Four things stand out for me of my time in Norwich, the first was the ravaging effects of Marek's disease on the poultry industry, the second was the importation of the bacterium Arizona in a group of young turkeys, and the third was the setting up of a computer recording system for the diseases diagnosed. The fourth was the Swan Commission into Antibiotic Resistance.

Marek's disease must be the most important disease ever to hit the poultry industry and almost every day the post mortem room tables were just covered with dead birds. A hundred dead chickens in a day was not unusual and almost all of them had died from this 'tumour'. The problem that bedevilled the work to control this dreadful disease was that there were several conditions that all looked the same, although they affected birds of different ages, but it was assumed that they all had the same cause. It was finally ascertained that Marek's disease was an infection caused by a herpes virus. Herpes viruses in humans cause chicken pox and the cold sore that is such a nuisance at the edges of the lips. Once these viruses gain entrance to the body, they never leave. On first exposure to chicken pox the child or adult develops an acute fever and spots appear in various parts of the body. As the person develops immunity to the virus so the virus retreats along the nerves to the ganglia, those little bundles of nerve tissue rather like a traffic roundabout where the nerves leave the spinal cord, and there they remain dormant sometimes for life. In other people, when they are stressed or suffer from some other infections, the virus leaves the ganglia and migrates up the nerves when it is responsible for the condition known as shingles. A similar picture is seen with the cold sore agent. As the body builds its immunity the scabs dry up and fall off and the virus retreats down the nerves to the ganglia, only to emerge again when the person has a nasty cold or other infection, when up they pop again. It seems that while the virus is within the nerve cell it is resistant to the body's immune mechanism.

Lesions in Marek's disease are most commonly seen in the liver and spleen but, in addition, can be seen just about anywhere. Histological examination of these 'tumours' shows that they are not tumours at all, but a chronic inflammatory reaction to the virus infection. For some reason, unlike the human infections, the bird was unable to develop sufficient resistance before the lesions were so big that the bird died. Once the scientists realised this fact, the hunt was on to find a vaccine. One group of workers were trying to attenuate the virus; that is, to make it less virulent so that it could be used to produce resistance without killing the bird. The second group were looking at herpes viruses from other birds, to see if they could find one that would provide resistance to the agent that caused Marek's disease. It was the latter group that won. The vaccine was an instant success and made the developers a great deal of money; it also reduced the level of disease to almost nil. Marek's disease is rarely seen today and only in those flocks that do not use the vaccine. Once Marek's disease was controlled, Avian leucosis in its various manifestations took its rightful place as conditions of minor importance; they are true tumours with altered cells growing out of control. They are rare. I was taught a valuable lesson, or rather I should say that a lesson learnt was reinforced.

The similarities of shipping fever and contagious bovine pleuro-pneumonia confounded the problem of sorting out the diseases. CBPP has been known in Britain since its first introduction in 1840. In those far-off days vets had difficulty in separating rinderpest from CBPP despite the former producing lesions mostly in the alimentary tract and lesions of CBPP being normally confined to the lungs. Rinderpest had occurred sporadically in Britain since it was first recognised in 1715 but the importation of cattle from Russia in 1864 led to the great epidemic that changed the face of farming in Britain for ever.

There was no doubt that the major livestock industry in Norfolk was the poultry industry; it was certainly the fastest growing. The post war austerity was disappearing fast and people had more money in their pockets: as Macmillan so rightly said, 'You have never had it so good!' New poultry units were springing up over Norfolk, the largest of which was Bernard Matthews. His chicken ventures were so successful that he was branching out into turkeys. And new hybrids of turkeys were being imported. One farmer had set up a new turkey slaughter house for the Christmas trade. By slaughtering, dressing and freezing the turkeys he could even-out production throughout the year. Turkeys take between twenty and thirty weeks to fatten. The first time he used his new slaughter house the machines broke the wings of every bird that passed through. The owner was worried that some nutritional problem was affecting the birds, and we were presented with six oven-ready 20-lb turkeys together with a variety of internal organs selected at random. Both wings on each bird were neatly broken in the same position. A simple way to test the quality of the bones of birds is to try and break a limb bone. When the bones are inadequately calcified then it is very difficult to break them, because they are all rubbery and they bend and twist but do not break. With adequate force it is easy to break a healthy bone. These bones were very healthy. But we checked them for calcium and phosphorus levels and all was well. There was no doubt that the defeathering machine was incorrectly set. The carcases were divided among the staff and made very good eating. This was not my case, but I suggested to John that he should report that our tests were inconclusive and that further samples were required! He did not take my advice.

'Roger, you had better come to reception,' This was a call I always relished when I was on duty, because it meant that there was something interesting afoot. And sure enough this phone conversation led to a most interesting investigation. The Americans were way ahead of the world in breeding hybrid animals, particularly pigs, chickens and turkeys, and consequently the farmers were always clamouring to be allowed to import birds from the States. The Americans were good at improving the genetic quality of livestock, but their disease control was years behind ours in Britain. The reasons for this were the huge size of the country and the high costs of eradicating diseases as well as the practical difficulty of controlling movements on such a large scale. Consequently they were draconian in their import regulations to prevent disease gaining entrance. By contrast, Britain had eradicated rinderpest, CBPP, foot and mouth disease, rabies, and sheep pox; TB eradication was nearly complete and the Brucella Eradication Scheme was about to start.

I do not altogether approve of what has gone on in turkey breeding, as they have produced these strains of 'broad breasted' birds with such huge breasts that they cannot mate naturally; the male has such a massive breast that he is unable to introduce his penis into the female and so he has to be 'milked' and the female has to be inseminated. However, this was the early days and this farmer had imported a thousand day old chicks of the grandparent lines to set up his own breeding unit.

'I am not sure exactly where these birds were produced,' he said. 'They come from a major breeding company in the States which has units in various states. All the documentation is with the Ministry and, since I was not particularly interested in the specific origin, I did not keep copies. However if you need to know, the information is available. We lost one or two in the first days but probably less than I was expecting and I was delighted with their progress for the past eleven weeks, until a couple of days ago when they started dying. Again I thought nothing of it at first, we had recently changed the food and we usually get the odd one dying. But this is different and there were ten dead this morning and so I have brought them to you.'

'Have you moved the birds at all and have you noticed anything odd about the way they are behaving?'

'No, they have not been moved from their original pen, but I think that some of them have a little diarrhoea and others are blind.'

'Why, are they bumping into each other? They should have no difficulty with finding the food because they know where it is.'

'No, there are no signs of blindness but the eyes of some of them look opaque.'

This was something new.

'And something more this morning, the food intake has gone down.'

'Have you brought anything onto the farm since the arrival of these birds?'

'No we are not allowed to by the Ministry until they give us the all clear.'

'Well, we will have a look and I will be in touch, once I have done the examinations.'

Post mortem examinations were not done until after the coffee break, as we had to clear up the work from the day before and get our reports dictated for the secretaries to get typing. The birds were in excellent condition and had obviously been doing well until the lurgy had hit them. The cloudiness of the lenses in the eyes was quite striking and all were affected. There were signs of mild diarrhoea but nothing else was seen before they were nailed onto the dissecting board. We nailed the birds with their wings stretched out, as if being crucified, to prevent the carcase moving about. They were well feathered and there were no external parasites to be seen; the bones appeared good and strong. When we looked inside there was not much evidence of disease. Some congestion of the sub-cutaneous tissues and lungs was seen and the intestines were brighter than they should have been – although I had never examined such young turkeys before and was not sure what they should look like! We split the heads of some of the birds longitudinally and put the entire opened head into formalin for histological examination, I opened some of the eyes to look inside but only the lenses appeared

89

abnormal. Samples were taken for cultural examination and all vets were called to the PM room for a pow wow, nobody had seen anything like it and no suggestions were on offer.

Back to the drawing board, or in this case Biester and Schwarz, the poultry vet's Bible, which encompassed all avian knowledge. Since I had no idea where to start I was flicking idly through the pages, when I came across a photo of a turkey with an opaque lens in its eye. It is the classic sign of Arizona infection in turkeys. It looked as if the problem was solved. The description in the book fitted the picture on the ground to a 'T'. It seemed as if the Americans had exported yet another of their foul diseases to us. Arizona is a type of salmonella which was first isolated, well you can guess where. The birds had obviously brought the infection with them and I wondered what the 'trigger factor' was. I never did find it: the disease normally makes its appearance at that age, even though it is transmitted through the egg from its mother. I phoned the owner and explained the problem to him and pointed out that the diagnosis needed to be confirmed. I informed him that I would be notifying the Ministry vets and that he should contact them to see if they would permit him to treat the birds. I also pointed out that he probably had a good case against the supplier since the birds were infected from the mother through the egg.

We phoned the Ministry vets and they all trooped over to see what it looked like. We were lucky, we had a good bunch of vets in Norwich who took their cue from the Divisional Veterinary Officer, Martin Roe. I was surprised to see Bill Pratt walk in, as the last time I had seen him was at his farewell party in Nairobi. He and his wife had bought a guest house in Ipswich. How the mighty were fallen! He had been the Assistant Director of Veterinary Services in Kenya in charge of Meat Hygiene Services and now he was a humble veterinary officer, the same grade as me. I went through the description of the disease and its epidemiology that I had just boned up in the 'Bible' and was able to trot it out like a real expert: of such things are reputations made. We suggested that they should make a tentative report to Tolworth, the headquarters of the State Veterinary Service, and inform them that we thought we were dealing with Arizona, but that confirmation would have to await the outcome of the cultural examination. What we did not know, but should have guessed, was that this was only part of a large consignment and turkeys from this source had been shipped all over the country.

Martin was very pleased when he called in the next day to see how we were getting on, as he was able to tell us that his report was the first and, to date, the only report of the infection in the turkeys. From our tissues we had isolated profuse pure cultures of what appeared to be a salmonella that agglutinated with anti-Arizona sera. We now needed to confirm the identity with biochemical tests and carry out an antibiotic sensitivity test. We also set up culture media to send to the Central Veterinary Laboratory for them to confirm the identity. However, despite being the first to identify the infection we were not allowed to visit the farm – that was a Field Service prerogative as it was a farm quarantine. Martin was most apologetic but could not overrule the powers-that-be. Had we not made a diagnosis they would have wanted us on the farm yesterday. Sadly it was the shape of things to come. Slowly but surely from around the country came reports of the infection and almost all the farms were involved. Treatment was permitted but I do not know the outcome. The irony was that when the scientific paper was published, the Norwich Veterinary Investigation Centre was not mentioned.

I suppose that the introduction of any new system is bound to be traumatic but the Veterinary Information and Diagnosis Analysis (VIDA) computer scheme, also imported from the States, was a disaster. It had obviously been thought up by some idiot with nothing better to do. It was ill thought out and there was a serious basic flaw in the design which was that every sample that was received in a diagnostic laboratory should be included in the analysis. When it was not possible to make a diagnosis (a not uncommon problem when only a single tissue is received) then the pathological process had to be recorded. The code for a disease was eight digits long and the code book was about the size of the London telephone directory, only the print was larger. The problem in the early days of computing was that the programmers started at the wrong end. Instead of asking 'What do we want out of this system?' they used the opposite premise, 'What can we put into the system?' This led to that wonderful and apposite acronym of early computers 'GIGO' – garbage in, garbage out – and that perfectly described VIDA.

We spent hours and hours trying to complete the coding boxes. For many specimens it took longer to fill in the coding form than it did to carry out the work. One of the major problems was that there were no specific codes for specific diseases. To give just one example, there is a gangrenous disease of cattle that is known by different names in different parts of the country: black leg, black quarter, garget and a host of others. In the coding book it could be referred to as any of these; it could also be classified by the tissue affected, in this case only muscle, but it could also be classified by the causal agent *Clostridium chauvoie*. It could also be caused by other clostridia such as *Clostridium septique* and nobody knew all the different combinations used by different vets. Analysis was impossible and the system was unworkable. Nevertheless it took five years before the system was scrapped – five years of massively wasted manpower. People did not want to admit that they had made a serious cock-up.

A working party was set up to produce a new system, VIDA 2, and this was a superb streamlined system which realised that in practice there are only few diseases that are worthy of analysis and these were given a three figure code. And so in the example quoted above there is one three figure code for all the different combination of names and agents. There were specific codes for an unlisted diagnosis, and for where no diagnosis had been made, and it had the flexibility in that new diseases could be added if they became important. For example, when I was working in the Cambridge centre and streptococcal meningitis caused by *Streptococcus suis* type 2 became a significant disease problem, the disease was given a specific code. Each year the 'Unlisted Diagnoses' were examined to see if there were any 'new' or emerging diseases being missed: each centre received a list of their case numbers and they had to reply giving the diagnosis that had been made, and occasionally as a result of this exercise a new specific diagnosis was added to our code sheets. A simpler, yet much more valuable, system had been set up, which has lasted more or less unchanged until the present day (thirty-five years – a long time in the computer world). I was later able to introduce this system to the INTA laboratory in Salta, Argentina; the National Veterinary Laboratory in Gaborone, Botswana; LABVETSUR, in Arequipa, Perú; and I recommended it for the regional laboratories in Vietnam, the National Laboratories in Laos and the Central Laboratory in Kabul, Afghanistan.

As can be seen from the VIDA fiasco, being a detective can involve much humdrum, time-consuming and extremely boring work. Another such task befell me in Norwich: Sir Michael Swann (later

Lord Swann), Vice Chancellor of Edinburgh University, was appointed chairman of a government commission to investigate the development of resistance in bacteria to antibiotics. From the start I suspected that this was really set up to try and stop vets from using antibiotics in animals. The Veterinary Investigation Service would obviously provide the body of evidence in the animal world, while the hospital laboratory services and Public Health Laboratories would provide the majority of the evidence from the human world. Being one of the newest recruits to the service, and having a degree in bacteriology, I was a prime target to be the dogsbody, and so it happened. I was asked to compile the figures for the English and Welsh centres (the Scots had a separate service – thank God). Each month I received the results of antibiotic testing from each centre. One strength of the service was that we all tested bacteria against the same antibiotics and the manufacturers made up testing discs especially for us: one disc for Gram Positive organisms and another for the Gram Negative bacteria. This did not preclude us from testing against other antibiotics but we had to carry out the routine tests as well.

The bacteria that were of special concern were *Staphylococcus aureus* (Gram Positive) and *Escherichia coli*, a common cause of neonatal diarrhoea, *Salmonella typhi*, the cause of typhoid fever, which rarely affects animals but its cousin *Salmonella typhimurium* affects both man and animals with great frequency. These last three are all Gram Negative organisms. The centres from Newcastle to Truro and Carmarthen to Cambridge had to send me the sensitivity results of all the *Staph. aureus*, *E. coli* and *S. typhimurium* that they had isolated and I had to compile these results into a single table that could be sent to the Swann Enquiry. It was tedious work but I suspect it had some merit. It took hours of boring time each month, but I consoled myself with the thought that every job has its mind-numbingly boring tasks; at least I was sitting in a comfortable chair in a warm dry office when I might be standing in the freezing cold and pouring rain carrying out a routine tuberculin testing of a 200-cow herd.

I am not sure that these figures added much to the debate but the Commission decided that greater control over the use of antibiotics was required. Few would disagree with that: antibiotics were being used in the feed of pigs and poultry, as they were said to be growth promoters, but whenever animals are kept in close proximity in large numbers then the opportunities for bacteria to develop their ability to kill or maim increase. There is a perennial argument between doctors and vets about who is responsible for bacteria developing resistance. My position is that farmers have to pay for the drugs they use and so do not use them indiscriminately, whereas the taxpayer pays for the drugs that the doctor prescribes and many people do not complete a course of treatment prescribed for them; once they feel better they stop taking the medicine. You have only to look at what is happening in hospitals at the moment with *Clostridium dificile* and MRSA, two organisms of little veterinary importance, to realise that it is the medical profession who are the authors of their own misfortune.

I found us a house to live in: the Georgian wing of Heydon Hall, a Tudor manor house set in 180 acres of parkland in north Norfolk. The house was owned by the Bulwer Long family who had temporarily fallen on hard times and so had rented it out to H. Gordon Parker, an entrepreneur of some style who, as a retirement hobby, purchased the rundown Felixstowe docks and turned it into the largest container port in Britain. Mr Parker lived in Stoke Ferry Hall during the week but had rented Heydon for the shooting. He and his wife moved into the house each weekend and their daughter looked after the hall during the week; she, however, was getting fed up with living alone in this huge pile when she had her own lovely cottage in Stratton Strawless. Under the terms of his lease the hall had to be occupied at all times and, since we had impeccable references, Miss Parker agreed to rent us the east wing of the hall for £4 a week, payable in advance. There was one additional clause in our verbal lease, which was that I had to stoke the boiler – which was not a problem since it required only one scuttle of coke morning and evening and it only required cleaning once a week. This was an advantage to us in that the boiler was just outside our bathroom, which was always warm. We took possession of the unfurnished east wing and since we had no furniture we had to set about acquiring some. Luckily the post war boom was starting and people were sick of their old comfortable armchairs and solid mahogany furniture; they wanted the new Scandinavian furniture, light colour, light weight and light on comfort. Nearby was Rackheath Hall, the great antique junk shop, which had furniture stacked from floor to ceiling throughout its rooms. We purchased a Victorian solid mahogany extendable dining table for £14, and a glass-fronted dresser in mahogany for the same price. Four oak dining chairs cost £5. We bought an American spring rocking chair for £4 and then felt cheated when we bought a second one in a different shop for £2. Luxurious great armchairs cost next to nothing. Our bedroom was thirty feet square and the ceiling was about twenty feet high and so curtains had to be made by Maxine – material was purchased by the bale and stair-carpets by the roll. Our families lent and gave us stuff, and soon we had enough to live comfortably although I am not sure by modern standards the word comfort properly applied because there was no central heating.

Our bathroom was always warm because we had to go through the boiler room to get to it. The kitchen, which was only twenty-five feet square, was heated by a coke-fired Baxi boiler which also provided the hot water in the kitchen. This was a lovely room that looked onto the lawns leading to the front door with their attendant peacocks. We were at breakfast one morning listening to the fore-runner of the 'Today' programme, when Brian Redhead said that an African hoopoe had been spotted in Norfolk, miles away from its normal summer haunts in southern and central France; imagine our surprise when we looked out of the window and there it was, strutting around on the lawn! Having just come from Kenya we had no difficulty in identifying it. The dining room was small; I suspect that it had originally been a butler's pantry. It was next door to the sitting room, again about thirty feet square with a very high ceiling. We had a single guest bedroom which was like a corridor being thirty feet long by only twelve or fifteen feet wide. And why did builders in those far-off days always put the fireplace at the long end of the room when its effects would only be felt a few feet away?

We had no refrigerator (in the summer we bought a small box made of diatomaceous earth over which we poured water and the evaporation kept the milk, butter, cheese and bacon cool), no television, no telephone, no hi-fi system and our sole source of sound entertainment was the radio. (We are still fervent supporters of the BBC.) But we had a wonderful life. No debt, no mortgage, and just the two of us. An old girlfriend of mine from school days lived in Norwich and she and her husband became firm friends; Maxine met an old school friend and the circle kept expanding and expanding. It was the era of the dinner party, there were concerts in Blickling Hall and Norwich Castle, there was the Theatre Royal with plays and opera, the Maddermarket Theatre, where actors from Anglia

95

Television put on plays for their (and our) entertainment, The Scientific Anglian and a host of other second-hand book shops were there to be plundered and you could still afford to eat in a good restaurant.

We had permission to wander in the parkland and in the spring the whole estate was ablaze with daffodils. It was a wonder to watch the ducks laying their beautiful blue eggs in their nests round the lovely old pond. There were at least fifty such nests and one day they all disappeared: once the requisite number of eggs had been laid the ducks covered over the nests with leaves and grass and so when they were not sitting on them they could not be seen. Soon the pond was full of fluffy ducklings. In the summer there were wild strawberries growing in the hedgerows. We could go and bathe in the sea or we could just wander round the park looking for red squirrels which were in abundance, and there were song birds everywhere.

However, soon the dread words foot and mouth disease were heard on the radio and in the laboratory. It was talked about in hushed tones: was this going to be the big one that had long been predicted as herd sizes had grown and grown and the cattle population in the west midlands was the greatest ever? The disease had first been seen in the livestock market in Oswestry in Shropshire and fanning out to the north and east as the wind blew the virus.

It was now November and we drove down to London to a dinner party hosted by an old school friend Richard Crouch and his wife Carol in their flat in Little Venice. We were in the middle of a superb trout niçoise when the phone rang. Richard answered it and looking rather surprised he said, 'Roger, it's for you!'

I was equally taken aback. 'Roger Windsor speaking.'

'Roger, is that you boyoo? Leslie Hughes here.' He was the Deputy Regional Veterinary Officer for Eastern Region. How the hell did he get this number? He must have had my parents' phone number from the next of kin records. My mother (she normally answered the phone) must have given him the number of my in-laws, where we were staying, who had the Crouchs' number. This must be important.

'You have to report to the foot and mouth centre in Edale, Derbyshire and you must leave straight away.'

'I cannot possibly go there this evening, I have been drinking.' (Maxine always drove home after parties.) 'Anyway I will have to go back home to Heydon to collect clothes.'

'Well just you get there as soon as you can. I am sorry to have interrupted your evening with such news.'

'How long can I expect to be away for?'

'Sine dei, Roger, sine dei; you'll be there until there is no more work for you to do. I cannot even guarantee that you will be home for Christmas! Anyway I will interrupt your evening no further; good night.'

What a bugger. But I was to learn a great deal about disease control during the next few weeks: how to do it, and even more definitely, how not to do it. There were commiserations from the assembled throng but the evening continued with no further interruptions. In the car going home, Maxine said, 'I think I will stay here while you are away. I cannot live alone in that house without a car.'

It was a quarter of a mile to the village and a walk of a mile and half to the main road where she could have caught a bus; too far to carry groceries and too expensive to take a taxi from Norwich.

'I can get some jobs temping in the city or West End, which will give me some money but you will have to collect some clothes and send them to me as I cannot exist on what I have brought down for the weekend.'

And so early next morning I set off for Heydon in glorious autumn weather: cold with clear blue skies. I had been given a list of the clothes that I was to send and so I packed a suitcase with Maxine's clothes on the top and set off for Derbyshire – it was almost due west across the country on not the best of roads. As I drove down into the valley the sky was lit up with huge fires – the dead animals were burning. It was about 6 pm when I arrived at the Church Hotel in Edale, an old country hostelry with a few bedrooms. There were not enough rooms for all the required staff and so beds had been brought in and we were three to a room. I was to share with Chris Randall and Brian Spence, two senior veterinary officers from VI Centres. They were both in the room preparing for dinner when I walked in: I was shown my bed and the place for my clothes. I opened the case and out fell Maxine's underwear! I have never lived it down and to this day whenever I see Brian, almost his first remark will be, 'Are you still cross dressing?'

It was pointless to try and explain. The next day I found a box and sent the clothes off to London.

Dinner was a jolly affair with excellent food and some good beer. The man in charge of the centre, Andy Wilson, was a Regional

97

Veterinary Officer but came from a different mould to many others of his grade: he believed that all vets had valid contributions to make; he enjoyed the company of younger men and he believed in communication, that people perform better if they know what they are doing and why. Over dinner he gave us a lecture on foot and mouth disease control, only he made it seem that he was seeking information from us.

There were several VI staff, including me, who had had no experience of epidemic disease control. He pointed out that sheep were a major problem in foot and mouth disease control as they often carry the virus but show no signs of disease, which makes life very difficult. Cattle almost invariably show signs of disease and so it is very useful to have some cattle mixed with sheep as marker animals. However, up on the moors there were no cattle. They had identified how the disease had got into the valley and to date all four infected farms were mixed cattle and sheep. However, he was worried about the farms up at the top which were purely sheep, and that was why he had requested us youngsters, who would be able to climb to the top and walk all day! He was a worried man – worried because he knew that if an outbreak was seen on top of the moors he would have to slaughter all the animals in the valley; this he was loath to do. A public meeting was to be held the next day in the market square. In the morning we were to go to the Peaks National Park Centre, where we would be issued with protective clothing and all the necessary gear and we would be shown all the forms and have them explained to us.

The eradication by slaughter of a disease is as much a legal exercise as it is a veterinary one. Because you are slaughtering a farmer's animals, it must be done in a strict, legal manner. If foot and mouth disease is suspected then 'Form A' has to be issued which prevents people entering or leaving the farm. If the disease is not confirmed, then 'Form B' is issued removing the restrictions. However, if it is confirmed then the full force of the law comes into effect. The vet has the authority to shoot all animals showing signs of the disease. A valuer comes to the farm and values all the stock, including those shot, and this valuation is agreed with the farmer and then a team of slaughtermen come to the farm and shoot all the susceptible animals (cattle, sheep, pigs, alpacas). The vet has to follow along behind to ensure that the animals are dead. In those far-off days it was thought much better to bury the carcases where possible: the ground was too rocky in Edale and so great funeral pyres had to be constructed according to well laid down principles, so many old railway sleepers and so much coal per animal.

Once the animals are all burnt or buried the great clean-up begins. As soon as disease is confirmed a policeman takes guard at the entrance to the farm and forbids all entries and exits other than official personnel. The children cannot go to school and the wife can do no shopping. This continues until the preliminary disinfection is completed when the draconian restrictions, designed to prevent the spread of the disease, are lifted and life can start to return to normal, if things can ever be normal again on a farm with no animals. Things do not stop there, the farmer's neighbours are all visited, all the stock on their farms are examined and these farmers are served with a 'Form D' informing them that they are in quarantine and they remain so for the next fourteen days. For the first few days the farm is visited daily and the animals examined. If at the end of fourteen days the animals are still healthy then 'Form E' is served which lifts the restrictions on the farm. That does not mean that normal life can be recommenced because there will be area restrictions on movement: these do not apply to a single farm but to all the farms within the area. At times during the 1967 outbreak there were national restrictions affecting the whole country.

In the Centre itself there was a wall of maps (six inches to the mile) showing the whole area and even the fields were marked. The infected farms were marked in red. The vast majority of the vets were employed 'on patrol'. We were given a number of farms to visit and we had to identify on the map the boundaries of each farm and indicate the number and species of animals in each field. This was not possible on the moors as not all the grazing areas were fenced, or more accurately walled, since in those areas the demarcations were dry stone walls. The farmers knew whose sheep were whose but no one else did. This instruction lasted most of the morning and it was time for lunch. The Church Hotel, while not providing the most luxurious of accommodation, made up for it by the quality of its food which was truly superb. Bed, breakfast, lunch and dinner for 45 shillings (£2.25) a night and the meals were excellent. Lunch was a different affair to dinner the previous night because Sandy Lowe, the Assistant Chief Veterinary Officer was with us – he had come to address the meeting, and could not dine with humble veterinary officers. Many of the senior veterinary staff, at the time, hid their ignorance behind their authority. After lunch it was time for the meeting. Andy and the ACVO stood on the steps of the war memorial and addressed the huge gathering of farmers, wives and hangers on. Andy spoke first and explained the gravity of the situation and how important it was to keep the disease off the tops of the moors.

'If it gets loose on the top, we'll no stop it afore it gets tae Scotland. We must nae let this happen, or we will lose all control throughout the whole country.' His worry and concern came through in his south-west of Scotland voice and the people responded. It was then the turn of the ACVO and where the previous speaker had tried to get the farmers' support, it was now the voice of authority: you will do this, you will do that, or we will know why. I thought that he might get lynched. Public relations it was not. This was the mentality of the old style State Veterinary Service, where the show was run with full military authority and the more senior you were, the more you knew. This was the service where no humble veterinary officer dare question a decision of a Divisional Veterinary Officer, let alone an RVO or an ACVO: and veterinary officers did not dare speak to the Chief Veterinary Officer. 'All power corrupts, and absolute power corrupts absolutely,' so said Lord Acton and it was true of the SVS. Not that the senior staff were corrupt in the moral sense, just that they were unable to see that they were playing with people's livelihoods and their lives and were unable to go about it in a humane way.

Later in the outbreak I was working in the Crewe Centre which was run by the authoritarian Regional Veterinary Officer, Tom Stobo: I was talking to a senior veterinary officer who had just completed the slaughter and disinfection of a farm. He was retelling what had happened when he was first on the farm. He had diagnosed the disease and had phoned Tolworth (the headquarters of the State Veterinary Service) to obtain their confirmation of the diagnosis: since they were paying the bill they liked to give the final verdict, although how they could make a diagnosis from a distance of almost 200 miles I will never know. He had contacted the centre and asked for valuers and slaughtermen. All the paperwork had been done but nothing had happened, nobody had turned up and so he phoned the centre.

'Crewe Foot and Mouth Centre,' came the reply.

'I am on Buttermilk Farm and I have been waiting for hours for action: what the fuck is going on: what are you idle bastards doing down there?'

'Do you know who you are talking to?'

'No, I fucking don't,' the VO had said.

'This is Tom Stobo, RVO and head of the centre.'

'And do you know who I am?' the VO asked.

'No, I do not.'

'Thank Christ for that,' said a relieved VO and put the phone down. Such was the fear of authority, as careers have been broken for less.

For the next fortnight I spent the days tramping the hills. Each day dawned bright yet freezing cold. Over breakfast we switched on our car engines, to thaw them out and get the ice off the windows. At 8.30 we were at the foot of Jacob's Ladder to meet the farmers and their dogs who were to take us on patrol on the hills. We donned our thigh-length wellington boots, our long black rubber coats, our rubber sou'westers and black gauntlets. We washed them down with disinfectant to the satisfaction of the farmers and began our ascent. I was reasonably fit in those days but the climb in that gear was something else. I was not helped by the farmer who told me, 'The last time we had a problem on the moors I went up with one of yon vets all dressed up like 'ee, it were a fine summer day and when we got to the top 'ee had a heart attack. I 'ad to go back down and get the pony to bring 'im down.'

I would have been fine without all the clobber but I was really sweating by the time we reached the top. I then realised that this was what the surface of the moon must be like. 'All to left and right the bare black cliff clanged round him' (Tennyson, *Morte d'Arthur*). The rock being limestone, the water percolates rapidly, leaving insufficient moisture for plants to grow. There was grass and heather in places but no bushes or trees. I knew nothing of hefted sheep in those days, but I soon learnt that the sheep have an inbred knowledge of where to find water and food all the year round. You can bring in sheep to join the heft. But if these animals were to be slaughtered, any new sheep would have to be taught by the shepherd where to go for shelter from the wind and rain and this is a very tedious and long-term business. The farmers were petrified at the thought of all their sheep being killed and they were angered by the insensitivity of the ACVO.

'It's all right for him living in his posh house in Lunnen, what does he know, or care, about the likes of us?'

Sandy Lowes had not gone down well in Edale. I had had my first real lesson in people management and those first few days in Edale changed my whole attitude to disease control. Disease control must be done for the people and not to them. If we have to kill animals, it is not for that farmer's benefit but for the good of the community. In some ways the farmer is a hero, giving up stock to save those of others. Consequently the opinions of the farmers must be incorporated in all policy decisions. Thereafter my motto has been 'For farmers, not to farmers.'

Once at the top of Jacob's Ladder we split up and departed in all directions of the compass: a vet to a farmer. We walked until we found the sheep. It would have been easier had the sheep been brought down off the hill as they do for shearing, dipping, vaccinating and all the other procedures to which we subject our animals. There were crushes in the farmyard which made it easier to catch animals for examination. However the risks would have been much greater: there might be virus in the valley, and mixing the sheep which would have occurred had they been brought down would be a stressful and risky activity.

My shepherd on that first morning had a three-legged dog. 'What happened to that left foreleg?' I asked.

''Ee got a tumour. The vet said it wor a sarcoma and it wor the leg or the dog. It broke my heart because 'ee's the best dog I ever owned. I would 'ave preferred 'em to take my arm.' And there was no doubt he meant it, because there were tears in his eyes as he spoke.

''Ee can still run and jump the dykes but 'ee's not just as sharp as 'ee wor and sometimes 'ee tries to jump more an 'ee can, and falls.'

A few lame sheep were seen, and with some difficulty on top of the hill they were caught and examined but none had the telltale signs of foot and mouth disease. Each evening we were briefed over dinner by Andy Wilson, and we watched the news on the hotel television. Each night Gwyn Beynon the CVO, a Welshman, spoke to the nation, and each night the news was getting more gloomy with the daily tally of new cases ever increasing.

However, there was no spread from the initial four outbreaks and so the hill sheep were saved. The centre was cut down in size and just a few vets remained to ensure that all the work remaining to be done, was done. I was instructed to report to the Worcester Centre which

102

was just starting up. No longer did I feel such a new boy as I had a basic grounding in the methods of control.

Worcester was a model centre, run by Alec Brown who was later to become the CVO and he was another of the new wave of SVS senior staff. However, the centre started badly: it was based in the basement of the headquarters of the Worcestershire constabulary at Droitwich. The centre had opened the day before my arrival and all the stores arrived by lorry: boots, coats, brushes, buckets, disinfectant, the lot: it had been unloaded and stacked up in the centre store, beneath the police station. That night the whole lot was stolen! It had to be an inside job but the culprits were never caught, much to the embarrassment of the Worcestershire police. It was here I met up with many old college friends including Anthony Gill of Bath Club fame. He was still wearing the same old sports jacket he had worn throughout his college days. He was in practice in Moreton-in-the-Marsh, near where the family farmed, and the disease was getting close to home.

This centre was a much bigger one than Edale with many more dairy farms and many more outbreaks, and so many more vets. There were regular briefings at 8.30 in the morning and 4.30 in the afternoon. These were usually by Alec Brown himself and they started with the national picture which was followed by what happened the previous day in Worcester and what the plans for the day were. All very well handled, and questions and complaints were addressed. After the disease briefing there were questions on domestic issues. We were divided into teams headed by a senior veterinary officer who knew his or her stuff, and they portioned out the work for the day. As in Edale my job was patrolling, and each morning I was given my list and went to the common room, and with the aid of the Ordnance Survey Maps planned my work for the day. I was sitting there one morning when the great Annie Littlejohn sat down next to me: I had never met her, but she had the awesome worldwide reputation as the queen of footrot in sheep. She worked at the Central Veterinary Laboratory but travelled the country sorting out problems. She introduced herself to me; I told her that she needed no introduction but I introduced myself.

'Ah,' she said, 'I have heard of you already! What do you think of that?' and she handed me a letter from a farmer in Nottinghamshire. It was the classic description of foot and mouth disease in sheep and there were also cattle becoming lame.

'I don't think,' I said, 'I know! You have to go and show this letter to Alec Brown, so that he can get things moving in Nottinghamshire.'

This was the first outbreak of the disease to the east of the Pennines.

Although it was not a major milk producing county such as Shropshire and Cheshire, there were many small dairy farmers scattered round Worcestershire and many of my visits were to such smallholders. It was policy not to go onto farms without the permission of the farmer. If he refused we went away and returned with a policeman, who pointed out that they were obliged to allow us to enter. If they still refused then 'Form A' was served and the policeman remained at the gate prohibiting the entry or exit of people or vehicles. After the milk tanker had been turned away a few times and the farmer had poured his milk down the drain for the second day, they usually allowed us on to examine the stock. Signs were appearing at farm gates: 'BE OFF OR BE SHOT'. Blood was running high.

'But it is you vets who are spreading the disease, going from farm to farm and infected farm to clean farm. You take the disease with you!'

I explained to him that any vet who had been on an infected farm was not allowed onto a clean farm for three days, during which time every item of clothing the vet wore on the farm went to the dry cleaners and he was kept on office duties. I also pointed out that we were clothed in rubber from head to toe and we disinfected going onto the farm and again before we left. I always invited the farmer to wash me down with disinfectant – it was easier to get them to do the back – they almost never refused. I also pointed out to the farmer that although I had been working on foot and mouth disease for a month, I had yet to see a case of the disease.

On this particular morning I had to go to a smallholding run by a woman who kept about twenty cows. Her steading was close to the road and so I parked on the verge, put on my gear and tooted the horn. The woman came out, looked me up and down and nodded her head.

'I am glad it is not the man who came yesterday,' she said. 'I was milking the cows when he came: he was the first of your lot that I'd seen. Anyway I came out of the shed with a bucket of milk in each hand. I put them down and asked him what he wanted. Before saying a word, he put one foot in one bucket and the other in the second bucket!'

Had it not been ten gallons of milk down the drain, she might also have thought it funny. The poor man had thought that she was bringing buckets of disinfectant for him to wash in, and it is easy to confuse milk for White Fluid, the disinfectant that we used until the new iodophores came into use, especially when the milk is frothy from recent milking. Her animals were all healthy and I went on my way.

The driver of a milk lorry had been careless and not disinfected his lorry properly between farm visits. Special dispensation had to be given to dairy companies to collect milk because the country needed the milk even if there was an outbreak of foot and mouth disease. Abattoirs also remained open because people need meat. Animals ready for slaughter need to be killed and not kept eating away on farms. It was easy to see the route of the milk tanker as one after another the farms on his route went down with the disease. The routes reflect the needs of the industry and do not respect county boundaries, and so the disease was taken into Warwickshire. A sub-centre to Worcester was set up in Stratford-upon-Avon and I was on the move again: I was able to make a couple of visits to the Shakespeare Memorial Theatre and I also went to the cinema with a colleague to see some undistinguished Western. Sitting in the cinema, there was definite sniffing coming from behind followed by a voice saying, 'There is a dreadful smell of disinfectant in here. I wonder what's been going on?'

The centre was in the Stratford-upon-Avon College of Agriculture and members of the college staff often dropped in to see how things were going. The weather had still not broken and we were having a glorious, if cold, autumn. On such a morning I set off on a round of visits near Henley-in-Arden and as I came over the brow of a hill I saw at the bottom a narrow humpback bridge. I gave a light touch on the brakes and the car set off like a maniac; the road had not been gritted and I was in a tail spin, going round and round absolutely helpless to control events. I saw the bridge looming ever nearer and saw my beautiful new Renault being wrapped round the parapets. However, I came to a stop on the very hump of the bridge, having touched nothing en route. I think it was a fifteen-point turn that was required to get me off the bridge which was barely wider than the length of the car from nearside front to offside rear. My greatest preoccupation during these manoeuvres was that another car would come over the top of the hill, see my predicament, touch his brakes and come crashing into me. However, I escaped unscathed and carried out my calls without incident.

Perhaps the strangest visit that I made was to the chocolate pigs on a farm near Bournville; the farmer had a contract with Cadbury to collect all their food waste up to seventeen tons a week and there were penalties if he defaulted. Sadly the pigs looked remarkably ordinary despite being fattened on chocolates and chocolate products. They were also completely healthy. The farmer was desperately worried lest he should get the disease and have his pigs slaughtered, and have to default on his contract. I assured him that if his animals were to be slaughtered then he would be compensated for all incidental losses. This reassured the worried farmer, but I wondered how Sandy Lowes would have handled him.

During this same visit I had to inspect several abattoirs. I never knew that so many small abattoirs still existed in view of the competition from the production line abattoirs. However, many of these small units were owned by butchers who killed, dressed and hung their own animals as they wanted to make sure that they got top quality meat, unlikely to be produced on a production line. It is a sad fact of modern life that quality is regularly sacrificed for profit. People today, despite the increasing affluence, are not usually prepared to pay for quality in their food.

The conditions around Stratford-upon-Avon were not conducive to the spread of the foot and mouth virus. Livestock farms were often separated from each other by fruit farms and there was little contiguous contact. The outbreak was rapidly brought under control and I was on the move again to my fourth centre, and I had still not seen the disease!

The Crewe Centre, the largest and most important of all, at the centre of the still developing outbreak, was housed in what had been the main police station (previously two police stations ago) and appeared to be an old Victorian church hall. Mr Stobo and his team of thinkers and planners occupied the whole of the ground floor, and the workers, a hundred or more, were relegated to the first and higher floors. This was the worst-organised of all the centres: it could be argued that it was the biggest and fastest growing, with many new outbreaks to be handled each day. There were no briefing meetings and no teams; there was a delightful DVO (also of the old school) who tried to instil some sense of order, but without support from the top he was fighting a losing battle. I was told to report to the Map Room to be given a job to do. On the wall was a massive map with many areas of red and in charge of this was this imposing looking chap wearing a thick three-piece tweed suit, with a pair of brightly shining brown boots. He was smoking a huge Sherlock Holmes pipe from which emanated more smoke than many a factory chimney. Before I could make a fool of myself, this 'chap' introduced herself as Gwen Shollick: a real case of having been born the wrong gender. She turned out to be a great teacher, and was always willing to help her charges. I was told that since I had not seen the disease I needed to be 'blooded', and so I was put into the group of vets who sat around the centre waiting for the phone to ring. A farmer or vet would call to say that he/she suspected that they had a case of foot and mouth disease and one of us would be dispatched by Gwen. First we were shown the farm on the big map, by this time many of the farms had been visited by a patrolling vet and so its boundaries were known. If this were not the case then the farm had to be checked first and its boundaries established on the map before the suspect animals were examined.

The first farm that I visited had been patrolled previously and had been visited several times before the 'Form D' was lifted, which had happened more than two weeks previously. I gowned up and disinfected myself before entering the byre. This was an old fashioned farm where the cows were tied up all winter and mucked out and bedded daily to keep them comfortable. As soon as I walked into the byre, I knew that the animals had foot and mouth disease: I could see that some animals were uncomfortable, not standing quietly but moving from foot to foot and some were gently drooling. Despite having lived in Kenya for two years I had never seen foot and mouth disease, but without touching an animal I knew that that was what they had; I could even see blisters on the teats. I did not examine the animals very carefully – I did not want to handle those with lesions in the mouth because this would be very painful for the animal. Sometimes it is imperative to check mouths thoroughly, but not these animals. We lifted a few feet so that I could check between the claws and round the coronet, and there was no mistaking the lesions. Here was classic foot and mouth disease.

I made detailed notes of the animals and phoned Tolworth: they were happy with my diagnosis and gave me an IP (infected premise) number, somewhere about 1200. This number would head up all correspondence. I went and shot all ten of the affected animals, and then phoned Gwen and gave her the reference number and was asked for the farmer's phone number (there were no mobile phones in those days). I was told to do all the paperwork while she organised valuers, slaughtermen and a burial team. To keep the farmer from brooding while all this was set in motion, Gwen suggested that I take the farmer out onto the farm to select a good burial site. He was an old fashioned farmer and his cows were his life. He asked if we could wait until dark for the remaining animals to be shot because this could be done by expert marksmen and the other animals would not see it happening. It seemed reasonable to me and the slaughtermen told me that this is what they preferred as it prevented the animals from panicking at the smell of blood. We found a spot in the field which would make an ideal burial site and not interfere with the water table or watercourse. The valuer arrived and went through the animals one by one; the epidemic was now well underway and animals were increasing in value almost daily, so much so that at the end of the outbreak they had to go back and revalue some of the earlier animals killed because prices had risen so sharply. It seemed an honest valuation and the farmer was happy with the prices if not the fate of his animals. I counter-signed the sheets and the magic IP number was appended to each. The valuer would send these sheets to the centre where they would be checked against my list of animals and the form was then sent for payment.

Meanwhile back on the farm we were preparing for slaughter; the cows were released from their yokes and allowed to move of their own free will into the big collecting yard to await their fate. About 6 pm the shooting began; the marksman took up his position at the door and the lights were extinguished. The assistant then shone a lamp onto a cow and the marksmen fired a single shot to the head. The animal fell where it stood. I went in and with the aid of the assistant with his torch checked that it was dead, took its number and checked for lesions. We left; the assistant identified the next cow, shone his lamp; there was another single shot and another dead cow. Yes, it was slaughter but the animals died with dignity: there was no panic as one by one they fell. No animal required more than one shot. I was impressed at the efficiency and demeanour of the slaughtermen. The farmer was crying silently. We moved onto the heifers and bullocks and the same story was repeated. The calves in their pens were killed with a humane killer, and after the shot each animal was pithed, a stiff wire being passed through the shot wound to ensure that the brain was destroyed.

In less than two hours the work was completed. We cleaned up, I disinfected my boots and coat – I had removed the gloves and sou'wester earlier. I went into Crewe for dinner absolutely shattered, not just physically but also emotionally drained. This was the first large scale killing that I had seen. The next day I went back to supervise the burial and the start of the clean-up. By the third day I was finished. Other people took over supervising the major cleaning of the premises. I took my car to the yard and washed it thoroughly, bagged up my clothes and put them all into the dry cleaners for processing.

That was the only case of disease that I saw (and similarly in the 2001 outbreak I only saw one case). I was given the routine chores in the office and was moved from Gwen's ambit to that of Sheila Loxton, one of the brightest and best and destined for stardom. She was widely expected to be the first woman Divisional Veterinary Officer, but she never made it: she was killed in a car crash just outside Edinburgh from where she came. Sheila was another one of my teachers who made a big impression on me. She had this air of knowing exactly what to do and how to do it, and she made you feel that you too could do it; you just needed to put a bit more effort into it. She was definitely one of the boys and could drink and swear with the best but she completely retained her femininity.

I was billeted out in the sticks in a very depressing pub. The company was good and among the numbers was Keith Meldrum who was also destined to become CVO. He had been a couple of years ahead of me at college but I hardly knew him. I felt that I needed more comfort than this ale house could provide and found the ideal spot, the Crown Hotel in Audlem, a lovely village close to Crewe. The publican was Mayor of Crewe and his wife had been his barmaid, so knew her job and was a great cook. The place was warm, comfortable and friendly and I spent the remainder of my time there. As the last inn, I had the attic room at the top – just across from the church tower with its clock that struck regularly every hour: it seemed that the clock was actually in the room, but I soon got used to it. I was one of the few Brits in the hotel which was full of American, Australian, New Zealand and South African vets who had come to see how a real outbreak should be controlled. It was obvious that I was going to be settled for a few weeks at least and so Maxine came up for a weekend to join me and it was great to see her again. She was having a high old time working in a variety of jobs in London and enjoying herself with her old friends.

The outbreak had definitely peaked and so there was hope that we might get some time off. We had worked non-stop, seven days a week for the past eight weeks. I was told that I could have Christmas Day and Boxing Day off but I had to be back by midday on the 27th. It was great to get away from the smell of disinfectant, the talk of animals, disease and problems on farms if only for forty-eight hours. On my return it was obvious that the worst was over. From the peak of thirty outbreaks a day handled by the Crewe Centre alone the number had fallen to below ten and there was an air of inevitability that, while not over, the battle had been won and it was just a matter of time. We worked under less pressure and there were fewer visits to make each day.

The epidemiology team visited the centre, among whom were Gareth Davies and Sherwin Hall, both of whom were later to become colleagues. They were there to record the details of the outbreak for future historians and possibly a government enquiry. While the epidemiologists were in town there was great excitement as a result of the action of the tranquilliser team; their role was to visit farms where there were unhandleable animals and, with the use of the rifle, inject a sedative. They had sedated a bull on a farm along the side of the newly finished stretch of the M6, at which point the bull had taken off, jumped the fence and decided to go to sleep on the southbound carriageway of the motorway. All traffic had to be halted while the animal was examined, luckily it did not have foot and mouth disease: a truck had to be brought onto the motorway, the bull was given the wake-up injection and it was led into the transporter and driven home. The motorway then had to be disinfected and so the traffic was delayed for an hour or more.

I was en route to a farm and had ended up in the middle of Sale; I was driving the wrong way down a one-way street when I was stopped by a policeman. With my foreign car with its red French number plates I thought that I would bluff it out. When he spoke to me I answered in Swahili – to my horror he replied in Swahili. He had been in the Tanganyika police force in Moshi! We had a good laugh, I explained that I was lost and he set me on the right road. During this time I had had to apply for an extension to the import permit for the car: the magic words foot and mouth disease did the trick. I finally got to the farm which was run by a brother and sister who were both well into their eighties. It was a smallholding rather than a farm, with a few cows and sheep, a couple of goats, half a dozen pigs, a donkey and a small flock of chickens, all running indiscriminately round the yard. I had come to serve 'Form E' removing the restrictions on the farm. I examined those animals that I had to examine and found all to be well. We went into the kitchen for the paperwork to be completed over a friendly cup of tea. Before I could complete the paperwork I had to see the 'Form D' that had been served because I needed to copy the details. When asked, the farmer scratched his head

'Meg?' he called. 'Where be that paper the vet gave us?'

'That young chap didn't give us no paper.'

'You must have received a Form D when you were first inspected,' I said.

The farmer went to a roll top desk in a far corner of the kitchen and pushed back the lid revealing a massive pile of documents through which he began to rummage. Eventually with a cry of delight he said, 'I've got the bugger!' and handed me the paper.

It looked very strange but it was a 'Form D' all right. However, it was written in ink in a beautiful script. What was more it was signed by a policeman, Sgt John Longstreath. Stranger still; policeman, even sergeants, are not allowed to sign such documents. Only vets are now allowed to sign 'Forms D'. Then I looked at the date: July 17th 1924 – 43 years ago! Without more ado I completed the paperwork, finished my tea. I took my leave and the ancient 'Form D' and returned to the Centre. Sheila thought it was a huge joke that the smallholder had been under restrictions for more than 40 years and nobody had noticed. My paperwork was duly accepted and I heard no more about it.

Another amusing incident occurred when lifting restrictions on a farm: this was a slightly bigger one than the previous case, a dairy herd of about thirty cows that had been infected with foot and mouth disease. I was carrying out the final inspection prior to serving 'Form B'. As there were no ruminant animals or pigs on the farm, I was there to inspect the buildings and make sure that the cleaning and disinfection had been properly completed: there is nothing worse for a farmer than to restock only for the animals to develop foot and mouth disease a week later. The farm was pristine. We went into

111

what had been the calf house which also was spick and span. The farmer turned to me and said, 'I was born in that farmhouse, and I have lived on this farm, man and boy for the past 84 years, and when them soldiers cleaned out this house, it was the first time in my life that I saw it had a concrete floor!'

By the end of January my work was done and I was returned to the Norwich Centre after almost three months' work with just two days off. Later, in recognition of our work we were given a tax free gratuity of £300. We spent it all buying an early Victorian silver bullet tea service, which still sits in pride of place on the sideboard.

During my time in the west Midlands I had barely given a thought to our return to Kenya. I had learnt several important lessons during this epidemic. The first and most important was that while such a campaign had to be run on military lines it did not have to use military methods. When you are destroying a person's livelihood, it must be done with compassion and not just as force majeure by the state. Many farmers have a deep emotional attachment to their animals and this has to be factored in to any slaughter policy. It is right and proper that the state should eradicate major epidemic diseases, but in its turn it must acknowledge that it is the individual farmer who makes the sacrifice for the majority. I was taught the importance of team work to success and the value of communication from the top, informing the staff of what was going on. Too many of the senior staff thought that knowledge was power and thus that the less they disclosed, the more important they were because they alone knew; a stupid philosophy in the modern world. Well informed people are better motivated and better able to perform their job well. It was also obvious that people work better in small teams where they can know everyone: even the army breaks its units down to platoons.

I also thought about the value of the slaughter policy. Over the years it had served Britain well in keeping our island free from the infection: Europeans vaccinated. However, a cost benefit analysis of slaughter against vaccination had shown that since the First World War the slaughter policy had cost, at today's prices, about 12.5p per animal per year. The cost of the vaccine then would have been at least £1 a year for the two doses and on top of that would be the cost of administering the vaccine. At that time there was no competition.

It was back to the Centre and family life in Heydon, during the worst of the cold winter. However, it was good to be home even if it meant I spent most of my spare time sawing up the undertakers' offcuts. John Simmons, who had also returned, came round one Saturday morning as I was sawing up the elm and remarked, 'You get double your money's worth with that wood, as it makes you warm twice.'

All official recruitment activity had ceased during the epidemic and it would be some time before a recruitment board would be put together to interview candidates. I thought it ironic that I still needed to be interviewed for the post of Assistant Veterinary Investigation Officer Grade II, when I had just worked non-stop for three months for my potential employer. However, bureaucratic rules are bureaucratic rules, and it is all supposedly designed to prevent corruption. Until I was an established civil servant I could not be seconded back to Kenya, and so I waited. Eventually a board was constituted and I made my way down to Kingsway in London for the interview. It was more of a chat, mostly about foot and mouth disease but also about how I saw my future in the service. Along with John and several others I was appointed. You normally have to serve six months from the date of appointment for your position to be confirmed, but because of the delays of the foot and mouth disease campaign it was decided that this would not be necessary.

It was now possible to start the secondment process for Muguga, and I had to apply for a further extension for the import permit on the car. Again it was granted. We had planned to be in Britain from June until December 1967, but it was October 1968 before we were on the plane to Nairobi.

7

A Lung Time in Kenya, 1968–1973

'You know my methods, apply them.'
Sir Arthur Conan Doyle *The Sign of Four*

I had completed my basic training in clinical and diagnostic pathology, I had been taught how to investigate outbreaks in the field and I now had had first-hand experience of controlling a major disease epidemic in the field. All that was required to complete my basic education in the diagnostic, detective world was to learn how to plan, organise, execute and write up a research project; that was what I was going back to Kenya to do.

The East African Veterinary Research Organisation (EAVRO) at Muguga, Kenya had been set up in the last heady days of Empire; the Europeans were moving towards setting up regional groupings of countries and we thought that it would be good for our colonies to do the same. The East African Common Services Organisation later to become the Community (Kenya, Tanzania and Uganda), the Central African Federation (North and South Rhodesia and Malawi) and Malaysian Federation (Malaya, Sabah, Sarawak and Singapore) all came from the same drawing board. Not one has survived because the people concerned were not asked what they thought; it was just another bright idea from Whitehall. There were undoubted merits in the idea of pooling resources for the common good. But what the people wanted was to be free to do their own thing, not to have Uhuru, as Independence was called, circumscribed by people in a country that they did not like: there were enough people in their own country they did not like without going looking for more. Without including the Europeans and the Indians brought in by them, there were more than fifty tribes in Kenya belonging to four different ethnic groups. More than enough groups to dislike each other!

There was a common customs organisation, there was the East

African Railways and Harbours that served all three countries, East African Airways flew under the flags of the three countries and so research bodies were also set up to look at regional problems: EAVRO and the East African Agriculture and Forestry Organisation (EAFRO) were set up at Muguga, Kenya where we shared common facilities; The East African Trypanosomiasis Research Organisation was set up in Tororo, Uganda. They were all established to solve problems common to all three countries and EAVRO worked on the major diseases causing problems: the epidemic diseases of rinderpest and contagious bovine pleuro-pneumonia (CBPP) together with East Coast fever, the big killer in all three countries all the time. In addition there were smaller sections devoted to parasitology and animal nutrition.

The laboratories were all new, as was the equipment, and the money rolled in from round the world to support this splendid concept in disease control. There were world-renowned scientists heading up the sections: Walter Plowright CMG, FRS – the man who had produced the tissue culture vaccine which made feasible the concept of eradicating rinderpest from Africa and the world – was the head of the Virology Section; David Brown (later to become the Deputy Director of the Tate Gallery in London) headed the CBPP Section; and David Brocklesby (future head of the Centre for Tropical Veterinary Medicine, in Edinburgh) headed the Parasitology Section. I was destined for the CBPP Section. By the time I arrived David Brown had left to become Director at the Federal Laboratory in Vom Nigeria, and his place had been taken by Gareth Davies from the CVL, in Weybridge, whom I had met when on foot and mouth duty in Crewe. Like me, he was on secondment from MAFF.

We all worked for the grandly titled Joint Project 16 that was to work on the laboratory tools required to eradicate CBPP. Joint Project 15 was for the eradication of rinderpest and it was almost a major triumph. They thought that they had succeeded and so the project was closed down. Sadly there were two tiny pockets of rinderpest left, one in East Africa and one in West, and within ten years the disease was almost back to its former glory.

Nobody ever mentioned Joint Projects 1–14 although I suppose they must have been set up. JP 16 was supported by a large number of organisations who put more or less money into the pot: FAO, the Food and Agriculture Organisation of the United Nations headed the list although they gave almost nothing. Then came the OIE, the

International Office of Epidemics (it is more euphonic in French) who gave us their blessing, but since they were in Paris and a disguise for French Imperialism and this project was in an Anglophone country they gave us nothing at all. The OAU, the Organisation of African Unity had no money to give. USAID weighed in with a big budget that was not at the disposal of the project but controlled by Stan Stone, the scientist they sent to work on the biochemistry of the organism: he was pretty generous. The OECD , the Organisation for Economic Cooperation and Development, made no appearance at all. The one name that was not on the letterhead was ODA, the British Overseas Development Authority, who provided all the expatriate staff apart from Stan – that is, three vets, one biochemist, and three laboratory technicians – stumped up almost the whole of the recurrent budget for the project, and behind the scenes was paying the basic running costs of EAVRO which provided all the facilities, maintenance, equipment and the wages of all locally employed staff.

To eradicate an infectious disease by 'stamping out', as the slaughter policy was called, requires little knowledge of the disease to succeed. Rinderpest and CBPP were both eradicated from Britain before the agents that caused the diseases had been identified. However, the policy is expensive, because the owners have to be compensated for the animals killed, and their loss of income, and disposal of the bodies does not come cheap. In some countries and cultures, slaughter of animals is unacceptable: the Masai people in East Africa and the Fulani in West Africa have emotional and religious ties to their animals, and a further complication for the Fulani is that most animals have no real owner, but are held in trust for the owner's sons or brothers, and so with whom do you negotiate about slaughter? Consequently, alternatives to slaughter have to be found and the major plank is a good vaccine. A vaccine was therefore necessary against *Mycoplasma mycoides* the tiny microbe without a cell wall that causes CBPP.

In his book *King Solomon's Mines* the author Rider Haggard describes an early method of vaccinating against CBPP in South Africa and the term used was 'salting':

As for 'lung sick,' which is a dreadful form of pneumonia, very prevalent in this country, they had all been inoculated against it. This is done by cutting a slit in the tail of an ox, and binding in a

116

piece of the diseased lung of an animal which has died of the sickness. The result is that the ox sickens, takes the disease in a mild form, which causes its tail to drop off, as a rule about a foot from the root, and becomes proof against future attacks. It seems cruel to rob the animal of his tail, especially in a country where there are so many flies, but it is better to sacrifice the tail and keep the ox than to lose both tail and ox, for a tail without an ox is not much good, except to dust with.

The first objective of JP 16 was to look at the existing vaccine and work out just how good it was. It was at EAVRO that the $T_1 44$ vaccine had first been produced. The strain had been isolated from an outbreak of disease in Tanzania in which only a few animals had died. This led the workers to believe that it might be less pathogenic than other strains. It had been shown with other organisms that growing them in eggs reduced their virulence for their host animal and so they started passaging the T_1 through hens' eggs containing embryos: the 44 indicates that it was passaged forty-four times. It was thought that by then the virulence would be sufficiently reduced to provide the basis of a good vaccine: adequate protection of the animal with little risk of disease. The vaccine was shown to protect but little was known of its properties. This egg-adapted vaccine had been used in field trials, killing thousands of animals: however those animals that survived the anaphylactic reaction caused by the egg protein had complete protection against the disease. It was shown that it was the egg proteins that caused the severe reactions and deaths in the animals, and so a broth culture vaccine was made to remove the risk of anaphylactic reactions. In the field this proved very successful at controlling the disease.

It is very easy to test for protection given by a vaccine against rinderpest or foot and mouth disease: you give the animals a dose of vaccine and several weeks later you challenge that immunity by injecting the real thing. In the case of rinderpest a sub-cutaneous injection of the virulent virus will produce clinical disease and death in the unvaccinated animal. In the case of foot and mouth disease, the virus is injected into the tongue and the classic lesions in mouth and feet can be seen. Sadly you cannot do this with CBPP; as we have seen with the virulent *M. mycoides*, injected into the tail by means of a piece of lung, there is a large reaction in the tail but the animal does not get pneumonia. If you inject the organism under the skin over the chest, a nasty abscess is produced but no pneumonia. In desperation workers tried anaesthetising the animal, passing a tube into the lungs and pouring a broth culture of the organism directly into the lung. This worked very well; the typical disease could be produced and the results varied just like the normal disease from acute death to animals with a walled up sequestrum in the lung. Unfortunately it did this whether the animal had been vaccinated or not! It was such a coarse technique that the defences of the animal were overcome even if the animal was adequately protected against natural infection. And so the idea of an 'in-contact trial' was hit upon, using artificially infected animals as described above and putting them in direct contact with vaccinated and unvaccinated animals. Using wondrous techniques, statisticians calculated that a minimum of forty-eight animals per trial were required – sixteen artificially infected, sixteen vaccinated and sixteen unvaccinated.

CBPP was a serious problem in Australia, and so the workers there had pioneered this method of 'in-contact trials' and had worked out a satisfactory means of evaluating the results. The Australian work was repeated in Muguga. The vaccine used in Australia was the V_5 a strain isolated in Victoria: this had been tried in Kenya but had been discarded because the vaccine caused too many tails to fall off – we still vaccinated in the tail. The Australians used this vaccine to great effect, and with movement controls they brought the disease under control and it was declared eradicated in 1973.

The preliminary trials had been completed when I arrived at Muguga and had shown the $T_1 44$ vaccine to be very effective vaccine in the short term. A series of trials had been arranged to test the level of immunity at six, twelve, and twenty-four months; a vaccine dosage trial was planned to determine the minimum number of organisms that were required to produce immunity. The broth vaccine was bulky, it was produced in the eight-ounce bottle from which it was dispensed, had to be transported in cold-boxes, was required to be kept cool at all times and had a shelf life of only three weeks, which meant that it had to be made to order and could not be stock-piled, or adequately tested before it was used. Despite these short-comings, once we had shown its value we sold many millions of doses throughout Africa – Kenya, Tanzania and Uganda, Zambia, Southern Rhodesia, Sudan, Nigeria and Cameroun. The French workers were using the broth vaccine but were trying to produce a lyophilised (freeze dried) vaccine in Addis Ababa in Ethiopia and Fort Lamy in Chad. A lyophilised vaccine was included in our trial schedule.

Our knowledge of how the disease behaved (we call this epidemiology) needed to be greatly expanded: how did the disease spread from animal to animal? Could it only be spread by direct transmission from animal to animal? How did new outbreaks arise? A serious problem was that we had no adequate serological test to identify animals that had been vaccinated, or had had the disease and recovered. A serological test is when you take a blood sample from an animal (or human), let the blood clot and then separate the serum: this serum is then tested for the presence of antibodies to a specific agent and by this means you can tell whether or not the animal has had contact with the infection. When an animal was vaccinated against CBPP, a fortnight after the vaccination there were detectable antibodies in its blood and the level rose for a few weeks and then fell to nothing, although the animal was still resistant to the disease. Animals that became infected developed antibodies a minimum of six weeks after exposure, the levels of which then rose rapidly and, if the animal recovered, proceeded to fall so that by six months no antibody was detectable even though there was a sequestrum in their lungs. Could an animal suffer twice from the disease? We needed to look again at diagnostic techniques. Sequestra can be found in many parts of the body, bone, liver and lung among others. It occurs when a part of an organ or tissue is deprived of its blood supply. When the blood supply is resumed the body cannot resuscitate the dead tissue and so it walls it off instead with a layer of fibrous tissue. Such sequestra can persist until the animal dies.

There was a good deal of work to be done but there was a great team eager to get stuck in. The technical staff were Cliff Boarer, Wilf Read and Geoff Turner, all from the Central Veterinary Laboratory at Weybridge. Gareth was the vet in a charge and there was myself and my old friend, Roy Gilbert from Norwich making up the veterinary team. I was allocated a Type 2 house next door to Roy.

The house, which had been unoccupied for 18 months but had been redecorated, was set in a garden of almost two acres, part of which had reverted to bush. The day we moved in, Oxford, a marmalade cat, came to join us. He had been living in the house with the previous occupants and they left him to fend for himself when they went: he had done well and seemed in good shape when he came to

119

us, and was very friendly. The house was a delight: raised about three feet above the ground to prevent flooding in the rainy season, with a small veranda leading into the sitting room, off which was the dining room, which in turn led into the kitchen and the back door. Doors from the sitting room and kitchen led into the passage to the bedroom area with two moderate and one large bedrooms. It was more than adequate for the two of us. At the bottom of the drive by the road were the 'servants' quarters' with rooms for two members of staff, a shower and common cooking area. There was a large vegetable garden which was soon put into production with the aid of Mzee Kamau, an old white-headed and white-bearded Kikuyu gardener whom we shared with Bill Taylor. Bill had been in the year ahead of me at college and preceded me as President of the Veterinary Students Committee; he lived next door to Roy and was a very keen gardener, which was not surprising since his father had been the Director of Kew Gardens.

Before we were allocated a house and before our luggage had arrived we stayed in Muguga House, a club/motel which was an oasis to visitors to both the veterinary and forestry institutes. For almost a month we lived in a rather pleasant chalet in the delightful grounds of the club, and had a small living room, bedroom and bathroom. Food was provided by Mrs de Souza in Muguga House itself. There was a dining room, a bar in which was a small, but well stocked, library and a large meeting room/dance hall. There were tennis courts, a squash court and a bowling green. Just down the road was a small, beautiful church built by public subscription: it was Christian, but non-denominational and used by Anglicans, Baptists and the Presbyterian Church of East Africa (which had been established by the Church of Scotland, which had founded two excellent schools for local children at the nearby town of Kikuyu).

The estate was enormous and had been carved out of the virgin bush and some of the original forest still remained just outside the boundary. Much of the land was given over to experimental forestry, looking at improving indigenous trees and experimenting with imported trees, and they had one stand of Australian eucalyptus that grew by twelve feet a year. There was a large area of grassland for raising the experimental cattle that were required for research purposes. All was set in an area of great natural beauty with undulating pastures alternating with stands of trees; from one side of the estate you could see Mt Kilimanjaro and from another Mt Kenya. There were fifty or more senior houses all grouped together like a small village, with houses ranging from the Type 3 up to the two palatial director's houses. On the other side of the road near the church was the African village (junior housing), with its neat rows of terraced houses set around the shop; they were small but well designed, with sanitation, running water and electricity, and a definite step up from the usual African hut with no services. There was a massive building programme in train when we arrived to house the educated young Africans who had been recruited as trainees. These intermediate houses and flats were eagerly snapped up as soon as they were completed.

Soon after arriving at Muguga I had a phone call from the British High Commission to say that the Aid Attaché wished to see David Radley, who had also just arrived to work on East Coast fever, and me, in his office and would Friday at 9 am be suitable? It was. At nine David and I presented ourselves at the British High Commission and were asked to go to his secretary's office. This was actually a large room occupied by four British women.

'Sorry to keep you waiting, the boss will be a little bit late so please take a seat.'

We waited for an hour and a half, during which time not a scrap of work was done. First they all had to view one of the women's holiday snaps which called for many oohs and aahs. One, who was obviously unmarried, proceeded to make her arrangements for the forthcoming weekend, which required a great number of phone calls. Another woman spent a long time on the phone to the local supermarket, putting in her order for the weekend. Finally the great man arrived; he had undoubtedly been drinking. He ushered us into his office and sat us down.

'Well, what was it you wanted to see me about?'

We pointed out that it was he who had asked us to come and see him.

'Oh, well, it was just to wish you all the best and hope you have a profitable stay in Kenya. Thank you for coming and if you need any help, just give me a call.'

I thought to myself, 'You will be the last person I call in an emergency.'

We bad our farewells and, hardly able to conceal our mirth, left the British High Commission. A good place to avoid.

It was too far for Maxine to travel to Nairobi to work but there

121

were plenty of jobs available to highly competent secretaries, and she started in the Physics Section at East African Agriculture and Forestry Research Organisation (EAAFRO) where she learnt a great deal about hydrology. Her first boss was Matt Dagg, a very go-ahead scientist who soon went on to become the Director of Agriculture for Northern Nigeria. But not before he had wangled an invitation for me to speak at a large international meeting discussing 'Limitations to Agricultural Production in Africa', in Zaria, Northern Nigeria. It was the first time that I had been asked to speak at a major international meeting and so I went to a great effort to make sure that my talk was well prepared.

EAAFRO was a walking distance from our house but EAVRO was a couple of miles away on the estate and we worked from 8 am till 12.45 and from 2 pm to 4.30, well that was the theory. However, on most days we were able to be on the tennis court before 5 pm. This gave us an hour and a half to play because it was always dark by seven o'clock and at certain times of the year it was already too dark to play by 6.30. Tuesday and Thursday afternoons were 'Mix-In' sessions, when we were all mixed up, good and bad, and just one set was played before changing partners. Muguga Club was a welcome diversion and so important because we were a long way from town.

The great worker in the field of CBPP, J.R. Hudson, an Englishman who had made his name working on the disease in Australia, was sent to Muguga by FAO to help us set up our research programme. This plan was revised regularly and the list of priorities was kept up to date. Resources were directed primarily to the major targets of the project. But in those halcyon days there was money and staff to do anything within reason. Regular meetings of staff were held. At the start the only African senior enough to attend these meetings was John Senyango, who was a man of little education but great ability, with a natural talent for handling animals and the junior staff. He knew what was possible in terms of staff and facilities and was a vital member of the team. These meetings planned out in some detail what was going to happen the next month: this was important because we had to work with a huge number of animals: when planning for experiments with forty-eight animals up to two years in the future there had to be a fair few extra animals to make up for those that would die in the interim. There were four such trials planned. All these animals were examined daily and were bled once a week and their sera examined for antibodies to CBPP. Massive

122

amounts of equipment and reagents were required for all this work and it was Wilf Read who had to arrange the purchase and importation of all this material: it was some undertaking.

It was decided that, as a trained microbiologist, I should be responsible for the scientific work associated with the production of the vaccine and attempts to improve the shelf life. One of the many problems of working with mycoplasms is that they grow so slowly; on a nutrient plate it takes a week before the colonies are large enough to be seen. If they grow in broth then it takes a week before you can see the turbid growth. Working with *E. coli* or *Staphylococcus aureus* you get the results the following day. A clever dodge was developed to speed it all up when someone had the bright idea to relate optical density to the number of organisms in the bottle: the more organisms present, the cloudier the culture. Of course, this does not work with mycoplasms, as you have to have a thousand million (10^9) of them in every millilitre of medium before the machine measuring the density can detect any change from the blank medium – and by the time you have those sorts of numbers, they have almost stopped growing.

What we really needed was a test that would allow us to calculate the numbers in a rapidly growing culture of between a million (10^6) and a thousand million (10^9) organisms per millilitre. People working with fungi have a similar problem, and they solved it by measuring the amount of a specific enzyme in the culture. Enzymes are wonderful works of nature; they are made from proteins and are designed for specific jobs – one to split the sugar molecule in half, another to join two proteins together to make a different protein, and so on, and there are hundreds probably thousands of them: all good trade unionists and only doing one single job! We decided to see if we could do the same as the mycologists. Wilf developed the cultures systems and Cliff worked out techniques for measuring the quantities of different enzymes in the culture. With almost the first enzyme that we tried we hit the jackpot and we were able to accurately relate the amount of enzyme present to the number of organisms in the culture. This could be done in a little over an hour instead of a week! It was major breakthrough, a real achievement, because it gave us almost instant knowledge of what the culture was doing. The development of this technique gave us the key to looking at prolonging the shelf life of the vaccine, which was our next project.

123

First of all we had to find out why the cultures stopped growing and the organisms started to die. Was it lack of food? Perhaps it was lack of space, or perhaps, like humans, they were polluting their environment? We examined all possibilities and concluded that pollution was the problem. All forms of life require energy for growth and we provided energy in the form of glucose in the broth we used for vaccine production. There was still some left when the mycoplasms stopped growing. The organisms gain the energy by breaking down the glucose and one of the by-products of this breakdown is lactic acid, and so with growth the medium goes from being slightly alkaline to acid – and with increasing acidity more and more mycoplasms die.

The next question was how could we stop the medium from becoming acid? We were not the first to confront this problem, it was vital in many industrial and chemical processes and as a result a whole range of 'chemical buffers' had been developed, which were usually a mixture of two related chemicals. As acid was produced it was used to convert one of the chemicals in the buffer into the other, using up the acid in the process. Cliff calculated how much acid was being produced and how much buffer would be required to neutralise this acid. We tried all three of the buffers in common use: phosphate, barbitone and bicarbonate in that order. The phosphate buffer worked perfectly while the vaccine was in the incubator at 37 degrees and as a result the pH remained above 7 – the acid to alkaline levels go from 0 to 14 and a pH 7 is neutral, neither acid (less than 7) nor alkaline (greater than 7) – just what we were aiming for. However, we had to put so much buffer in the vaccine that when we put the culture in the refrigerator the buffer precipitated out of solution. Back to the drawing board. Neither of the other buffers was much better. And that was that; plan scrapped. Scientific research is littered with failures: people have bright ideas which when put to the test do not work, but that is what research and science is about. It is just as important to document the failures as it is to trumpet the successes, because you stop others from making the same mistake again.

And then I had a bright idea. I had noticed when we were doing the enzyme studies that the vaccine normally reached a count of 10^9 well before the acid level of the broth had fallen below a pH of 7. For some reason the magic count for the vaccine was 10^9 although nobody seemed to know why. Possibly the reason was that

124

invariably the T_144 strain of *M. mycoides* reached that count. We had not yet carried out the dosage trial to establish the number of organisms required to produce a good level of immunity. That was to come later. Perhaps what we were doing wrong was to leave the culture too long in the incubator?

A trial was set up to see what happened if we removed the vaccine before its allotted time. By checking the mycoplasmal count every six hours using our enzyme technique we were able to determine at what time the count would reach 10^9: it was a bit of a nuisance this one, because we had to take samples at six o'clock and twelve o'clock – including midnight and 6 am – but we took it in turns. Once we had a rough idea of when the vaccine would reach the magic figure, we took samples every hour around that time and we started the vaccine growth at a time when we could take these samples during the working day.

The vaccine was taken from the incubator and put into the refrigerator when the tests showed that we had 10^9 organisms and before the pH had dropped below 7. Each week for three months we took samples of the vaccine and checked how many organisms still remained and we were delighted that over that period the level kept above 10^9. We had found a way to keep the mycoplasms alive.

We now had a bevy of young and enthusiastic East Africans working in the lab. They were recruited from the three countries and only the best of the applicants had been selected: they were bright, intelligent and moderately well educated. We had young Enoch, an Abaluhya from near the Uganda border, and he was the solid dependable type. By contrast there was John, also an Abaluhya, who was more the 'Flash Harry' type with an eye for a deal and who never missed a trick; despite this he was a good worker. From Tanzania was Brenda Mtui, a tall Chagga girl from the mountain, whose father was a senior chief and almost 100 years old. She was to develop into one of the most beautiful African women that I have seen, and to go with her looks were her ability and industry. Later, when her husband's job took them to Botswana, I was delighted to recruit her to work in the National Veterinary Laboratory in Gaborone. Those three made up the bacteriology laboratory staff of the CBPP Department where Wilf and Geoff soon had them sorted out and working well.

Len Ivins, from the CVL in Weybridge, joined the biochemistry team but I am not sure he strengthened it! But two young Kenyan girls certainly did: Catharine Kariavu from Meru and Madeline Kinyanjui, a Kikuyu, both with a bent for biochemistry, and under the eyes of Stan and Cliff they developed into first-class technicians. Catherine became a senior technician and was later recruited by an international consortium to work in their laboratory. Madeline married and had children, and was lost to veterinary research. There were also two old boys of limited education but great skill: our vaccine maker, Harun, was reputed to have been employed as an executioner by the British during Mau Mau days; David Kinyanjui carried out all the serological testing including the complement fixation test (CFT), which is a fearsomely difficult test to get your head round but, at the time, it was the only really effective test for CBPP. I am not sure that David ever really understood the principles of the CFT, but he knew how to carry it out and record the results. He was a gem, ever ready to assist me in my work. I remember, many years later, visiting EAVRO and I went to find David. I saw him sitting on a rock outside the laboratory. Long before he saw me, I stood and watched him from afar and eventually he looked up and saw me – from thirty yards he recognised me and sat there as if in disbelief, shaking his head from side to side; when I got to him he jumped up and we embraced.

'It has been a long time Dr Windsor, too long.'

'Almost ten years, David,' I said. His hair was beginning to turn grey but his eyes had lost none of their sparkle.

'You have come back to work with me, to teach me some more?'

'I am sorry, but no. I am just here on holiday but I could not return to my old laboratory without coming to see my old friend, colleague and helper.'

'Things are not good here, no more. The *wazungu* [Europeans] have nearly all gone, there is no money for work and laboratories lie idle. Equipment finished: no one know how to repair and so we sit and do nothing. When you come back to help us? You know I like to work, to help my people and make my country better.'

It was a sad reflection on 20 years of independence. We really had screwed up, giving the nation its freedom without giving them a system that would enable that freedom to work.

We also had a batch of washers-up, cleaners and animal attendants that John had well under control. The EAVRO buildings were at the far end of the estate with an open gate leading to a small African village. I never did discover its name, but there was an illegal shebeen in the village to which John took us after work on Fridays. From the outside it was a normal rondavel – the typical Kikuyu thatched hut (the estate was in the heart of Kikuyuland) – but inside it was a different story. In the centre of the hut was a circular pit where the brewing occurred and which could be covered over if the law was about. This was a harmless place and the police left it well alone. The two local brews were pombe, a cloudy beer made from maize meal which always gave me diarrhoea, and honey beer in which our landlord specialised, which was a sparklingly clear drink with a good flavour. At a simuni (6 old pence, or 2.5p) a glass it made a pleasant end to the week's labours. Two glasses were enough and only one if we were going out that evening. It was a pleasant place for an informal chinwag over the week's work.

Having been able to stop the organisms from dying, the next step was to try bulk production of the vaccine. The vaccine was currently produced in eight-ounce medicine bottles and the 200-ml contents were enough to vaccinate 400 animals. There are great disadvantages in producing vaccines in small containers, the most important of which is that you have no idea if the contents of one bottle are the same as another, and so it is impossible to carry out significant testing of the batch. There is also a greater risk of a contaminated bottle going unnoticed. That this did not happen was down to Harun's skill. We looked at the possibility of buying a small commercial fermenter in which pharmaceutical companies make vaccine but decided that this was too great a jump. Instead we purchased a unit that would provide stirring of the broth, a means of passing oxygen (as the more oxygen there is available the less lactic acid is produced, as the sugars are used more efficiently) and 'ports' through which we could add nutrients if required and take samples without contaminating the cultures, which was essential to us. This unit was fitted into a rubber bung with which we could seal a forty-litre flat-bottomed flask in which we put twenty-five litres of culture broth (about five gallons, or enough vaccine for 50,000 animals.).

Making the broth was a pantomime in itself and it was a wonder that we ever produced sterile media for our organisms to grow in, as it required ten percent of serum. Earlier workers at EAVRO had come up with this wonderful recipe known as Newing's Tryptose Broth which contained everything that a mycoplasm could wish for in terms of nutrients. The basis was tryptose which is a breakdown product of protein; it also contained yeast extract (the mycoplasms like their vitamins), glucose and a host of other goodies topped up with ten percent serum. The serum was obtained from the Uplands Bacon Factory: we had to use pig serum as bovine serum might contain antibodies to *M. mycoides* and so kill the growing organisms. One hundred litres of broth requires ten litres of serum and so the blood was collected in buckets, albeit sterile buckets. It is one thing to start with a sterile bucket, but holding the bucket under a dead pig whose throat has just been cut, to collect the blood, is not the most sterile of procedures. There was a regular run to Uplands on a Monday morning and sometimes we had to make a repeat visit if the medium was running out. This was another reason why the vaccine was only made to order.

Once back in the laboratory the buckets were stood in the cold room for the clot to retract allowing us to separate the sera. This serum was then passed through a continuous flow centrifuge. In most centrifuges the material to be spun is put into cups and the machine set in train. A continuous flow centrifuge cuts out the stopping and starting. The serum containing some red blood cells feeds into the machine and the pure serum comes out the other end. Once made, the medium is put into an incubator at 37° C for forty-eight hours to check that it is not contaminated, and it can then be stored in the refrigerator until required.

Our first attempt at bulk production of the vaccine was a total disaster and we produced a wonderful culture of fungi! We had not sorted out the correct way to take samples from the sampling port and had obviously introduced the fungus at one of the samplings. Out came the instruction book for the equipment yet again, and we had another go. Our next attempt was greeted by success and we produced two flasks each containing twenty-five litres of culture vaccine, one of which was taken to the cold store, the second was dispensed into our regular vaccine bottles and sealed. They were also put into the cold store. Each week thereafter, five bottles of vaccine were taken from the store and checked to see what was happening to the organisms. We found that for several weeks the numbers remained the same and then they began a gentle decline associated with an increasing amount of acid in the broth.

It would be fascinating to know what actually goes on among these organisms; do they continue to multiply even in the cold temperatures of the refrigerator, the numbers remaining constant because the new organisms are balanced out by those dying? Or do the organisms remain in a state of limbo just 'ticking over' and expending the minimum amount of energy to keep them alive and hoping for better times, until finally weakened by inactivity they succumb? We now knew that we could keep this vaccine alive for up to six months, a great advantage over three weeks. However, we did not know if this vaccine would work. We injected animals and they responded in the same manner as they would to the conventional vaccine, and there were no untoward reactions to the vaccine even if it was given under the skin behind the shoulder instead of the conventional tail tip. We knew it was safe and we knew animals responded in the same way as to the conventional vaccine but we did not know if it actually protected animals.

We asked the Director of Veterinary Services for permission to use the vaccine on an experimental basis in the field. Permission was refused. That last interview with him came back to haunt me: 'If you go and work at Muguga you will receive no cooperation from me.'

The Director wrote and asked him to reconsider; I was then asked to go and visit him in his office at Kabete. He was quite cold: he did not like people not doing what he told them.

'I warned you, that if you left my department I would do nothing to assist you. Now I am forbidding you to go out and do any field work.'

He was piqued and hitting out in the only way he knew, having no regard to the benefits of his country and to the animals in Kenya if the new vaccine were to be successful.

'Do you really think that your decision is in the best interests of your country?' I wanted to ask him, but I did not, thinking that I might still need his help for something else.

Salvation came from a different direction. Graham Duncanson who had been the District Veterinary Officer in Nyeri, had now risen to be the Provincial Veterinary Officer, Coast Province. Despite annual vaccination campaigns against CBBP, there was a constant problem with disease in animals coming out of the north. They had tried to solve the problem of trekking the cattle to the abattoir by commissioning a boat to take the cattle from the northern coast on the border with Somalia down to Mombasa. However, there were no proper unloading facilities at Mombasa and so the boat sailed along the coast to the abattoir. There all the cattle were herded into the sea and they swam to shore, where they were rounded up. It sounds barbaric but I suspect that it might have been much less stressful

129

than unloading from the ship and into trucks for the short journey to the abattoir. There were almost no casualties from this method which is more than can be said of the lorry journeys.

Trekking the cattle was still the favoured method of the traders and they were bringing a mob of 40,000 when they were stopped at a quarantine where CBPP was diagnosed among them. Graham needed 40,000 doses of vaccine urgently and did not want to wait the three weeks required from order to dispatch. I told him the story of the vaccine, and the problems that we had had with Muriithi, and suggested that we could bottle up one of the flasks of twenty-five litres which would provide 50,000 doses. He could bluff it out with the Director, saying that he had obtained the vaccine in the usual way but there would of course be no charge as it was an experimental vaccine. That was good for his budget, although the cost would only have been £2000 and the cost of administering it would be much greater. We bottled up the vaccine and packed the bottles into our special boxes which Graham took away with him.

He reported that there were no reactions to the vaccine in any of the animals. He was also impressed with the speed with which the outbreak was brought under control. It seemed that we had cracked the problem of stockpiling the vaccine. However, it needed to be properly tested before we replaced our current production. This account has taken a short time to relate here, but the work had taken several years and the project, and in particular my part in it, was coming to an end before the tests could be set up. This is an example of the problems of scientific research: a really exciting discovery is made which then requires funds to take it to a commercial product.

The most incredible loss of all time concerns the discovery by Fleming of the bactericidal properties of the fungus *Penicillium notatum*. Florey and Chain isolated the active principal penicillin and showed it to be a revolutionary life-saving drug, but Britain was at war and it was said that the drug used in Britain had been purified by passage though the Oxfordshire Constabulary! The drug was given to volunteer policemen and their urine was collected as it was much simpler to purify it from urine than from culture! And so it happened that the Americans undertook the purification work and it was they who took out the patents on its commercial production and made all the money from it!

I took part not only in my specific work but also in the day-to-day work of the vaccine trials. These were a complicated business. For each trial eighty yearling animals were purchased from areas of Kenya known to be free from CBPP and brought to Muguga. Once they had settled down, those with horns had them removed by one of the vets, as you cannot have horned animals housed with non-horned animals: to do this each horn had to be given a local anaesthetic, a tourniquet was applied round the base of each horn and then with a pair of horn cutters, resembling giant garden shears, the horn was chopped off and some antiseptic powder was applied. It is hard work and, if the tourniquet slips, a bloody operation, as the blood sprays everywhere until the tourniquet is replaced. The animals were housed in a fly-proof building for a couple of days until the healing process had got underway. Each animal was given an ear tag with a unique number and a blood sample was taken and checked for antibodies to CBPP; positive animals were discarded back to the general farm stock and became available to other sections. Using a deck of playing cards the animals were randomly put into the three groups, sometimes more. For instance, for the trial to establish the minimum number of organisms required to produce immunity we had three vaccinated groups; one which received a dose containing 10^5 organisms, one receiving 10^7 and the third receiving 10^9, and so we had to increase the number of animals in the control group and the group of those to be artificially infected. The date the animals were to be vaccinated had to be counted back on a year planner from when the trial was scheduled to start.

It all seemed to go without a hitch. Each week a blood sample was taken for David to check the antibody status. Of course the animals had to be dipped each week to keep the ticks under control and they received a worm treatment on a regular basis but apart from that they were all grazed together until the fun began.

Many people have asked me, 'Does it not disturb you experimenting on all these animals and causing some to be very ill and even to die a dreadful death?' (That never really happened because any animal *in extremis* was humanely dispatched.) Also, 'How do you reconcile this with being a vet whose primary aim should be to prevent suffering?' I have never varied in my reply which is that I believe that animals were put on this planet to be of benefit to man. They are there to be used by us, but with this right comes the responsibility to ensure their welfare. We were not experimenting on animals for vicarious ends, but to help control a major epidemic disease which in its time had killed millions of cattle. If we could eradicate CBPP from Africa as we had done from most of Europe and as the Australians had done, then many bovine lives would be saved from disease and death. Our experimental animals were no different from the animals that were slaughtered on farms infected with foot and mouth. They died to prevent the deaths of others. I felt no conflict of interest as I was working in what I considered to be the best interests of animals. All the animals on the farm were well looked after, and received food and water on a regular basis which is more than can be said for many animals in Africa with its regular droughts. I also believe that animals do not have *rights*: rights involve a concomitant responsibility.

On the appointed date, the donor animals that were to be infected were taken to the experimental pen: we had two, the main one was a single building large enough to hold fifty animals in comfort. The house was down on the boundary of the estate just inside the fence outside which was the indigenous forest. The house was in a cleared area with a security fence round it that was kept securely locked. The house was bright and airy with a small crush along one side for sampling and an office in one corner in which we kept the equipment for sampling together with all the temperature charts: each animal had its own chart which was made up daily.

We set about anaesthetising the animals using chloral hydrate injected into a vein. The main reason for using this old drug was that it had a very short effective time and the animals were back on their feet within a few minutes. Once the animal went down on to the well-bedded floor it was put on its right side, a gag was inserted in the mouth and a tube of plastic with a bore of about one centimetre was passed over the epiglottis and into the trachea (the windpipe). This was the tricky bit because the tube had a knack of going into the oesophagus (the tube leading to the stomach) instead of the trachea: holding a small piece of hay at the entrance confirmed that air was passing up and down the tube. The tube was slid gently down into the lungs until it would go no further; a fine plastic tube with a bore of two millimetres was then passed down the larger tube until it too could go no further. Then the infecting broth (15 millilitres) was injected down the fine tube: we used the Australian Gladysdale strain which had the reputation of being the most severe strain ever seen and this was washed down with 100 ml of culture media. The tubes were withdrawn and the animal was put up onto its brisket, and watched carefully until it was back on its feet. From the time the animal went down until it was up on its brisket was rarely more than five minutes and within fifteen minutes the animal was back on its feet. And so on to the next one. We had an excellent team of animal handlers from the foreman, the military Gichuru, with his carefully trimmed moustache, to Kamau who was the usual butt of the jokes; they were a hard-working, efficient, well-trained team.

As soon as all the animals had recovered from the anaesthetic, the vaccinated and control animals were put in the building. There was no fighting because the animals had all been run together for at least six months. All the animals were bled and their temperatures taken, and the in-contact trial was underway. John and his team took the temperatures of the animals every day and reported anything amiss, but it was usually three to four weeks before the intubated animals started showing signs of disease and it was always six weeks before the control animals developed antibodies in their blood, indicating that they had become infected; never less but often more.

It was from these trials that we concluded that the incubation period was six weeks. Really sick animals were shot; if an animal died then a full post mortem examination was carried out. Six weeks after an animal first developed antibodies in its blood, it was killed and examined, All lesions in the lungs were measured and a large number of samples from the respiratory tract were put into broth to see if the organism was present. We noticed that animals that died from acute disease often had great purple blotches in their kidneys and we were able to show that the mycoplasm had escaped into the blood and then got stuck in the capillaries of the kidneys – this is known as an embolus and it produces the same effect as deep vein thrombosis which we are warned about now when flying. The blood supply to parts of the kidney are cut off and that part dies. We wondered whether or not the organism was passed in the urine and so we examined the urine: in some cases we found as many as ten million (10^7) organisms per ml of urine, and a cow can hold as much as a litre of urine in its bladder: that is a lot of organisms – ten thousand million of them – which will all be deposited in one place. It led us to think. A few of the animals were pregnant when they died and as the fluids in the uterus would make a good culture medium for *M. mycoides* we checked the fluid for the presence of the organism and found up to a thousand million per ml – the maximum that we were ever able to achieve in our cultures! It seemed to us not unreasonable that these massive sources of the mycoplasm might play some part in the epidemiology of the disease. We would have to investigate.

Six weeks after the last animal developed antibodies to the infection, the trial was terminated. The Director of Veterinary Services permitted us to send those vaccinated animals that had not developed antibodies to the abattoir so that we could recoup some of the costs. We went down to the Athi River and checked the animals in the slaughter house, and collected samples from the respiratory tract. Even where the results were completely clear cut we carried out a statistical analysis. We used the Australian system for quantifying the disease which made it possible to analyse the results; it also made it possible to compare the results from different laboratories round the world.

The results of the trials indicated that the vaccine provided total protection for a year but that by two years the immunity was waning. We had demonstrated that a vaccine dose of ten million organisms (10^7) was required to produce immunity and that the dose we supplied of 1000 million (10^9) organisms gave a good margin for error. What was really interesting in that trial was that the animals that received a vaccinating dose of a 100,000 (10^5) organisms were not protected at all and might even have been made more susceptible to the disease.

The heifer 'St Bees' was the animal responsible for taking CBPP to Australia, where it was first diagnosed in Melbourne in October 1858. She was taken in a mob of cattle that sailed from Cockermouth in Cumbria and the voyage took just over eighteen weeks. She was healthy when she was put on the ship and again when she was off loaded, but a few days later she developed signs of CBPP. It had been assumed that she was actually infected when she had been put on board and that she had been incubating the disease for the whole of the voyage. The evidence from our trials indicated that, in the vast majority of cases, the incubation period was six weeks. Another possibility is that she was a 'lunger', as an animal with a chronic lesion of CBPP is described, and that the stress of the journey caused the lung lesion to break down and become reactivated, and the animal to develop acute disease. Everyone believed this, because it was in all the books!

We now had the ability to test this theory, as we had a collection of animals that had been intubated and recovered from CBPP: some were bound to have a sequestrum. We carried out an in-contact trial with these animals and put them in contact with an equal number of healthy animals. All the animals were subjected to a series of stresses such as they would encounter in northern Kenya; lack of food and water coupled with walking long distances to try and find them. Our animal attendants did not like this work because they had to keep the animals walking round for four hours a day. We reduced the hay allowance and cut down their access to water. We were totally unable to produce any disease in our control animals. As replacement intubated animals became available we slaughtered the originals and found about a third of them had good-sized sequestra, and we were able to recover *M. mycoides* from the sequestra for up to twenty-seven months after infection. In a desperate attempt to break down a sequestrum, we treated some of the new additions with cortico-steroids but we were totally unable to induce a breakdown. It is impossible to prove that something never happens, but it was our conclusion that we had to look elsewhere for the source of new outbreaks.

Matt Dagg had left for Nigeria. His replacement was Fred Wangati, a delightful Kikuyu, and Maxine remained working for him until the birth of our first child, Richard. She received a welcome gratuity from the East African Community and we decided to spend the money on a matched pair of Kirman carpets: they were beautiful and when we saw them in the window of the Carpet Emporium we knew that we had to have them. The price was the equivalent of £1800 but we knew you could always bargain, and we did, for six months, and ended up paying ... £1800!

When the baby decided to arrive we were ready and off we went to the Nairobi Hospital for the delivery. Maxine had a torrid time and was in labour for hours. Richard was coming shoulders first but they thought that he would work his head into the birth canal: they did not know Richard! After two nights of pain and discomfort for Maxine they decided to call it a day and carry out a Caesarian section. Dr Mary Robertson Glasgow would stand no nonsense; Maxine was so tired and in such discomfort she was lying on her side to ease the pain.

'Mrs Windsor will you please lie on your back as I need to make some preparations?'

'I can't,' came the reply.

'Mrs Windsor, get on your back, remember you're British.'

Maxine rolled on to her back.

135

I was informed that Maxine was going into the theatre immediately and that she should be back in her room at 10 am. I went out of the hospital and sat on a rock on the side of the road, and wondered how Maxine was getting on, and whether the baby had survived the ordeal unscathed. I have to say that Richard's heart beat had been monitored on an hourly basis and I believe that it was when he showed signs of problems that they decided to operate. At ten I was back in the ward. Maxine was wheeled in looking a lot better than when she left, and we had a son, a healthy baby boy. Seeing that all was well I left to get some sleep. I called in at Kabete on the way home to tell Elma Sayer, the wife of a colleague Paul Sayer and the secretary to the veterinary faculty, the good news. She took one look at me and said, 'Bed,' and I was taken to the guestroom. I slept solidly for six hours, showered and went home. The next morning I sent a telegram to the families:

'Another bloody Caesar. A baby boy 8 lb, mother and baby well.' Maxine's sister had produced a baby by Caesarian section about three months earlier and at the time Richard had no name.

Maxine's recovery proceeded apace and soon she was back in the house in Muguga and Richard was ensconced in his cot in the new nursery. Her parents were coming to visit us and we arranged the christening in our own little church; Raymond Smith came from Limuru to take the ceremony. We had a great party after the do at which much champagne was drunk. Maxine was feeding Richard at four hourly intervals and when it was time for the six o'clock feed Richard could not be wakened. Maxine's father was a doctor and so was summoned; the explanation was simple, Richard was drunk! The alcohol in the champagne that Maxine had consumed had passed into her milk and into the baby. Was this to be the pattern of his future?

An ayah, Rosemary, was recruited to look after Richard, and Maxine returned to work. Her post at EAAFRO had been filled, but the Texan veterinary scientist Gale Wagner was looking for a secretary and after she had obtained the necessary clearances from the American Embassy, Maxine was employed as a scientific secretary. Gale had been seconded from the United States Department of Agriculture, Plum Island Animal Disease Center, to join work on the East Coast fever project which had been set up by FAO, with the aim of making a vaccine against this disease. Although nominally working for Gale, Maxine was involved with all project members and enjoyed the variety of work.

Life at Muguga was fun. There were many sporting activities and competitions, and when there were no leagues playing on a Saturday afternoon, Maxine and I and Gale and Beverley Wagner had a friendly four, which often ended with dinner at our home or at the Wagners'. There were trips to the theatre to see the professional Donovan Maule Company, or the amateur City Players or Theatre Group, and I made my African directing debut with 'The Prime of Miss Jean Brodie' which was a wonderful success. There was much theatre and I was asked to play the Jimmy Edwards part in 'Big Bad Mouse' although I never managed to get the pocket watch into the pocket with the style of the master. There were trips to game parks with family and friends, and trips to the coast to swim and snorkel, and a wonderful safari to Lamu where we slept on beds on the roof and were wakened each morning by the mullah on the roof across the road calling the faithful to prayer. Lamu is an island off the north-east of Kenya; you drive to a small port where your car is guarded for a small fee while you are on the island. You take a dhow across to the island. I had noticed on the way up that the car seemed to be going more and more slowly. I thought little about it. When we began the return trip the car would hardly go at all. It was decided that I had to be towed the 150 miles to Malindi. Maxine and Richard joined the Wagners and I 'drove' the Renault on the end of a twelve-foot towrope on a dirt road. I was shattered at the end and I think that Gale had found the ordeal of towing almost as stressful. We then had to find a mechanic at 4 pm on a Saturday afternoon. We finally tracked one down to his home and found him playing volleyball on the green outside his house. We told him the story and without more ado he stretched himself on the ground under the car and started making violent agitating movements with his hands. After about thirty seconds he got up, brushed himself down and said, 'You will find it is all right now. It is a common problem with front wheel drive cars that sand works its way into the gear box causing the drive to slip. You will have no more problems.'

And we didn't. He would take no money for his trouble and so we thanked him profusely and left. We were again thankful to that spirit in Africa where you always help the traveller who has a problem.

Back in the laboratory we turned our attention to urine and uterine fluids. Another unproved dictum with CBPP is that the disease is only transmitted by 'nose to nose' contact. We had watched animals at water holes in northern Kenya and there was almost no mixing of animals from different herds. The herdsman took the animals down to the water in the order that they arrived and the first herd left before the next one entered; a ritual developed over the centuries. However, we did see a calf born while we were watching, and a tussock of grass was liberally covered with uterine fluids and a large healthy-looking placenta. What if those fluids and tissue were rich in mycoplasms?

A group of four control animals were housed together and fed hay over which had been poured urine laced with 1000 million mycoplasms, and this was repeated for three days. After six weeks, three of the animals developed antibodies in their sera but none of them ever showed a rise in temperature. Six weeks after the development of antibodies all four animals were killed and examined. Three of the four had a small sequestrum in one lung from which we were able to isolate *M. mycoides*! In our work the incubation period was almost invariably six weeks. We had been unable to breakdown sequestra, but we had shown that indirect transmission could take place.

Walter Plowright was head of the Virology Section at the time and he had a bevy of young vets including Bill Taylor working for him on the relationship between rinderpest and wildlife. However, he always had time to help us with the planning of the work and give us his thoughts on the priorities. There is little point in undertaking research work if the results of that work are not published. Here again Walter was invaluable to me. I remember the first manuscript that I gave to him for his approval: I handed it to him with great pride. It returned with more red ink than the original print. Walter sat me down and took me through it point by point until there was an article ready for publication. He always chided me that I did not get to the laboratory until the official starting time of 8 am.

'You can get so much more done between seven and eight, when there are no distractions.'

But then, he was a morning person and was always away from the laboratory at 4.30 in the afternoon to get to the tennis court. He could not understand people like me who prefer to stay on at the end of the day for the same peace and quiet.

Much of the epidemiology work was done after the return of Walter Masiga from the London School of Hygiene and Tropical Medicine where he had just completed his studies for the Diploma of Bacteriology. The Dip Bact, as it was affectionately known throughout the tropical world, was considered to be the highest taught medical qualification that you could get. Walter was a large, bluff Abaluhya, with connections. His wife Elizabeth was teaching at the Aga Khan High School but ended her career as the Minister of Education. Walter had been sent to London by the project and was also destined for stardom. His first step was to take over the CBPP section when Gareth returned to the CVL. It was not long before he became Director of EAVRO as a stepping-stone to the post of Director of the Inter African Bureau of Animal Health (IBAH), which later broadened its scope to Animal Resources. This was the conduit through which much of the aid to the livestock sector in Africa was channelled.

I have never been known for my diplomacy and I have always believed in treating all people as equal. Walter was the first African to realise that my having a full blown row with him was an indication of my respect for him: I was treating him as an equal. We became firm friends and remained so throughout our professional lives. Later, when I was undertaking a field trial in northern Nigeria, of a test that he and I had developed at EAVRO, I was sitting on my veranda reading one Saturday afternoon when I saw a motorcycle approaching with Walter riding pillion, his suitcase perched precariously in front of him. He had managed to raise the money to come and join me, and had hitched a lift for the fifteen miles from Jos. So he moved into the house and I had someone to help with the work.

Halfway through our time in Muguga we went on leave and I was invited to undertake my first two consultancies: on the way home we went to Cairo and on the return to Addis Ababa. The Egyptian government had been keen to improve the genetic make-up of its beef cattle and to this end had imported cattle from the Sudan – and with them they had imported CBPP. Luckily all the cattle were on a feed lot in Alexandria. I was invited by Dr Al Haji Sabri, the leading worker on mycoplasms in Egypt and one of the founders of the International Mycoplasma Society, who later came to Muguga to see our work. I was taken to the feed lot and we examined the situation: the Egyptian government were keen to slaughter all the animals on the feed lot. However, Dr Sabri and I persuaded them that since the animals were in a confined group there was no need to take such drastic action. Vaccine was ordered from Muguga and it was decided to seal the place until there were no more clinical cases. None of the animals that were on the feed lot at the time of the outbreak were to be allowed to leave the premises alive and only animals born after the outbreak ceased would be allowed to go to new farms. This technique worked well, the disease never spread outside the feed lot.

The trip to Addis Ababa on our way back to Muguga was much more eventful. The Veterinary Research Laboratory was based at Debre Zeit about thirty miles from the capital and the site of the Emperor's Summer Palace. The Director of the Institute was Dr Woldegiordis and the man in charge of CBPP work was Dr Fikre with whom I became firm friends. The laboratory was the main veterinary vaccine production unit in the country, making a wide assortment of animal vaccines. In this they were being assisted by a team of French veterinarians from Maison Alford (the Parisian Veterinary School, and the then seat of the Institut d'élévage et de médécin veterinaire des pays tropicaux. The team leader was Dr Philippe Blanc, who had many years of experience in Africa. There was no adequate hotel in Debre Zeit, and so we stayed in the Ras Hotel in Addis and travelled daily in the car of the Assistant Minister of Agriculture, with the minister's personal driver. Personal maniac more like: I am surprised we were not killed. This was the Assistant Minister's car which meant it was more important than any other car on the road save those of full ministers or the Emperor; the driver drove as if he owned the road and overtook whether it was safe or not! On one occasion he pulled out to overtake, despite there being a Mercedes coming straight towards him. When I remonstrated, after the Mercedes had swerved off the road, he merely shrugged and pointed out, as if that was all that mattered, 'I flashed my lights at him'.

After the first day Maxine and Richard came with me because there was a large expatriate community, mostly working with the veterinary laboratory or the Animal Health Training School, and although we did not know any of the staff many of the people there were friends of friends. Stuart Watson in particular was a close friend of Andrew Bygrave as they had been at the Liverpool School together. Stuart's wife Patricia was on the verge of a nervous breakdown: expatriates were advised not to drive in Ethiopia because they were considered fair game by the locals. Pat had ignored this advice and on driving home one day, a small child had deliberately run at her car and hitting the side, receiving a broken arm and leg in the process. Pat was carted off to the police station and only released after money had changed hands. She had to pay for the treatment of the child and then came the court case where again she had to pay compensation to the family. However, that was not the end of the matter because court cases are never completely closed in Ethiopia, and while we were having lunch the police arrived again, to say that the family had decided that the compensation was inadequate and they wanted more. Pat had had enough and soon after left the country, and Stuart followed not long after that.

That evening driving back we had an interesting experience: when the Emperor is on the road everyone else stops, and not only stops, but the passengers have to get out of the car and stand by its side. One would have thought this would have made things even easier for an assassin. We stopped and as instructed got out of the car. The Emperor's car drew to a halt and out he got and came over to us: he wanted to know what we were doing in his country and was pleased with my answers. Sadly we had used up the last of our film in Debre Zeit as I am sure that he would have been delighted to pose with us!

Dr Fikre had heard of our work with the vaccine trials and was most interested in the dosage trial, particularly as we had found that when a culture of *M. mycoides* was freeze dried, ninety-nine percent of the organisms die: and so a vaccine which starts life with a dose of a thousand million organisms ends up with a dose of ten million organisms – still a good number but on the margins of what we found to be the minimum dose. We discussed this with Dr Blanc and his colleagues, who informed me that they were unable to quantify the organisms in their cultures. He asked if we would be prepared to undertake the enumeration and I was delighted to oblige. On our return I was armed with several ampoules of freeze-dried CBPP vaccine from several different batches. We carried out the work as soon as I returned and showed the numbers of the organisms to be on the borderline – between one and ten million with some batches right down at the danger level. I sent a purely factual report –and the shit hit the fan. What was I doing impugning the work of the French – Dr Blanc was not a happy man! Dr Woldegiordis put a stop on using the freeze-dried vaccine which I guessed made Blanc unhappy. To this day the problem has not been resolved. There are still doubts about the efficacy of the freeze-dried vaccine.

We still lacked a really coherent story to explain why the heifer St Bees became sick more than eighteen weeks after she left Britain We did not really understand why the disease was mostly confined to the lungs, and we had no idea what caused the body to react so violently against the mycoplasm. What separates research from investigation is that for a research project you put up a proposition and try and knock it down: 'If I vaccinate these cattle and challenge them six months later all the animals will be immune and will not get the disease.'

When mycoplasms grow in broth culture they produce the compound galactan which remains attached to the cell like a sticky cloak. Galactan is made by the mycoplasm from the sugar galactose which is very similar to glucose: the mycoplasm possesses an enzyme which joins molecules of the galactose in long chains and this polygalactose compound has many of the properties of another similar compound found in nature – starch. We suspected that the galactan protects the organism from the body's defence mechanisms in the same way as the waxy coat on the TB organism. The difference between the two is that galactan is closely related to a material – pneumogalactan – which makes up much of the cell walls of the lung. Does *M. mycoides* trigger off an auto-immune disease? This would account for the very severe lesions seen in the acute disease. The body produces cells and antibodies against the galactan of the mycoplasm which then turn on the body itself and start destroying the cells of the lung. This could account for the severe reaction to the infection, and to the body trying to halt the damage by walling off the affected part of the lung.

The serology and biochemistry teams were looking at this problem aided by Dai Roberts, who had been sent out from Weybridge to replace Gareth, and two able young Ugandan veterinary surgeons, Ibrahim Kakoma and Fred Rurangirwa: both were sent to the States for further training and both remained employed by their American universities, although Fred spent several months each year back in Africa. There was much convincing evidence that the body's response to CBPP was the result of an auto-immune reaction. Unfortunately we did not have the genetic tools available to research workers today and no conclusive proof was obtained.

Why do some animals get big lesions and others only small ones? Every time we answered one question it threw up a whole host of new ones. Why did the animals infected by the ingestion of infected hay all have very small lesions? The idea occurred to us that it might require multiple exposure to infection to produce big lesions and disease that can be seen. Many animals in which we saw lesions in the post mortem room had shown no signs of disease other than the presence of antibodies in their sera.

Walter and I decided to repeat the experiment with the infected hay, but we fed it more times and we put uninfected animals in contact with the infected ones to see if such artificially infected animals would be able to transmit the disease. They did. And what was most interesting was that the lesions in the naturally infected animals were larger than those that had been infected by the contaminated hay. The idea began to take shape which would explain the St Bees mystery. There were likely to have been thirty or more animals being transported. If one of them had been incubating the disease at the time, then somewhere during the voyage it would have been puffing out the organisms in its breath, although it might not have been seen to be sick. Let us say four weeks out on the journey this animal is spreading the organism and infects six animals within a couple of weeks. By week twelve there are six animals putting out the mycoplasms and these in their turn infect six animals each; the chances are that some animals are infected by more than one animal as there is much more infection about. And so nineteen or twenty weeks out from England and there is enough infection to produce clinical disease in St Bees.

If this picture is projected on to Africa you can envisage two herds having a chance meeting at a waterhole and just one animal becomes infected as a result. They go their separate ways. The animal with the acquired infection develops the disease but it is not detectable and so it infects six animals, and in six weeks or so they become infective and each infects six more, and then six weeks later there is a sudden explosion of clinical disease. By then the animals could have moved several hundred miles: Who is going to associate two outbreaks of disease four months and several hundred miles apart? It is a different story with rinderpest and foot and mouth disease, and it is not difficult to understand why the history of CBPP is bedevilled with myths. It was going to take more than a good vaccine to eradicate CBPP from Africa.

The serological tests that we had were excellent for monitoring the progress of disease within a herd but they were not really adequate for use in the absence of clinical disease. If you knew an animal had been infected then you could follow its progress through to death or recovery. But in a herd of unknown status a negative result could mean that the animal had never had any contact with CBPP, or it had been vaccinated and the antibodies had dropped to an unmeasurable level, or that the animal had had the disease and recovered and it might still be harbouring an infected sequestrum. A positive result on the other hand might, in the absence of clinical disease, indicate that the animal had been vaccinated or it might have sub-clinical, undetectable disease.

Earlier workers had tried to detect cellular immunity by means of injecting antigens of *M. mycoides* actually into the skin; not under the skin but into it. If the animal is infected then cells (especially the white blood cells) and antibodies invade the site, producing a swelling, and this is the basis for the Mantoux test for human TB and the Tuberculin Test in cattle. Earlier workers had tried to produce such a test for CBPP but there were too many false positive results to make the test worthwhile. Walter and I decided to have another look at the intra-dermal allergic test to see whether we could improve its accuracy. It seemed to us that it was the galactan, because of its presence in normal bovine lung cells, that was causing the non-specific reactions. We set about removing it from the cells. We grew large quantities of the cells in our broth, and by repeated centrifuging tried to wash away the galactan. That did not work. The next attempt was to repeat the washing and then break up the mycoplasmal cells using high-intensity sound and washing, and repeat the centrifuging in an attempt to produce pure cell walls. Even that failed to remove all the galactan. It was later shown that galactan, as well as being a slimy coat on the outside of the cell, was an integral part of the cell wall. We gave up!

The next idea was to carry out a comparative test using our cell wall extract and compare the results to an injection of a similar dose of pure galactan. Pure galactan was easy to produce as it could be washed off the cell walls.

We selected our animals to test: first we used animals that had been artificially infected and which had recovered. We clipped the hair from two sites on the neck of the animal, measured with calipers the thickness of the skin and with a very fine needle injected 0.1 ml of our cell wall antigen into the skin on the upper site – the same quantity of pure galactan was injected into the lower site. The thickness of the skin was measured daily for three days (the TB test is read after seventy-two hours) and the presence of oedema fluid at the site was noted.

The animals were then killed and a detailed post mortem examination was carried out. Those animals that had shown an increase in thickness in the skin injected with cell wall antigen that was greater than that of the galactan all had lesions of CBPP, whereas those with no reactions showed no lesions. We had a test. The next step was to see whether it worked on a large scale and what happened to vaccinated animals and those that had never experienced any disease or vaccine. The test was subjected to large scale trials in the laboratory and our excitement grew as the results came in. There was no doubt that under laboratory conditions the test worked.

We had produced a test which we thought might just work in the field and so we asked the DVS for permission to carry out a field trial in Kenya. Amin was at the height of his powers in Uganda and the country was in turmoil, and Tanzania only had the disease in Masailand on the border with Kenya. Muriithi refused.

It was soon after that I received my recall to Britain. Once established in Cambridge, I got to work to set up a field trial with the test, and thanks to Mark Philpott, a Cambridge vet who had been at Kabete during our time there and who was now working in Vom, northern Nigeria, I received an invitation to carry out the trial in Nigeria. ODA agreed to underwrite the costs of the trial and I started to put together a list of equipment for the work: we would have to prepare all our antigens in Nigeria.

In January 1976 I was off to Vom with my heavy load of equipment. It was while sitting on the veranda there one Saturday afternoon that I saw the cheery face of Walter on the back of that motorcycle. We worked in very exacting conditions in the bush of Nigeria, but the work was well worthwhile, as the test worked admirably under the harsh conditions of Nigeria. We now had to sell the test to the field workers in Africa.

I received my instructions to report to Cambridge. I wrote and explained that I was in the middle of some exciting work and I would need time to wind it down. I was given an extra six months. The project JP16 had played an invaluable role in the control of CBPP. It had answered many different questions concerning the disease. We knew the vaccine worked and provided excellent protection for at least one year; we had established the length of the incubation period and had started unravelling the pathogenesis and epidemiology of the disease.

The success of the project can be measured by the number of distinguished workers who came to see what was happening and to become involved with the work. They included Mohamed Ali Sabri from Egypt, who happened to be in the laboratory when Shmuel

Razin arrived from Jerusalem; it was most opportune as they always wanted to meet but Middle East politics prevented them from speaking, even when both were present in an International Meeting. Here in Muguga there were no prying eyes to report back to governments! Dr David Taylor-Robinson, the renowned worker from the Centre for Communicable Diseases, Colindale, England, spent a very useful week with us. Alain Provost the expert on rinderpest and CBPP from Fort Lamy, brought a bunch of his young colleagues to see how it should be done. Provost and Plowright were the two most distinguished veterinary scientists working in Africa. Not only was Provost a brilliant scientist and a member of the Légion d'honneur, but he was also a Maître de fromage – that distinguished body of men who meet in Paris to taste and discuss cheese and wine. (Alain offered to take me to such a meeting but I was never in Paris at the right time and now he is dead: God rest his soul, a great scientist and a lovely man.) When I was in Nigeria he drove from Cameroon in a Citroen 2CV to see our field trial in northern Nigeria and we had a wonderful few days together before he and his colleagues drove back. Luckily they had brought wine with them because it was almost unobtainable in northern Nigeria in those days.

And then there was Dr Santini, the Italian playboy but first-class scientist, who was the Italian Mr CBPP, with a base just outside Rome but a roving commission from FAO to sort out CBPP wherever it occurred in Africa. He was responsible for eradicating the disease in Italy after it had been imported from Spain, the last remaining focus in Europe. He was to turn up regularly throughout my later life and it was never dull working with him. Muguga was a very special place in those days with its successes in the control and eradication of rinderpest; with the production of a vaccine against East Coast fever; and the major studies on CBPP. Subsequently anyone who had worked at EAVRO in those halcyon days was referred to as a member of the 'Muguga Mafia'.

But it was time for us to pack up home and leave Africa for ever, and to start a new life in Cambridge. I had completed my apprenticeship as a detective and could now consider myself as a full-blown journeyman, working and training to become a master. We did not make a direct journey back to Cambridge but visited Israel, and Cyprus, Beirut in the Lebanon and Istanbul in Turkey before arriving at Heathrow. Hostilities had again broken out in the Middle East and there had been a terrorist attack on the Israeli Embassy in

Nairobi the week before we were due to fly to Tel Aviv. I visited the embassy to check that we did not require visas, to find an armoured car at the entrance and sandbags in front of the door. When we boarded the El Al plane to Tel Aviv it felt strange to be completely surrounded by soldiers in full military gear and holding automatic weapons at the ready.

We had a great holiday although Maxine's pregnancy inhibited her from really enjoying the sight-seeing and the travel. We arrived home to a new job, a new house and a new life.

PART 3
Journeyman, 1973–1981

8

The Milk of Human Kindness

'As a rule,' said Holmes, 'the more bizarre a thing is the less
mysterious it proves to be.'
Sir Arthur Conan Doyle, *The Red-Headed League*

From the first day it was obvious that I was going to enjoy the
Cambridge Veterinary Investigation Centre. Sherwin was a great
boss, provided you could stand on your own feet. He expected his
staff to be responsible for their own work, to make their own decisions and, while we worked as a team, we had to seek our own
niche. There was no doubt that the major livestock industry in our
area was pig production but there was enough dairy work to keep
Jock, the infertility man, in business. Where there is infertility there
is mastitis and so I set myself up to learn how to control and even
more to prevent mastitis outbreaks.

I do not know why God gave cows udders divided into four when
they normally produce only one calf, and sheep udders divided into
only two when they normally produce two lambs and sometimes
more. Most species have the udder in the posterior abdomen, save
for man, the great apes and elephants who have them on the chest:
this is understandable because as the great apes got up onto their
hind legs, the mammary gland would have been out of reach of the
baby, and it would have been most inconvenient to have to hold the
baby at groin level: far easier to cradle the infant in the arms while it
is sucking at the breast or teat. But then why do elephants have their
udders on the chest?

An udder is that organ in the body that produces milk for the
young: the four glands of the cow are separate and are called
quarters and deliver the milk through the teat. Although the sheep
only has two glands they are still called quarters! But it becomes even
more complicated when you think of the camelids, the alpacas and
llamas of the Andes: these animals have four quarters like a cow each

151

delivering through a teat, but each quarter has two glands making a total of eight – and they never produce more than one calf.

Mastitis, or inflammation of the udder (mainly the bovine udder), has held a fascination for me from the time, as a student, that I read Hutt's book *Genetic Resistance to Disease in Domestic Animals*. In this slim volume he opened my eyes to the fact that disease is not a simple concept of 'animal plus pathogen equals disease', but that other factors such as feeding, management, overall health and not least genetics play their part in allowing a pathogen to enter and a disease become manifest. And so, each time there is a change in the management of animals then a new set of variables comes into play: this is what makes veterinary detection such an interesting occupation; farming systems are always changing.

As you know, soon after leaving college I went off to Kenya buzzing with the zeal of a prophet: I was going to bring all that was new and good to my fellow man in Africa and among those things was a milking machine. I was brought down to earth with a bump by an old English vet who said to me, 'Roger, in this part of the world hand milking is much better than machine milking, because it does not matter how thick the milker, how lazy or uneducated; he knows that when the milk stops coming out, he stops milking. Machines don't know that and they go on tugging away at the udder and causing untold damage.'

Milking machines have become much more sophisticated today with built-in sensors to detect the flow of milk so that they remove themselves when milking is complete. But that old vet was right, because there is no doubt that the machine has played its part as the major cause of mastitis down the years, although modern technology is solving the problems of man's idleness or inefficiency.

Cambridge is not the centre of a big dairy industry: the land is too valuable for growing the more profitable crops of wheat, barley, sugar beet, field beans or oilseed rape. And surprisingly the climate is too dry for the best growth of grass. However, the vet school had a pedigree herd of Ayrshire cows and in Essex there were numerous big herds run by farming companies: these were a hang-over from pre-refrigeration days when all London's milk was brought in by train from farms all round the city.

Before getting stuck into the work we had to set about finding a house to live in, and move in as quickly as possible because Maxine was growing larger by the day with our second child, and the sooner she was settled in a house the easier it would be for her. There had been a steep rise in house prices and the deposit we had saved (£3000) suddenly seemed very small. We saw a house that looked just right, at a price we could afford, in Willingham, a village to the north-west of Cambridge: being just outside the maximum distance for university and college staff, prices were that much lower. We phoned, but sadly an offer had been made for the house; I gave the owner my phone number and asked her to be sure to contact me if the sale fell through. We continued looking – nothing at a price we could afford really attracted us, but one Friday afternoon I bought the local paper and there was a photo of the house in Willingham. I phoned straight away and said I would be out that evening with my wife. Joan Hind apologised for having forgotten my earlier phone call with the request.

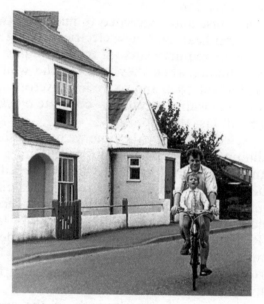

Outside our house, The Old Dairy in Willingham;
Richard is on the crossbar seat.

We just loved this odd little house; two old Cambridgeshire worker's cottages knocked together and a staircase put in: previously each had had a trapdoor and a ladder from the room below. The house was built from bricks of uncooked Cambridgeshire clay and I was able to tell friends that in Africa we lived in a brick house but in

153

Cambridge we lived in a mud hut. Down the side of the cottages ran a building 100 feet long by 12 feet wide, which had been the old dairy (which became the name of the house) where they had pasteurised and bottled milk, and made butter and cheese, and at the end was the stable for the horse that pulled the cart.

John Hind had been born in the cottage and as the milk delivery business increased so they stopped pasteurising milk and making butter and cheese. John had married and he moved into the dairy part of the house while his mother lived in the old cottages. As his family increased the dairy building had been converted piecemeal into living accommodation. John had been kept on short commons by his mother who owned the business, but on her death they had built their dream house in the garden, a large, square, double-fronted box. Having lived in the house all his life he could not see the possibilities for conversion.

We bought the house and proceeded to make the two houses into one, to put in central heating, a new electrical wiring system and as part of the mortgage requirements an injected damp proof course. That was a pantomime: when they injected the wall of the sitting room, the whole lot collapsed and so we had 'Acroprops' holding up the first floor until the wall was rebuilt – concrete blocks laid on their side, that house will last till doomsday!

It really was perfect for us; by the time we had finished we had five bedrooms, a dining room, sitting room, study and a playroom for the children, and a wonderful kitchen which was really a lean-to on the back of the cottages, and two bathrooms. Maxine was able to start sorting out the house before the arrival of our second child. She knew she would not have to undergo the turmoils of labour that she endured with Richard because her obstetrician had decided that she was to have an elective Caesarian section. Once I knew that the house was sorted and Maxine installed in our new home, I could concentrate on my work.

Mastitis problems were fairly common in the area and so the laboratory received a steady stream (if that is the right word) of samples. Although Jock was the infertility man he turned up his nose at investigating mastitis cases and because of my interest it fell to me. Liz was the duty technician for the day and so was assisting Joan in the office, 'booking in' or registering the samples that had arrived in the post. She knocked on my door and entered, carrying a small bottle of what looked like blackcurrant purée. She held it up and said, 'What is this? It says on the submission form that it is a milk sample.'

'And that is exactly what it is,' I replied. 'And I suspect that the cow is now dead: I'll wager ten to one that we will isolate *Pseudomonas pyocyanea.*'

And that was what we isolated. *Pseudomonas pyocyanea* is a water-borne organism that rarely causes disease, but when it does, the animal has little chance of survival. The organism is resistant to most antibiotics, and causes such intense damage that even if we found a drug that did work, the animal still died from the damage caused by the toxins. *Pseudomonas* mastitis indicated serious management defects and not just a single problem: things were going badly wrong; a visit was required to put this one right. I phoned Peter Jackson who ran a very smart pig practice deep in the fens. Peter had been at college with me although several years ahead; he was to become an academic, specialising in training students in pig diseases first in Edinburgh and then back in Cambridge where he was considered a leading expert on porcine reproduction (where he now has a building named after him). Cows were not a major interest of Peter's and they had precious few dairy herds in their practice. I phoned and sure enough the cow was dead, the fourth to die.

'Do you want her for a post mortem examination?' he asked.

'It's not necessary,' I replied. 'I think I know how to solve this one for you but we need to move quickly.'

'Can you get up here this afternoon?'

'I like to get to the farm two hours before milking, if I can, as that gives me a chance to get down all the details and have a look round before they start the milking.'

'Come to the house about one o'clock and Veronica will give us a bite to eat before we go off. Joe is a bit out in the sticks and he is a rum old cove who rarely uses us but he will listen to you.'

I had not seen Peter for a while; he was tall and thin with beaky features and a shock of straight black hair. Taciturn on first acquaintance, if he took to you he opened up and he was extremely knowledgeable. His wife Veronica was almost the exact opposite, small, blonde and bubbly. After an excellent if hurried lunch (vets and their wives were so hospitable) we set off for Water Meadows Farm and Joe Barnaby. He was not what I expected in a dairy farmer, as he must have been nearer eighty than seventy! Old, weather-beaten and gnarled, old Joe had been farming Water

Meadows Farm from before the Second World War. When investigating outbreaks of disease I do not usually use a proforma questionnaire, preferring to rely on one question to lead to the next: the exception to this rule is a mastitis investigation where there are so many variables that, if not prompted, I am liable to forget. Joe's was one of the few Jersey herds in Cambridge and the only dairy herd served by the practice. The new dairy herd had been purchased in Jersey in 1947 when Mr Barnaby had gone to the island to select heifers to form the foundation stock for his new herd. He was very proud of his cows which had won prizes everywhere and of the quality of his milk. 'Not like thaat Friesian roobish, why 'tis only fit for washing your hands in and if you take it straight from the cow then you get hot water.'

Despite his obvious addiction to Jersey milk and cream, there was not a spare ounce of flesh on him. He ran his herd of 45 cows with just a lad to do the heavy work of lifting the bales and shovelling the shit: this was not a modern farm; there was no big bale silage, and no yarding in winter on slatted floors for the effluent to be collected below. No, this was a byre farm, where the cows were tied up in winter and the dung and straw was barrowed daily to the midden. Joe was inconsolable about the loss of his four cows: they were part of his family and nothing like this had ever happened before. By the end of the questioning it was obvious where the problems lay.

'Can you tell me when the milking machine was installed?'

'That's no problem, lad: it was installed when I bought yon heifers in the spring of 1947.'

'And how often do you have it serviced?'

'What do you mean serviced? I top up the oil in the pump every week.'

Home in one! We now knew the source of the damage to the udder. Cows' udders are very delicate tissues and need to be carefully handled. Milking machines are just machines and they too need to be maintained very carefully to ensure that they are in perfect working order. If the suction is too high then the machine rips the insides out of the udder, causing all sorts of problems to the lining, and a damaged lining is a sure place for bacteria to enter. These observations were confirmed later in the visit when we examined the cows; most were suffering from 'extravasations of the sphincter'. The cow's teat, like the human anus, has a sphincter which seals it shut when it is not needed to be in use. This stops the milk from leaking out during the inter-milking period. The high pressure from the machine was pulling the sphincter out of the end of the teat, so impairing its function, and drops of milk could be seen on the tips of the teats.

Part one of the problem was identified and so now I turned my attention to the source of the *Pseudomonas pyocyanea*. I mentioned that this organism is a water-borne organism, and much water is used in a dairy. Mains water is never the source, because it is purified and chlorinated before it is put out to the public. The usual source of this particular infection was a badly maintained water heater.

'How do you heat the hot water for washing the udders and the machines?'

'We've two separate systems, there's an old gas boiler that heats the water for washing the machine between milkings and one of them new-fangled electric tanks that keeps the water at a nice steady hundred degrees fahrenheit, which is a nice comfortable temperature to wash the udders and it is supplied through the washing hoses in the parlour.'

'And provides a nice comfortable temperature in which *Pseudomonas pyocyanea* can multiply,' I thought, but said nothing. We went to look at this 'new-fangled water tank' which must have been at least ten years old; the enamel was peeling off and the rust was beginning to take a grip on the metal. There was dried faecal material on its surface and it looked as prime a suspect as a source of bacterial infection as I could imagine. I took samples of the water from the hose and we opened the heating tank and I sampled the water inside.

We watched the milking process. I took copious notes and timed how long the machines were on individual cows. I was really going through the motions of doing a complete investigation because I was sure that I had the answers as to the source of infection and what was allowing the bacteria to get in. All I had to do was to sell the solution to old Joe Barnaby. The milking came to an end and Joe left the lad to clear up the parlour and yard and wash the machine while we cleaned up, disinfected and adjourned to the house for a cup of tea, waited on by Vera Barnaby in her wrap-round apron and her head scarf under which were large rollers. She apologised but said that tonight was the meeting of the WI which she never missed; I sensed that this was her one outing a week. We were regaled with individual chocolate cupcakes and a jam sponge with our tea.

I decided that brashness would be the best policy rather than circle the problems.

'I think that I know where the problems lie.'

'Well thaat's a good start lad.'

'Your milking machine needs a thorough overhaul and I suspect that you will need to buy a new pump. With your permission I will ask Robin Mackintosh a dairy officer with the National Agricultural Advisory Service (also a division of the Ministry) to come and carry out static and vital tests of your machine.'

Robin, like Peter and myself, was Edinburgh trained and he was a brilliant machine technician, who was never happier than when he was fiddling with milking machines, so much so that he could almost make them talk. When I was asked by the Food and Agricultural Organisation to set up a dairy laboratory in north-west Argentina it was to Robin I turned to teach me how to use all his wonderful machines for checking milking equipment. I told Mr Barnaby that I would ask Robin to get in touch with him and arrange a visit and if possible I would come with him.

'The next thing is that you must never use your water heater again: it is a culture vessel for bacteria and no amount of washing will ever get it clean. Your new-fangled machine is out and you must get yourself a newer-fangled heater. Before you use that washing line it must be cleaned with a good disinfectant such as the quaternary ammonium compounds. Until you get a new water heater, I recommend that you stop washing the udders. It is summer, the udders are basically clean and so I suggest that you wipe each udder free from dust with an individual paper towel and if any cow is really dirty wash the udder properly with soap and a bucket of water before drying it with a paper-towel.' I finally drew breath.

Peter who had been taking copious notes during my discourse popped up with, 'And what about future clinical cases what do we do?'

'Watch 'em like a hawk: by not using the water tank we should have taken away the source of *Pseudomonas pyocyanea* and almost any other bug will be sensitive to the drugs you normally use for Gram Negative bacteria (in this case *E. coli* or *Klebsiella sp.*). Do take samples of milk before you treat the animal and send them to us. So if you are having problems with the treatment we can isolate and identify the organism and test it to find out which antibiotics it will respond to. A further recommendation that I would make is not to leave the clusters on the animal for any longer than four minutes. We must get the machine problem sorted out as quickly as possible, because until that is done it will continue to inflict damage on the sensitive tissues in the udder,' I added

'You could try hand milking in the meantime!'

'Get away wi' ye lad, I be far too old to start hand milking again.'

On that exchange of pleasantries we bade our farewells and I told Joe Barnaby that I would organise the visit of Robin Mackintosh as soon as possible. In Peter's car on the way home we discussed the case and he was profuse in his gratitude for the way we had got to the bottom of the problem so quickly. When I pointed out to him that he could have done it himself he demurred.

'The problem with vets in practice,' he said, 'is that there is always the next client to go to. Unlike you, who can devote a whole afternoon to one client, I have to rush in, make a quick diagnosis, and off to the next one.'

'But you have just spent the whole afternoon and more on one farm!'

'Ah, but you are here and so I can put this down as Continuing Professional Development!'

By not allowing themselves time to think and investigate, practitioners make life difficult for themselves, and our job necessary. They 'never have the time' but I have almost never investigated a disease problem on a farm without the presence of the practising vet. I think that they become accustomed to treating the individual animal and are frightened of herd problems when they think that large numbers of animals may die, with the consequent opprobrium of the farmer and the possible loss of the client. It is a form of protection against the worst, this casting off of the responsibility for the case. With the increasing economic problems and pressures, more and more practitioners will have to become their own veterinary detectives. Indeed, one can see the trend in cattle practice with practitioners doing more and more routine visits for pregnancy diagnosis and looking after the herd health rather than the expensive health of a single cow. The advantage that we have is that behind us are the services of highly trained and skilled laboratory staff providing and doing the various jobs that form the links that make the chain that is veterinary detection.

To return to Robin Mackintosh, he was a big man with a strong east of Scotland accent, but he did not look like a lowland Scot, being tall with a mop of black curly hair: with an ear ring he could have been mistaken for a pirate, but there was something of the Italian or Gypsy about him. He had been born in Scotland and educated in Scotland, this was his first time out of Scotland and he was loving it. He loved his work and his blessed milking machines. He was a great Walter Mitty character who saw himself in the role of liberator of cows from mastitis, by the laying on of his hands on the machine. And he certainly knew his machines; whenever possible I tried to go to a farm with him because he had a great deal to teach me.

I wanted Robin to teach me how to use his testing equipment because most places do not have a Robin, and what a good teacher he was. He realised, at once, that there was no way that Joe Barnaby, at his age, was going to undertake the investment required for a complete renewal of his milking plant and that the best to be hoped for was to persuade him to replace the pump and a few smaller items. Thanks to Robin the machine was returned to a reasonable state and the new water heater looked great on the wall and tested sterile for the presence of bacteria. My case with the 'blackcurrant purée' was the last animal to die in that outbreak. I never saw Joe Barnaby again and by now he must be long dead. But Robin and I often worked together.

There were not only professional worries but personal ones too, with the imminent birth of our second child. Guy was born by Caesarian section in the Mill Road Maternity Hospital and mother and Guy were soon fit enough to return home. While Maxine had been in hospital, I had tiled and painted both bathrooms, with the help of dear John Hind, so that they were bright and cheery for her return. There was no ayah to help look after the babies and wash the nappies but Guy was an angelic baby and there were plenty of people in the village to assist us. Because the house prices were cheaper than in the city, Willingham was full of 'first time buyers', young people who had just got onto the property ladder. Doyenne of the young group was Polly Fawcitt, a real mover and shaker, who not only looked after her five children but ran a wonderful playgroup that was almost impossible to get into because the waiting list was so long; she and her husband Alan were both church wardens and ran a monthly charity lunch in their house at which we ate bread and cheese and met all the other new young people. Polly also organised the babysitting circle where you earned 'tickets' by sitting other children which enabled us to go out without the expense of a babysitter. With a new baby, Maxine was not happy to go out at first and so we amassed a great wad of tickets.

We made many long-term friends in Willingham and despite having left many years ago, we still go back on a regular basis to see them, although John Hind has passed on: he was a wonderful man who would do anything to help anyone and assisted us to settle in. He was known by all in the neighbourhood and trusted by all and as he was up at 3 am in the morning he was the eyes of the community. I can remember a tap on our ground floor bedroom window at four o'clock one morning, and there was John with a policeman. He wanted to know if all was well; he had been passing the house at 3.30 when he saw the front door close but had not seen who had been there. Dear John – it had been Maxine who, having fed Guy, remembered that she had not put the milk bottles out and decided to do it before returning to bed.

Claire was also born in the Mill Road Maternity Hospital a little over a year after Guy, which meant that Maxine had three children under the age of five to look after. On this occasion while Maxine was in hospital, I decided to decorate the dining room. John and I stripped off the sheets of paper down to the plaster before painting the walls white. Between us we got the ceiling paper up and painted, and most of the walls presented no problem. However the 'new wall', put in when the stairs had been installed a hundred or more years ago, gave us real problems. We put on the white paint and the pink colour showed through – we put on a further coat and the pink colour showed through. We then applied a couple of coats of oil-based paints, and the colour showed through. Whatever we did the colour showed through. More than twenty coats were applied before we gave up! We agreed that it added character to the room.

It was not long after we had sorted out the problems of cold-blooded type mycobacteria causing miliary lesions in the pig livers that I met another cold-blooded type, this time causing mastitis in cattle. This was almost the opposite in type – a rapidly-growing acid fast organism: my knowledge of the TB family was growing by leaps and bounds. We had a call from Flash Harry, who was a small animal vet (today they are called companion animal practitioners) on the outer London fringe between Hertfordshire and Middlesex. He was not a man who used our services very often. Over the weekend he had had a locum working who had visited a dairy farm which presented three identical cases of a very strange mastitis: the affected quarters were stiff as boards but not hot and inflamed as is normally seen in cows with the disease. Two had only one quarter affected but the third was affected in three quarters. The milk coming out was grey in colour, thin in consistency, with what appeared to be a sediment throughout. He wanted to send samples of the milk to us and I suggested that the sooner they arrived the sooner we could get cracking.

The samples arrived first post the next morning and Sherwin, John, Blackie, Peter and I had a look. They were certainly grey and they contained a sediment: we all referred to our respective memories but no concrete ideas emerged. Sherwin remembered reading about mycoplasms causing mastitis. I was on duty that day and it fell to me to decide what was to be done: Peter and I thought that in addition to the usual cultures we should centrifuge the milk and examine the deposit. This entails spinning the milk at high speeds (in excess of 6000 revolutions per minute) in a centrifuge which has armour plated walls in case the spindle breaks. When I was a student studying for my microbiology qualification in Edinburgh, this happened to an old-fashioned centrifuge where the massive head was not enclosed: the spindle broke, the whole head flew off, went straight through a brick wall and killed a technician working in the adjacent lab. Such is the power of centrifugal force. This force is used to deposit particulate matter suspended in a liquid, and a good example in medicine is the centrifuging of blood to separate the red and white cells from the plasma when they are preparing it for blood transfusions. We were using it to concentrate the bacteria in the milk so that we stood a better chance of finding them.

One of the problems with mycobacteria is that they have a thick waxy coat: this is why they are so difficult to treat with antibiotics. To be effective most drugs have to enter the bacterium to get at its works and put them out of action. The wax prevents the drug from getting in. It also prevents the dyes in the stains that we use from attaching to the cell and so the mycobacterium does not take up either of the different colours that we use to make a Gram's Stain; without the stain they cannot be seen under the microscope. The Ziehl-Nielsen stain overcomes this problem because the slide is heated until the staining solution almost boils, which softens the wax and the stain can get in and stick to the cell wall.

Peter was triumphant. 'Roger, come and look at this,' he called

162

out. The smear was hooching with acid fast bacteria stained red by the carbol-fuchsin dye. We knew that this was not the typical bovine TB mastitis because the clinical findings were wrong. With bovine TB infection, the quarter becomes shrivelled with knots or small areas of hard tissue.

Peter went into our library and came back some time later with an article about mastitis caused by the 'rapidly growing acid fast bacteria'. Normally the growth of mycobacteria is so slow that it can only be seen in culture after about three months but these little creatures could be seen after a week. 'Set 'em up Peter,' I said (he was never called Pete in the same way that few people ever called me Rog).

The organisms were isolated and the cultures sent to Weybridge for identification. Long before that I had visited the farm and we had sorted out the problem. I phoned Flash Harry and told him what we had found, and asked to visit the farm with him.

'You are welcome to go to the farm but you won't want me about, I'll just be in the way. A spare prick at a wedding, if you know what I mean. I'll phone Perkins and tell him you will contact him to arrange a visit and you can then tell me all about it.'

According to the Royal College of Veterinary Surgeons, all vets must be omni-competent and able to treat all species. In a fast-developing world with science moving forward at an ever increasing pace, such a view is becoming outdated. But I do not know what Flash Harry did when he had no locum to bail him out, or what he would do when it came to resolving this problem. I am unable to recall the name of the farm but I will never forget the name of the road it was in – Trotter's Bottom. (Such names always caused me to double up: near Cambridge is Steeple Bumstead with its Smellie Bottom. We had an American veterinary student working with us in the lab and he was from Big Tits, Georgia!)

For this visit I had a student with me called George who was a delightful character. Tall and languid, George was the grandson of the man who developed the gramophone and was very wealthy. He incurred the wrath of college authorities when he took off in spring term to go skiing for a week: I am not sure why he was never sent down. He had managed to pass the first major hurdle of the course, and had obtained his BA in natural sciences and had passed the first of his final three years of clinical studies. Sadly he never qualified and I feel that it was a loss to the profession, as George had great charm and a striking intellect that could get to the bottom of a problem in a flash. In an earlier age he would have qualified, and so we lost a man who might have made an outstanding contribution. George was full of himself that Monday morning as he had spent the weekend at Cowdray Park playing polo although not happy with his handicap of + 6. He was highly amused by the problem before us and even more amused when we heard the full history.

When we arranged a farm visit, if there was time we put up a notice on the vet school notice-board inviting the students to come along and saying how many we could take; it was rare when the places were not taken up. Mr Perkins, a man in his late forties, did not seem unduly perturbed by his problems and was surprised that we should be interested. His farm kept the encroaching London at bay; to the south of his land it was all buildings and he was slowly being encircled. He was not worried about the demise of his farm because he knew that when its turn came he would be able to buy a much larger farm once he had sold his land for development. However, he was sad because for generations Perkinses had farmed the land and developed the beautiful copses of trees that almost obscured the urban landscape.

I went through my proforma questionnaire and an interesting picture emerged. The three affected cows had all calved on the same weekend and all of them developed milk fever at more or less the same time. Milk fever is not a fever at all but a disease similar to eclampsia in women, in which the cow suffers from an acute deficiency of calcium. After the cow has calved and commenced its production of milk there is a huge demand for calcium, which pours out of the blood and into the milk: calcium is stored in the bones. If the body is unable to mobilise the stored calcium quickly enough, milk fever follows. The cow develops a weakness in its muscles and finally can stand no more and collapses, unable to get up. There is a simple remedy, the injection of calcium into the vein of the cow which usually produces a spontaneous recovery. In the old days the vet would have been called and the advantage of this was that the vet would often notice additional factors that might delay the recovery and give various other treatments with the calcium. However, today economics are the determining factor and so the farmer keeps a few bottles of calcium in his parlour cupboard and treats the animals himself. On this occasion none of the cows got to her feet and all stubbornly remained recumbent.

Mr Perkins senior, the former farmer, was staying with his son and recommended an old treatment for milk fever. In the days before the nature of the disease was understood, it was thought that stopping the flow of milk on a temporary basis would solve the problem and for some reason, on occasions, it did. The remedy, and the method of stopping the milk, was to take a bicycle pump and pump up each quarter in turn! When the cows failed to respond to a second injection of calcium and remained on the ground, this bicycle pump method was used. All three cows regained their feet, seemingly no worse for wear! It was about ten days later that Mr Perkins was checking the milk in the quarters before milking (a legal requirement more observed in the breach ...) when he noticed the strange colour and appearance of the milk. He did not put the machine onto the affected quarters but milked them by hand into a pail. Although the milk had a strange appearance he did not think that the yield from the quarter was markedly reduced. He had not considered that the bicycle pump was to blame.

The usual remedy for mastitis is to inject a syringe of a special preparation of antibiotic directly into the quarter and to repeat this for several days. If the cow herself is sick then she may be given injections of the same antibiotic into her muscle. Mr Perkins had treated the quarters affected with intra-mammary preparations but they seemed to make no difference. I said to Mr Perkins that unless he was going to use the bicycle pump method for milk fever again, then there was little risk of the infection spreading to other cows. The problem was how to eliminate the infection from the affected animals. I suggested that it was not worth his while to use more tubes of intra-mammary antibiotics but that he was committed to stripping out the affected quarters twice a day for several more weeks until the animal self-cured, by eliminating the infection herself.

In the car returning to Cambridge I told George about Flash Harry and his lack of interest in the farm.

'But he is happy enough to sell him calcium, antibiotics and other drugs and things,' George said. I had to agree that it made a mockery of the Royal College stipulation that drugs were only sold to farms where the animals were 'under the vet's care'. Flash was also in a quandary, his practice had been established long before he joined, when there were fields all round and it was a genuine mixed practice. With 'development' the farms had disappeared one by one, and it was no longer a viable proposition to keep up to date and purchase all the instruments and equipment needed for a large animal practice. Luckily Flash would not be required to do anything towards the eradication of the mastitis problem. I would send him a written report of the visit and indicate that I would like him to keep his eye on the farm for the next few weeks and let me know how it turned out.

George was off to Kenya for the summer, to pass the time on the estate of a distant relative who like many of the White Settlers had decided to remain in Kenya after independence. He would see a little of the rancher's life and work; he would probably shoot a little and fish for brown trout, imported from the Annan Water in Scotland and now well established in the Aberdare and Mount Kenya streams, and he would almost certainly go down to Nairobi to play polo in Jamhuri Park. He knew that I had lived in Kenya and was eager to hear of my experiences.

'They were very different from what yours will be,' I said. 'The landed gentry in Kenya are probably even more aloof than the average British landowner. You will have heard of the Lord Erroll murder just after the end of the Second World War, and read the book *White Mischief*. Things are different now but all the families involved still live in Kenya and they still keep themselves to their clique.'

'But what did you get up to?'

'On arrival at the laboratory we were allocated a delightful little bungalow set in about an acre of garden in a road known as Millionaires Row because at the end of the cul-de-sac was the director's house and before that the houses of the brass. I was recruited as a bacteriologist but that lab had not yet been built and so I was put into the Diagnosis Section, and although I did not realise it, it was to change the course of my life. Within a few weeks I found myself as Head of Diagnosis! I knew nothing of Africa and little of African diseases, but what a challenge for a young man. And so I got stuck in: I had some good expatriate and African technicians; all the other vets in the vet lab were keen for me to succeed and gave me their time when needed, and I have an aptitude for organisation and so we streamlined all activities and we made that laboratory a real live place.

'But it wasn't all work. There was the club for tennis and social life, Nairobi was only seven miles down the road with its cinemas, restaurants and nightclubs, and there was the whole of Africa to explore at weekends and holidays. The climate was wonderful and the country was full of young expatriates who had come out after the birth of Independence to replace the old colonials who could not live with the idea of African rule. We all had the desire to help. I was a Kennedy baby, stirred by the fiery oratory of the tragically slain President. Kenya was still in the first flush of its freedom and its politicians were still free from the corruption that later engulfed them. For this I blame the Cold War with both the Americans and the Russians vying with each other to win the sympathies of the emerging countries and their votes at the UN. Whenever one country made a bid the other upped it and so it went on. I believe that it was these two countries that started bribing politicians to win favours and so the virus trickled down to the officials and then finally to the clerks and the man in the street. We destroyed a golden opportunity to build a society that cared, and look at the mess it's in now. I went out to Africa to help my fellow man, it did not take me long to realise that my fellow man didn't want my help on my terms, but on his, and I could accept that.'

'You're quite an idealist, aren't you?'

That stopped me in my tracks, and I realised that I had been pontificating again.

'Sorry,' I said. 'Let's get back to mastitis.'

9

More Milk and a Little CBPP

'We will devote an hour to glancing a little more closely into the details.'
Sir Arthur Conan Doyle *The Beryl Coronet*

When an udder suffers damage of any kind, from a kick by a neighbour to the excessive sucking of a machine, it responds in the way of all tissues, by a process we call inflammation which is an extremely complicated set of actions, usually ending in the repair of the damaged tissue. An early sign of injury to an udder is an increase in the number of cells in the milk. The cells come from the lining of the glands that actually produce the milk and from the blood that increases in flow when injury is sustained. Counting these cells provides an interesting indicator of the health of the udder and so the science of milk cell counting was begun.

At first it was laborious and time-consuming: part of the problem is the fat in the milk which makes it difficult to stain the cells or even to see them in a counting chamber. To count the cells, the milk fat must be removed; even so it is a tedious business counting large numbers of cells, and it means sitting at the microscope for hours on end. It was not until the development of the electronic cell counter in the 1960s that this method became a useful tool in mastitis control. The method is simple in concept but extremely complicated in the execution. The milk passes through a very narrow aperture in the machine and a beam of electrons is passed across this aperture; every time a cell passes through it breaks the electron flow and these breaks are counted. It all sounds very simple but it is much more complicated than I have described. For a start, it is designed so that you can state the size of the particles you wish to count and so you can set the machine to count red blood cells, white blood cells or the somatic cells from the udder.

Once the value of this type of machine was realised, huge sums of money went into their development and today there are automatic machines where you put your samples of milk from the farms in one end, the machine does all the processing and the number of cells per ml of milk is reported at the other end. Hundreds of samples per hour can now be processed and today farmers are paid on the numbers of cells that their milk contains. When the tanker from the milk company pulls up at the dairy and connects the farmer's bulk tank to his tanker, the driver takes a small sample of the milk into a bottle containing a preservative and labelled with the details of the farm. The fewer cells the better, and year on year the milk companies are demanding milk with ever lower counts. They produce for the farmer his results in the form of a graph so that he can see what is happening to the udders of his cows. Perusal of these graphs is now a very useful technique for the veterinary detective as it shows what is happening on the farm: Does the figure remain steady from week to week or is it on the rise?

A further development that went in parallel with the cell counting was the demonstration that cows could have chronic infections in their udders without showing the clinical mastitis that would alert a farmer to the idea that there was something wrong. Elimination of this condition resulted in the cow producing up to fifteen percent more milk without requiring any more food. Now this was an idea that farmers liked! And so the practice of examining the foremilk began: before putting the clusters onto the teats, the farmer stripped a little milk from each quarter onto a strip cup, a large aluminium cup with a black plastic shelf two thirds of the way up which had an opening into the cup; after examining the milk the cup was tipped and the milk drained into the cup so that the next quarter could be examined. Cows with chronic mastitis often have tiny clots in the milk which can be seen by the trained eye. The farmer would not put the cluster onto the affected quarter but would milk it by hand and start treating. The better-trained farmers would arrange with their vet to send us milk from the affected quarter, for us to isolate and identify the offending bacteria and carry out a sensitivity test.

There is a general misconception about sensitivity testing: it is not about determining the drug to use, but determining those not to use. If a drug does not work on an agar plate it will almost certainly not work in the body where there are other factors at play.

Staphylococcus aureus and members of the genus *Streptococcus* are the bacteria most commonly involved with subclinical mastitis and all these organisms can cause infections in humans, so these zoonotic organisms need to be treated with respect. There was an amusing incident on a farm involving *Streptococcus agalactiae*, a bacterium that is a bit of a maverick among streptococci which are able to survive almost anywhere, human throats, dogs' ears, dirt on the floor, almost anywhere. Not *Streptococcus agalactiae*, it needs to live on the bovine skin or in the animal itself. Take it away from the animal host and within a few hours it dies. The great advantage of this to farmers is that the disease can be eradicated from a herd; such is not the case with most of the bacteria that cause mastitis.

We had demonstrated the infection in a moderate-sized dairy herd in north Essex and I had visited the farm with Patrick Flemming and carried out a whole herd culture test; that is, we examined the milk of every cow and more than thirty percent were positive for the organism. Patrick and I visited the farm again to discuss the situation with the farmer, John Barley. We sat in the dairy office and I went through the position. John sat there looking very worried. He was a small tubby man in his mid thirties with a wife and three small children. He was furious because he had brought in the trouble with a 'cheap' cow that a neighbour was selling because he wanted to reduce the size of his herd. The cow looked good, had a splendid conformation, a nice neat udder and produced a goodly yield. He had hummed and hawed about buying her and because of the price decided to go for it. My motto has always been 'buy a cow, buy trouble'. No farmer ever sells his best cows and usually has a reason for getting rid of the ones he is selling. We discussed the costs of eradication and they were high: all the animals in the herd have to receive intra-mammary treatment for three days, including the dry cows, and the poor old bull has to receive his treatment by injection (Mr Barley did not keep a bull). The cost of the drug is not the main cost, which is the loss of the milk that cannot be sold because it contains antibiotics. Balanced against this he could expect a minimum ten percent increase in production and lower vet bills.

'I just do not know Patrick, it is a great gamble without a guarantee of success.'

'I win either way,' said Patrick, 'because I get to sell you the drugs if you carry out the eradication campaign but my visits to you will reduce, and if you do not do it I will continue providing you the services. However, my advice to you must be to go ahead, but the decision is yours.'

'I'll have to think it over for a few days and discuss it with the wife.'

We set off back to Saffron Walden and in the car Patrick said, 'He will not do it; cash is a bit tight at the moment and they are spending a lot on their house.'

He was right: a few days later he phoned to say that Mr Barley had decided not to go ahead with the campaign.

'Thanks Roger for all your trouble, I am sorry that he is not going ahead because basically he is one of my more progressive clients. But as I said before, cash is tight.'

I thought no more about it and got on with the next case. Six weeks or so later, I was most surprised to receive a phone call from Patrick.

'John Barley has changed his mind and has decided to go ahead with the eradication, and you will never guess why!'

'No,' I said. 'Please tell me.'

'John's wife has been really ill for the past few days, with a bad go of cystitis, and the doctor has confirmed that the organism causing the trouble was *Streptococcus agalactiae*. She is now on the mend but poor old John is kicking himself again for not taking our advice, and sparing his wife the pain and discomfort. When can we start?'

'Whenever it is convenient for you two; shall we say Monday of next week because that will give me time to get a detailed plan to you?' I like to combine an eradication campaign with a general clean up on the farm and so I always produce an individual plan of campaign for the farm. 'If John starts the treatment on Monday morning, then I will come out to see how he is getting on, on Wednesday afternoon and check how the clean up is going, and I'll be out again the following Monday to sample the herd to check that the blitz has been successful. Tell John to let the milk company know that he will have no milk for them for the next few days. I would like to see you on the farm on Wednesday but don't bother to come out for the resampling.' I knew that he would not be charging John for his visits.

The student that I took with me on that first visit was the son of a Cheshire dairy farmer. Bill was astounded at the state of the farm when we arrived.

'My dad's farm has never looked like this since the day I was born, you could eat your dinner off the yard floor.'

Patrick and I were both suitably impressed as we walked round the buildings.

'How is the work going cleaning all the udders?'

'Done!' he said. 'There was no pressure to get the cows milked as no tanker was coming, and so we did them all at the second milking. It was not a big job because not one of the cows had a really dirty udder. They certainly looked a treat when we finished. But it fair broke my heart pouring all that lovely milk down the drain. My bank manager is very keen for this to succeed, and so am I. Poor old Joan was really sick with that bladder infection and so I only wished that I had taken your advice the last time you came.'

Bill and I took a few swabs from surfaces in the dairy and from the teats of some of the cows for bacterial examination back at the lab.

'We'll be back next Monday afternoon to sample all the cows,' I said before we drove off.

'May I come with you on Monday?' Bill asked. 'I have an equine surgery practical then but I am sure the Colonel will let me off.' The Colonel was Col. Hickman, one of the leading horse vets in the country. He was happy for Bill to be doing something useful and allowed him to come with me. The visit was uneventful and we collected the samples, which to my relief were all negative. Patrick was delighted with the news.

'John will be so relieved,' he said. 'It seems that the effort and expense has been worthwhile.'

'Hold your horses for a while more,' I said. 'You will need to keep an eye on him for a week or two and do let me have samples from all clinical cases of mastitis that he has.'

'You bet; I'll watch him like a hawk and we will certainly come running to you if we need help. And thanks so much Roger for your support; John Barley is like a new man.'

Veterinary investigation is sometimes more about people than the animals!

I did not see John Barley for more than a year, until one day he came to the lab to bring us a dead calf for post mortem and asked to speak to me.

'Thanks, Roger, for your help with that mastitis problem. The cows have gone from strength to strength and production is up by twelve percent and they look well.'

'I am delighted that it has all been so successful,' I said pointing to the new Range Rover at the door.

'It's been a good year and no more trouble with the missus!'

It would be great if all cases were so successful but sadly not all eradication campaigns go so smoothly and then you feel bad when the farmer has spent a great deal of money and the infection has not been eradicated.

Farm visits in many ways resemble a theatrical performance: you have to put on a show for the farmer. While I have never believed in bullshit, you sometimes have to convey the impression that you know more than you actually do! However, I have found in my career that you rarely suffer from admitting a lack of knowledge. Most people accept that you cannot know everything; the important thing is to know where to find the knowledge required, and that was the great strength of the Veterinary Investigation Service, there were experts in almost every field of veterinary endeavour and all are willing to help.

Willingham rejoiced in a newly formed amateur theatrical group – Willingham Amateur Musical and Dramatic Society (WAMADS) – which had been founded by Amy Robinson, the post-master's wife and a tartar for discipline in the ranks: she was a fine actress and a good director. I was able to hone my directorial skills when Amy asked me to stage an entertainment for the Queen's Silver Jubilee: the idea was to perform on the village green an open air show for all. Luckily we had a back-up in the form of the church hall as, on the day of our scheduled opening, it poured in torrents.

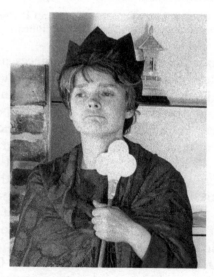

Anne Kirkman as the Red Queen, in 'A Royal Entertainment' devised and directed by Roger to celebrate the Queen's Silver Jubilee.

173

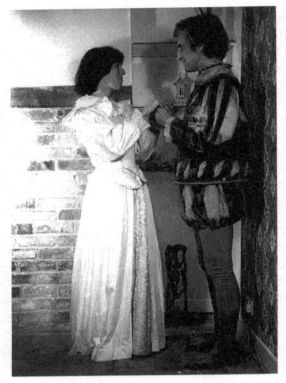

Hilary Barnes as Mary Queen of Scots and Robert Booth
as Bothwell in 'A Royal Entertainment'.

I assembled a pot pourri of theatrical pieces about royalty. We
opened with an excerpt from the Coronation Service itself, then the
prologue from 'Henry V', and the St Crispian's Day speech –
Richard II's famous speech when he realises that he has lost the
throne. These were interspersed with comic recitations, comedy
sketches, scenes between the queens in *Alice Through the Looking
Glass*; it was truly 'A Royal Entertainment' and it was amazing how
many villagers were prepared to have a go on the stage. It was a
great deal of fun and it did wonders for village morale: there were so
many newcomers that the old-timers had been feeling threatened,
but for the sake of the show old and new pulled together to produce
a triumph. 'Arsenic and Old Lace' was my follow-up and what a lark
that was – constructing a staircase so that Philip Carter, in the part
of Teddy Roosevelt, could blow his trumpet, shout 'charge' and rush
down the staircase (without killing himself). Again the old and the

174

new in the village pulled together to make the show a success. WAMADS played a great part in unifying the village.

Teaching also involves performance and I do enjoy teaching willing students, be they young or old, black or white; it gives me great pleasure to help people to understand. It was my teaching that led to another case with human involvement, which was brought to my attention some years later by a vet on the Suffolk–Essex border and involved a hobby herd of pedigree Dexter cows, the smallest British breed. They were owned by a retired banker called Roger Green: throughout the whole of his banking career he had dreamed of being a farmer and with the bonus he received on retirement he bought a small farm near Framlingham and established his herd of Dexters. Unlike Mr Barley, Roger bought wisely and had produced an excellent small herd of about forty cows. He sold his milk unpasteurised to the local cognoscenti who paid a small premium for the quality milk that they were buying and he never had any shortage of customers. His herd was tuberculin tested, brucella accredited, and we kept a regular eye on the quality by checking the butter fat, protein and lactose. We also carried out a regular cell count on the bulk milk and regular checks on the bacterial count in the milk. His cell counts were so low that we could never get a statistically accurate result and his bacterial counts were rarely within the limits of the experimental error.

He achieved this because his herd was small, and the attention to detail was absolute. Everything in the parlour was spotlessly clean. The overalls and hats were clean for each milking, the boots worn for milking were only used in the parlour and were properly washed with disinfectant after each use. The milkers, after washing their hands in disinfectant, donned rubber gloves which were washed in disinfectant between cows. The udder of each cow was washed clean and thoroughly dried with individual towels that Mrs Green had embroidered with the cow's name – and woe betide anyone caught using the wrong towel on a cow. Mr Green did not routinely do the milking but his wife did with a couple of assistants from the village. Mastitis was unknown in the herd, until one day I received a call from Dougie the assistant in the local practice.

'Roger, I have just been to Roger Green's farm and he has three cows with a raging clinical mastitis. He wants you to come down straight away as he says he knows you.'

I racked my brains but could not think where we had met.

'At this stage there is no point in my visiting the farm: please take samples from all affected quarters and get them to us as quickly as possible and then start treating.'

Two hours later Roger Green was in the lab. Not many farmers would drop everything and drive samples to a lab (although I do remember once many years later when working in Botswana, a farmer was so concerned about his animals that he took some samples, jumped in his plane and flew the samples 400 miles across the Kalahari to our laboratory in Gaborone; but then he had no vet within 100 miles). Roger was a small man with a round cherubic face and a bald head with a halo of white hair all round. He exuded humour and gentility and was 'frightfully sorry' to bother us 'but he had a wee problem': there was definitely Scottish blood in his background. I knew the face but could not place him.

'You will not remember me,' he said, 'but you taught me on an Agricultural Training Course on calf management.'

'So that's where it was. I am sorry I do so many of these courses that I do not remember the names of any student and only the faces of about half.'

'They were an excellent series of courses that I attended in the Writtle Agricultural College, in Chelmsford. When I started I knew next to nothing about farming and keeping cattle, and I think that we who keep animals for a profit should possess the latest specialist knowledge on the welfare. So I enrolled in every course on cattle going and a few more. It is such a pity that the ATB has been closed down because they organised such wonderful courses; I do not know what I would have done without them. But I am going on and I am not here to waste your valuable time but Dougie said you would sort out my problems.'

'I don't know about that but we will certainly do our best to help.'

'Well if the work going on here is anything like the teaching you gave us ...' He paused and then went on, 'But there I go again when all you want to know is the details of the problem. '

'I don't know about that,' I said, 'it's always nice to hear praise: the staff get enough brickbats from people who have waited three weeks before calling their vet and then the animals die before we give them the results. It would be a miserable world for me if we did not have time to exchange pleasantries, but the sooner we get started the sooner we can get your cows better.'

I took the details of the farm and the animals, and realised that here was a man who knew everything about his animals and believed that they were sentient beings and not units to be run for the maximum profit. This was the start of a friendship that lasted for more than ten years until Roger went to his well-earned rest in his eighty-fifth year.

The next morning we knew what the problem was: from all the milk samples we isolated profuse pure cultures of *Staphylococcus aureus*. This was a nice straightforward organism that was sensitive to all drugs tested. Dougie reported that all the cases had responded rapidly to treatment with penicillin.

'Nevertheless he still wants you to come and have a look: he is certainly a big fan of yours.'

'I don't know why, but I could certainly do with some at the moment.'

Sherwin, John and I were involved in a perennial battle with the Ministry bureaucracy. Jock and Blackie took no part in the battles raging in the Ministry concerning the future of the Veterinary Investigation Service. Big brother, the Field Service, was the police arm and law enforcers and so was not popular with the farming community. They tend to behave like PC Plod with astonishing insensitivity to the plight of farmers who were having restrictions or worse placed on their livestock, whereas the farmers looked to us as a source of assistance. Consequently the Field Service was very jealous of our relationship and thought that if they took us over some of the gloss would brush off on them. Hence the constant battle for our survival as an independent entity.

'Anyway I will not embroil you in Ministry politics but when do you want us to come, bearing in mind that today is Thursday and we would not want to set up cultures on Saturday morning? Would Monday be all right with you and Roger?'

'It's not me you will have to deal with: when the VI staff come then it's the boss Hugh Clay who handles the case. I will check with Hugh and Roger and let you know.'

'Soon as possible please, as I want to get a note on the vet school board to alert the students to what might be an interesting visit.'

Hugh Clay was a vet of the old school who believed that the red carpet should be put out for the lab boys and that they should deal with the partners rather than an assistant who was learning his trade. Dougie was in my year at college and knew his trade as well as anyone, but he had not yet been offered a partnership, which was only a couple of years away.

It being another mastitis visit, Bill quickly signed up and we set off for lunch with Hugh Clay. Hugh was really a horse vet and had limited interest in cattle but he had taken a liking to Roger Green and so we set off for the farm. This was my first view of the system. Bill was visibly shaken by the management of the farm, with cows treated as princesses, and he could not believe the individually named drying cloths. It was not like this at home. Since it was such a small farm we were able to take our samples and watch the milking at the same time – something I rarely do. What we needed was to identify the source of the infection, and so in addition to taking the milk samples I took nasal swabs from Roger and Eleanor Green and their assistants.

Bill could not stop talking in the car going home. 'How can he possibly make money with all that luxury for the animals and the human inputs?

'He does,' I replied, 'but he is a niche farm, selling milk at retail prices and a premium. However, I have always considered that the best maxim for a dairy farmer was "consider the comfort of the cows" which is so often ignored by busy commercial farmers. You should tell your father about this farm!'

'I most certainly will, and I strongly take your point about comfort.'

It was an interesting journey home.

The real surprise when we looked at the results a few days later was that the culprit was Roger Green himself. The cows from which we isolated the organism were all treated and Roger went to his doctor who put him on a course of antibiotics. It transpired that the weekend before the outbreak Roger had helped Eleanor milk the cows because the assistants had gone to a wedding.

Somewhere in the middle of this busy professional and personal life I fitted in a trip to Nigeria. The trip was a great experience in dealing with West African bureaucracy and inefficiency and not all of it African. I flew to Kano with British Caledonian Airways, whose flight to Lagos stopped there, and had a charmed entry into the country. It was the time of the Haj, and Kano airport was thronged with white-robed pilgrims. I had visions of a wait of hours before getting though immigration but, like the Red Sea, the crowds parted and I was able to walk directly to the counter. I was in: the next hazard was customs; I was looking for my suitcase when this scruffy

178

little man in a grubby T-shirt came up to me and said, 'Are you Dr Windsor, Saar?' I said that I was and he went on, 'I am the head of customs, Saar and I have been asked by the British High Commission to assist you, Saar. Where are your bags?'

I pointed to my suitcase, and with that he put a large cross on it and told me it was cleared. I informed him that I had some freight coming for my work and he gave me his name and told me to contact him when it arrived. I was through and there was Dick Best to meet me: we were into his Land Rover and off to his house which was right at the end of the runway. It had taken almost no time at all and we were sitting on his veranda drinking our gin and tonic when the BC plane took off for Lagos.

Dick and Rosie Best were both vets and had been working in the field in Kenya when we had been there. We were not close friends but they were very good to me during my stay in Kano, sorting out the various bureaucracies. The worst of which was the British High Commission; they had been asked to look after me during my stay. The first problem was my subsistence payment. I was to be in Nigeria for three months; this was too long a period to be paid a 'daily subsistence' and too short to be paid an 'overseas allowance'. They therefore were unable to give me anything. I sent a telegram to the Overseas Development Administration in London, telling them that I had come with £300 and, without money from them, when it ran out I was going home. It was agreed that I could have 'Actuals'; that is to say, I had to keep receipts of what I spent and could claim that back together with 10 Naira (about £20) per day. This was somewhat difficult when most of one's shopping was done in the market. It meant that instead of buying cheaply in the market, I had to go to Kingsway in Jos and pay their inflated prices. Nevertheless it meant that I could buy beer, gin and whisky and claim it on expenses as there was no upper limit on what I could spend. All that was needed was the receipts.

My freight arrived and the friendly customs boss had it cleared in a trice (I do not know what sort of retainer he was on from the British High Commissioner, but in Nigeria, nobody did anything without a 'dashee'). Once I had everything sorted out Dick gave me a Land Rover and driver, and I was off to Vom to start the work.

The nominal head of the Bacteriology Section was a Pakistani, Dr Al-haji M.A. Bhathi, a graduate of the London Veterinary School. During my three months' stay I met him in the laboratory on just one occasion: he was never there, but attended to his own business interests. The same could be said of Dr Sansi, the Director of the Laboratory, who had been a couple of years ahead of me at college – I only met him once, as he was forever travelling; what he was doing apart from earning subsistence was another matter.

There were some people that I knew working in the laboratory. Mark Philpott from Kabete, who was responsible for setting up the CBPP project, was carrying out research into breeding diseases; Bill Taylor from Muguga days was still carrying out his research on rinderpest; there was an excellent Pakistani, Dr Nawathi, who worked with Bill and made the rinderpest and pleuro-pneumonia vaccines and worked hard enough to make up for the idleness of his countryman. And here were some excellent Nigerians, almost all Ibo, who were slowly making their way back into the north after the ruinous Biafran War. There were three who had studied in Scandinavia and all three had returned with Scandinavian wives. And so there was a good crowd and the parties were plentiful. My counterpart was Dr Onoviran who was charm personified and very able. Unfortunately his business interests were more important than scientific endeavours and I saw little of him and even less once Walter Masiga had arrived.

The worst incident during my stay was when, luckily, I called round to see Ruth Philpott for some recipes as I was looking after myself. I walked into the house with the usual call of 'hodi', the African expression to attract attention, and noticed that there was no one to be seen, but there was a strange dog in the living room. One looked told me that the dog had rabies. I shouted to Ruth to remain where she was with her three children and the maid, and told her I would go and get help. I made sure that the dog could not get out, and went and got the farm manager, who had a gun. I explained the situation, he got his rifle and we returned to the Philpotts' house. All was as I had left it and the dog, which had 'dumb' rabies, was lying on the threshold drooling. Armed with a large broom I entered the sitting room and chased the dog out and when he was in the garden he was shot with a single bullet. When I told them the news, Ruth and the family came out and Ruth promptly burst into tears. It must have been a terrifying ordeal for her to be in the house with her three small daughters with no means of getting help: there were few phones in Nigeria and those there were, mostly did not work.

I was there to carry out the field trial with our diagnostic test. The antigen had to be prepared before we could start and that is when the first problem arose: there was no ultra-centrifuge in Vom and so I would have to take my cultures to Zaria where that great worker on malaria, Dr Brian Greenwood, was producing his vaccine. I set off for Zaria with all my materials and when we got to the boundary of Zaria about twenty miles from the city we were stopped by an army checkpoint. The sergeant approached me and asked me to give a lift into town to one of his soldiers; I explained that this was the car of the Director of the Federal Laboratory in Vom, and I had been instructed that we were to give lifts to nobody.

'Calm down,' said the sergeant.

'I am perfectly calm,' I replied, 'it is just that we are not allowed to give lifts.'

'Calm down,' he repeated even more loudly, and as I sat there he screamed at me, 'Calm down,' and the penny dropped. He meant 'Come down' or 'Get out of the car.'

I got out of the car as he was waving his gun rather frantically in the air. The standard Nigerian road block check ensued where they were more interested in inspecting my underpants than looking for weapons. The driver had a quiet word with me.

'I think it would be wise to give the soldier the lift, shall I speak to the sergeant, as he is my tribe? I think we will have no more bother.'

We gave the soldier a lift. I dropped my suitcase at the Government Guest House where I had stayed during the conference seven years previously, and set off for the vet school. On entering, the first person I met was David Shannon, the former DVO in Nakuru, Kenya. We looked at each other blankly for a few moments and then said simultaneously, 'What on earth are you doing here?'

David was teaching in the Large Animal Clinic and his next question was, 'Where are you staying?'

'At the Government Guest House,' I replied.

'Oh, no you are not,' he said. 'You are coming home with me'

And so we returned to the Guest House to collect my case and set off for David's house. Dorothy immediately made me feel very welcome and I was introduced to their young son Patrick. The Shannons' house became a pied-à-terre for me during my regular trips to Zaria and it was a wonderful place to relax. Dr Greenwood was my next port of call and he showed great interest in the work we were doing and immediately put all his facilities at our disposal.

Soon the antigens were prepared and it was time to return to Vom, but not before the Dutch had thrown a party for me: they had taken over the running of the vet school. I had met some of them in Kenya before but knew none of them well. The Shannons had a prior engagement and so I was the only Englishman among a sea of orange, all talking away in Dutch when I arrived. I was introduced to all, and I never heard another word in Dutch all evening: the very essence of hospitality and good manners. It was a great evening.

Walter arrived on the back of a motorcycle just after my return from Zaria. He had flown from Nairobi and had hitched a lift from Jos airport. He did not want to miss the fun. I never found out who paid his expenses. We slept under mosquito nets in Vom, and it was as well that we did because I woke one morning to find five scorpions on the net. I was living in a newly built house, whose only previous occupant was one Barti Singh, whom I assumed to be a Sikh but who was actually Barti Synge a protestant from southern Ireland and with whom I was to work many years later in the Scottish Agricultural College. Apparently when houses are built it upsets the ground and destroys the scorpions' nests and for several years they are a real pest. I developed a plan for dealing with them: I slipped out of the net on the side where there were none, grabbed my strategically placed squash racquet and then knocked them off the net onto the floor, picked them up with a pair of salad tongs and dropped them into a beaker of acetone: they died with their tails in the attack position. The only thing that I had found in the house was a resin kit to make paperweights and key rings, and so I made my children, my godchildren and my nieces and nephews a paperweight or a key ring containing a scorpion.

We had identified a source of diseased animals near the laboratory in a travelling Fulani herd: we were able to vaccinate cattle belonging to the laboratory and we travelled to a government ranch at Mokwa in the south, where the disease had never been diagnosed. The lack of a functioning telephone system made working in Nigeria such a problem, as we were unable to book accommodation in the Guest House in Mokwa. Walter and I arrived hot and sweaty after the eight-hour drive to find that there was only one single room available; one of us would have to sleep in the servants' quarters. We tossed and Walter won: the servants' quarters consisted of a room with a bed which had a foot of space round it, together with a closet containing a Western toilet and a shower. Despite being less than ten miles from West Africa's largest dam and reservoir, that night there was no water. We washed in soda water from the bar. The following day we spent working in the dust and heat and returned to find that there was still no water and soda water stocks were running low. Luckily on return from working with the cattle the following day the problem had been resolved and I was able to wallow under a cold shower – servants' quarters do not have hot showers.

The work was completed in a few days and all the animals were negative to the test. Since I was already half way to Lagos it seemed a good idea to continue the journey and go and visit David and Pam Field. David was an old friend from the Nairobi Theatre Group and we had kept in contact during his moves on behalf of the Singer Sewing Machine Co. I had managed to contact them by phone on my arrival in Vom and I was invited down to stay with them on a date to be fixed. It seemed a good idea to contact them to let them know that I would be travelling down. Unfortunately there was no phone in Mokwa, the nearest being in Jebba at the crossing of the Niger a mere sixty miles away. For three days I was driven to Jebba and waited at the phone office while they tried to put me through. Each afternoon I waited until 4 pm but no contact was made. The phone office closed at 4 pm.

Should I risk it or not? It was still a 400-mile journey and I did not know where they lived: Lagos is a large city! When the work was completed I set off by taxi – the famous Nigerian tafa duka (flying coffin). With a change of taxi in Kontagora, Ilorin and Ibadan I arrived in the centre of Lagos mid-afternoon on a Saturday, a perfect time for an expatriate to be at his club. I knew that David belonged to the Apapa Yacht Club and soon a local taxi deposited me at the entrance. I found the secretary's office and asked for the use of their phone, which was immediately granted. I dialled, and miracle of miracles, a connection was established at the first dialling. There was no answer. Obviously they were at the pool enjoying themselves. The secretary did not know them, but nothing daunted I walked round the pool listening for American accents (Pam is American and there were far fewer Americans than Brits in Lagos in those days). I stopped at the first American accent and the woman knew the Fields. She wrote their address on a scrap of paper, wished me luck, and sent me on my way. We arrived at the Fields' house, I paid off the taxi and knocked at the door. It was opened by a European who was definitely not David.

'He used to live here but he has moved to a larger house nearer the office. He's my boss and I would be happy to take you to his new house, but my wife has gone off with the children in the car. You will not have too much trouble getting a taxi.'

He too wrote down the address on a piece of paper. I finally found a taxi – it is a lot easier to get a taxi in the city than in the suburbs. The driver soon found the house, but I had learnt my lesson: I asked him to wait, while I approached the armed guard at the gate.

'Not here, Saar,' said the guard.

'Will they be back soon?' I asked.

'No Saar. Gone away Saar, not know when back, Saar.'

Bugger!

I had travelled all that way to see them and they were not there. I got back into the taxi and wondered what the hell I was going to do. I knew nobody else in Lagos and you could not get a hotel bed in Lagos for love nor money: it was the height of the Nigerian oil bonanza when people had money to burn and anyone with a job was earning almost more than they could spend. While I was wondering what to do the guard came up to the taxi, opened the door, popped his head in and said, 'Are you Dr Windsor, Saar?'

'Yes,' I replied, wondering how he knew my name.

'Missie Field give me letter for you, Saar,' said he, pulling an envelope from his ex-army greatcoat pocket.

I do not remember the exact words of the letter but it went something like this:

Dear Roger,

I have this dreadful premonition that you are going to come to see us this weekend, just as we have taken off to go and see you in Vom. We will fly to Jos on Saturday morning, the driver having set off in the car on Friday. Just in case you do come I have salved my conscience by arranging with some good friends for you to stay. You will like Jean Michel and Marie-Marthe and their two lovely children. However, I should warn you they do not speak English.

Love
Pam

Their address was at the bottom of the letter and the driver had me at their house in a few minutes.

Pam was correct, I did like Jean Michel and Marie-Marthe, they were delightful and their children were adorable. I had been away from home for almost two months and was missing Maxine and the children and so it was a real pleasure to be in a family and have young children to read stories to. They were French and so I had to read French stories, luckily my schoolboy French honed in a Parisian secondary school, although rusty, was up to the task. The family were from Bordeaux and they gave me a wonderful weekend.

All too soon it was time to make the 1000-mile journey back to Vom and put my life in the hands of the mad taxi drivers. There was no way that the journey could be done in a day, however, an old friend Martyn Edelsten ran the veterinary laboratory in Kaduna and having stayed with him before, I thought he would put me up. I did not expect to arrive in Kaduna at three o'clock in the morning though. I had to change taxi twice on the way to Kaduna, in Ilorin and Contagora; of course you have to wait until the taxi was full before it set off. I was happy to sit in the middle seat in the back, usually squashed between two large Yoruba ladies; I reckoned that that was my best chance of survival if we hit anything. It was slightly uncomfortable when a large breast was removed from its cavernous bra – so that she might suckle her offspring, but I considered it a small price to pay for survival. The standard of driving has to be seen to be believed and on the way down I had noticed many a lorry on its roof on a long straight stretch of road. And so to while away the long hours of boredom I decided to count the number of upturned vehicles that we passed. Unlike Kenya, the countryside in Nigeria is exceedingly dull – flat land with boring scrub bush consisting of short, broad-leafed shrubs with no hint of large trees or wild animals. There were twenty-two lorries upside down – not one was on its side!

We finally arrived in Kaduna and there was a local taxi to take me to Martyn's house – luckily I knew how to find it, although I did not know the address. I also knew which room he slept in and so was able to bang on the window – he saw my face and opened the front door.

'I thought you might turn up some time; you know the guest room, the bed is made up.' With that he returned to bed. Even today, many years after the event, I still cannot credit his sang froid at that time of the morning.

Martyn had an official truck returning to Vom the following day and I was able to cadge a lift. The Fields were staying in the Jos Hotel and we met up for a dinner together before they returned to the south. My trip to Lagos caused them great merriment but Pam was relieved that she had written that letter.

The final flourish was to travel to Bauchi in the north where there was an Argentine-run abattoir and processing plant. There was a good possibility that some of the animals would be infected with CBPP, but this was a real 'blind' run of the test. We would perform the test on the animals as they went into the abattoir to determine their status and then we were able to see how accurately the test performed when the animals were slaughtered. The manager of the abattoir was an Argentine with the unlikely name of David Churchill-Brown. He and his wife were most hospitable and insisted that Walter and I stay with them while the work was in progress. The work showed conclusively that the test was of value and could detect infected animals when other tests were negative.

On my return to Vom I found an invitation to dine with Dr Bukkar Shaib, a graduate of the Liverpool Veterinary School and now raised to the dizzy heights of Permanent Secretary of Agriculture in the regional government. It was a fascinating meal. Dr Shaib was a true Moslem and despite his wife being a qualified medical doctor, I did not meet her. Although she cooked the meal she did not eat with us and I only saw her through the hatch between kitchen and dining room. The meal was delicious, but HOT. I do not think I have ever eaten a meal with more chillies in it and I suffered the next day. It is little wonder that Nigerians have a high level of stomach problems.

Sadly the CBPP test never became widely used. It arrived too late on the scene. The fashion for field testing had passed: the new enzyme-linked tests which were carried out in the laboratory and gave a result to three decimal places (which must be good) were making their mark in the rinderpest field and of course anything that works with rinderpest was bound to work with CBPP! Twenty years on and there is still no test available to equal the intra-dermal allergic test, but we had missed the boat. Walter and I said farewell and we returned home. Not before I had a tiff with the customs' official when I refused to give him a 'dashee'. For some reason the crate of equipment was 'delayed' and all the beautiful mangoes were rotten on arrival....

There had been almost no communication between Maxine and I

186

since I had left – the telephones did not work in Nigeria and post always took a month, and of course there was an attempted coup while I was in Nigeria and the perpetrator took refuge in the British High Commission which aroused a great deal of anti-white feeling: it became so bad that Rector of the University of Ibadan had to issue a statement to the student body: 'Students should not molest the expatriate members of the staff, but should leave it to the police, who are specially trained for the job'!

The government closed the borders and they remained closed for almost a month. This had had a very depressing effect upon me. I missed my family and was worried about them. How much easier it is today with the Internet and mobile phones. Mark and Ruth Philpott and their three charming daughters kept me sane. But it is the one time in my life when I have felt severely depressed.

I had left in the cold of January snows and returned in spring-like April, to find the kitchen littered with beds, as the children were all infected with mumps. Poor Maxine was going frantic trying to keep them amused as well as fed and watered. This was not a time for the young friends to rally round as they had their own children, but as usual the Hinds were wonderful. It was good to be home. I had not even time to write up my Nigerian experiences when I was called for mastitis duties.

A practice in southern coastal Essex had several large dairies as clients and they were pioneers in the use of cell counts as a tool in the battle against mastitis. Sherwin was asked to assist in the development of their mastitis control schemes, and knowing my interest in mastitis he referred them to me. This was not a time to take a student and so I drove alone to the practice, where the first shock of the day awaited me: I had not realised that the name Neill on the practice headed paper was a man who had been at college with me. Hamish Neill had been in the same year as Peter Jackson and the infamous Sansi. Being several years ahead of me he had no idea who I was; you only know those senior to you.

Before going off to the farm I was seated in the practice office with a cup of coffee while their ideas were explained to me and they sounded great. The practice was receiving copies of the cell count reports and building up a picture of the different herds within the farming group. What they wanted from us was laboratory back up for their efforts. When a herd was experiencing a problem they wanted us to come out and sample each individual cow and carry out a cell count and a bacterial sample; in this way they would be able to identify the offending animals and sort them out. This was fine in theory but would entail the lab in a great deal of travelling, as it was a journey of seventy-five miles each way. We agreed that I would do the first few herd samplings and train one of their vets to take over.

The second surprise of the day was when we arrived at the farm to find that the manager was Peter Acton, the younger brother of Edward, a friend of mine from the village in which we lived. I knew that Edward had a brother who was a keen farmer but did not know that he was related to the owners of the farm. Peter, Hamish and I sat down in the dairy office and planned a strategy: there were ten farms in the group and two were experiencing problems at the time. It was agreed that we would begin the sampling on Tuesday the following week with the most seriously affected farm and then go to the second the week after. One farm with 200 cows was the most we could handle in a week with our facilities; we would need to establish a team in the laboratory to set this work on a production line. This was definitely a case for student labour but they were not a problem as there were a great number interested.

We decided to sample at the afternoon milking so that the lab staff would be able to commence work first thing in the morning. I had not done this type of work before and I did not realise what a massive undertaking it was going to be. Two hundred cows means 800 quarter samples, and two samples from each quarter, one for cell counting and one for bacterial culture, 1600 bottles per farm: we should have started with a smaller farm! It was not going to be possible to wash and dry all the udders and so we decided that they would be wiped with a dry paper towel and then the tip of the teat would be sterilised with spirit. I would supervise three students and Liz would be responsible for labelling each bottle and putting it in its right place. Our first attempt was chaos and I am not sure that more than seventy-five percent of the samples were correctly taken, but we learnt and developed sampling kits that worked efficiently and Liz became an excellent master-at-arms. The students enjoyed their contact with the animals and most of them came into the lab on a regular basis to see how the results were coming along.

That was another story. Peter and Denis had as many problems to solve, if not more. Denis was in charge of cell counting, Peter the cultures. But it was all hands to the pumps. It did not take us long to decide that it was uneconomic to work with quarter samples and it

188

was better to bulk up milk from all four quarters on the farm: this immediately cut the laboratory work by three-quarters and made it a physical possibility. It was agreed that a vet from the practice would revisit the farm and take quarter samples from all cows that seemed to have a problem. Hamish was the man we trained and he took to his task with great enthusiasm but he had to persuade Peter, the farm manager, to lend him staff to undertake the sampling; we had had five people and he had just the two and so he had to draft in help. However, the farm were happy to pay for the work as they realised the long-term benefits. With our electronic cell counter, 200 samples a day was the maximum that we could process and that required at least two staff members, one of whom had to be Denis.

Each milk sample cultured used a minimum of three different types of agar plates: after a time we cut this down to two, but our incubators were full to bursting. Each plate had to be identified and then a sample of milk was streaked across the surface and this took about two minutes per sample, eight minutes per cow when we were looking at individual quarters: 200 cows ... it took a great deal of time. The following day each plate had to be examined and the findings recorded. The plates were returned to the incubator until the following day when the final examination was made and those that did not show growth were discarded. We had to limit the work and so plates with only a few colonies of bacteria on them were also discarded. Those showing a significant number had to be examined and the bacteria identified. This could be a lengthy process in itself as a smear of the colony had to be made and a Gram's Stain performed and then the slide had to be examined under the microscope. Potential pathogens had to be subcultured onto more agar plates for identification and for an antibiotic sensitivity test to be carried out.

When the work was completed there was a report to be written giving all 200 (originally 800) cell counts and the results of the bacterial cultures. Last, and most important of all, was that an interpretation of the results had to be made and a statement of what the farm needed to do to improve the situation. However, the farmer knew if we were of value to him because he only had to look at the results from the milk company. Peter Acton was very impressed with the work, because lower cell counts meant more milk being produced, a bigger return for the farm and a larger bonus for him.

This work reminded me of the great C.D. Wilson, the mastitis king, who pioneered the work of mastitis control in the days of shortage just after the war. Duggie was a great man in many ways, small in stature but massive in character, without the bombast so often seen in small men. His height was the only small thing about him. During the war he had been a fighter pilot and had lost a leg in the process, but nothing stopped Duggie. When I first met him I was a student seeing practice in Oxfordshire, but he was only too happy to explain in great detail what he was doing and to ask my opinion on the theory of it. He was at the time in the midst of his great pioneering work to prevent the spread of udder infections in cows during milking. To this end he had designed and constructed a portable steam steriliser that could be moved from farm to farm. There was a definite air of Heath Robinson about this machine, which had tanks and pipes and cogs all over the place, and it gurgled and wheezed like a man with a smoker's cough, and steam poured out on every side. How the farm staff were not scalded when using this machine, I do not know. The work entailed the milkers rinsing the clusters after they had been on a cow and then putting them in the machine for a minute or so to sterilise them. Then they had to be cooled before they were put onto the next cow. It dramatically increased the length of time the milking took, and the idea never caught on, but the principle did: udder washing, individual paper towels instead of the all-purpose cloth, examining the fore-milk, teat dipping after milking with a bactericidal liquid, all stemmed from Duggie's work. It was seeing Duggie's enthusiasm for what he was doing that decided me that there was more to veterinary medicine than being in general practice. It was that that stimulated me to undertake a microbiology degree after I had finished my vet course and I resolved to follow in Duggie's footsteps as a bacteriologist; this resolve was changed by circumstances when I was in Kenya.

Duggie was still going strong at the Central Veterinary Laboratory in Weybridge when I went to Cambridge and he was a source of inspiration and a mentor to any who sought his advice. I remember the first time I phoned him for advice. I explained who I was and when we had first met.

'I've no forgotten ye Roger,' he replied (yet another Scot, they really dominate the profession). 'How could I? Ye naiver stopped asking me questions aboot that wee machine. Ye ken that it's noo gathering dust and rust in the department shed, but it sairved its purpose.'

He remained my teacher throughout my time in Cambridge and I never spoke to him without receiving help and advice: a lovely man. I hope that the work I did, helping to control one of the major causes of loss to the farmer and discomfort to the cow, goes some way to repaying my debt to Duggie.

This was a period of great inflation in Britain with the mortgage rate and prices for household goods going up almost monthly, and salaries not following suit: we were getting more and more into debt. When we returned from Kenya, we thought that the fun was over and that we would not work overseas again but now I was seriously thinking of it, not because I was unhappy in my job or my life, but because the family finances were so dire. I was having to go to London most weekends to undertake locums in small animal practice just to pay the bills. We now had three children and so paid work was out of the question for Maxine, who had more than enough to do in the house. Each time that I thought of seriously taking action, the Ministry would raise our salaries and so I took no action.

10

Naughty Boys

'It is my belief Watson, founded upon my experience, that the lowest and vilest alleys in London do not present a more dreadful record of sin than does the smiling and beautiful countryside.'

Sir Arthur Conan Doyle, *The Adventure of the Copper Beeches*

The great foot and mouth disease epidemic of 1967 changed the face of the British livestock industry for ever. Before 1967 the British farmer had produced the great breeds of cattle for which we were famous, the Hereford and Aberdeen Angus among beef animals and the famous dual purpose breeds such as the Shorthorn or Red Poll. We had even adapted the Dutch Friesian to being a British dairy breed along with the Ayrshire and Jersey. Almost every county in Britain had some breed of farm animal named after it: the Suffolk, pre-eminent among sheep bred to produce lamb; the Dorset, Hampshire, Romsey, Blue-Faced Leicester, Scottish Blackface ... the list is endless. All this came to an end in 1967 when farmers were restocking after the great slaughter. The government decided to allow the importation of the dairy breeds from Canada and the USA, and the rapidly growing beef breeds from the continent, Charollais and Limousin among cattle and Texel and Rouge for the meat sheep. Synthetics had replaced wool for clothes, fabrics and carpets and now the British wool breeds were worthless unless they produced good meat.

Britain was flooded with Holstein cattle, mainly from the United States of America, and with them came Holstein cattle disease agents: bovine virus diarrhoea, enzootic bovine leucosis, and *Mycoplasma bovis*. We were assured that the animals were all free from these infections! A cynic would say it is good for veterinary business, but there is little point in improving the quality of your livestock if it is riddled with disease.

The initial importations attracted great interest in the British

192

farming press and publications such as *Farmers Weekly* were regularly full of features on these new breeds with pages of colour photos. This had an unfortunate repercussion on one farm in East Anglia which had imported thirty in-calf Charollais heifers. The heifers all calved within a month of each other and amazingly produced thirty beautiful calves, without a single death. This herd had a double-page spread in the *Farmers Weekly:* there were photos of the heifers with their calves, the proud farmer with his stockman and even the vet managed to have his photo in the magazine.

A few weeks after the article appeared, the calves started to die. They presented a strange collection of signs: incoordination, trembling, falling over, and some stood with their heads pressed against a stanchion in the yard. The vet had no idea as to what was going on and the dead calves were sent to our neighbouring centre, in Norwich, for examination. All showed haemorrhages on the skull with seeming alteration in the blood. When the skull was opened there was a widespread haemorrhage. This was the cause of death but what caused the haemorrhage? A fungal toxicosis was diagnosed. A source of the toxin was sought and the farm was turned upside down but no fungi of significance were found. The food was checked and double checked; the producer was supplying other farms in the area and there were no reports of the disease elsewhere. The calves continued to die and the lesions were always the same. Rhys Evans the biochemist from the vet school visited the farm and took numerous blood samples but the red blood cell, and white cell counts were all normal and so Rhys did a platelet count: platelets are an essential part of the clotting process and diseases such as Vitamin K deficiency manifest themselves by causing a marked decrease in the platelet count. The platelet counts were all normal.

In desperation Edward Gibson the head of the centre phoned Sherwin and asked if we would accept the remaining few calves for examination. Sherwin agreed but said they had to bring us a couple of live calves as well as the dead ones. The next day five animals arrived, three very dead and two astonishingly healthy calves. We put the calves into a pen and Rhys came across from the vet school and we stood in a line watching the animals. Despite their journey, they ate with relish when we gave them some calf pellets. It was obvious that there was nothing wrong with these animals, they were bright, alert, interested in us watching them and not at all perturbed by their new surroundings.

Sherwin, John and I gowned up: Rhys had to go to a farm but asked us to leave the animals for him to look at on his return. We set about our task with a will: we wanted to solve the problem and we wanted to put one over the Norwich centre. The first stage in any examination is to examine the unopened body for any abnormalities and then to remove the skin. Ron reported that one of the eyes was bloodshot but until the skin was removed nothing else was noted. All three had large circular haemorrhages in the centre of the forehead. All three of us commented immediately, 'These animals have been hit on the head with a hammer.'

Peter was summoned to bring the laboratory camera and take photos of the evidence. Sherwin commented, 'There could be a court case in this one and so we need to dot all the "I"s and cross all the "T"s. There has to be an interesting story behind this. Perhaps it's a jealous neighbour.'

Despite being certain that we had a diagnosis, we continued with a full necropsy but there was nothing to see at all. It is essential to carry out a thorough examination, in this case it might have been required as evidence in a court case, although in my view one should always carry out a proper examination. In other cases the cause of the death might not be the most important finding, for example a sheep might have died from an inhalation pneumonia because the farmer had poured the medicine down the trachea instead of the oesophagus (a not uncommon, but usually isolated, happening); if the post mortem examination is stopped there you will miss the severe infestation with liver flukes, which could be a serious problem for the whole flock. As I always told my students, 'There is only one way to carry out a post-mortem examination and that is properly.'

We then opened the skulls and all three showed massive haemorrhages in the meninges – that wonderful membrane that covers the brain, providing protection from injury and infection, but not the sort of injury that had been inflicted on these animals. We carefully removed the brains and put them into the formalin jars for Cyril's later attention. The examination was complete and we were certain of our diagnosis.

Coffee was served in Sherwin's office while we discussed the next move. It was decided that Sherwin had to phone Edward and warn him of our diagnosis, because there was bound to be flak that he had not made this diagnosis with the fifteen or so animals that they had examined. Edward said that a diagnosis of malicious trauma had

194

been discussed with the farmer but discounted because it was not possible. My mind flickered back to the Sherlock Holmes comment, 'When you have eliminated the impossible, whatever remains, however *improbable*, must be the truth.' Having sorted out the political impact of our diagnosis on the Norwich Centre, we went on to discuss how the farmer should be told. He was coming to see us that afternoon. We decided that it had to be head on: he had to be told that this was the diagnosis and that he had better find out who was behind this before other things started to go awry on the farm.

When given the diagnosis the farmer became quite belligerent. Sherwin pointed out that had he listened to Edward when this first started, then he might have many more live animals. Three members of the staff including himself had carried out the examinations: all three of us on seeing the lesions on the skull had decided that it was caused by a blow from the traditional 'blunt instrument'.

'How many people are involved with the cattle?' asked Sherwin.

'There's myself, Biggie the head stockman, who has been with me for more than ten years and dotes on them Charollais, there's Bert who helps milking and doing odd jobs such as driving the tractor, and Tony who looks after the calves. He is a bit simple and I gave him the job to give him a bit of a lift; he is a real tiger for work and is a strong young man and able to do the lifting. That is all of us.'

'It has to be Tony,' said Sherwin. 'Can you put a surreptitious watch on him, so that he does not know he is being watched?'

'There's only two calves left; luckily he is off this afternoon but we will keep an eye on him.'

The farmer phoned the following morning to say that Tony had been caught in the act of hitting a calf on the head with a large spanner, unfortunately too late to save the calf from injury and probable death. Once an animal has come into the lab we do not normally allow it to leave alive, because of the risk of spreading infection. However, in this case the farmer undertook to accept the risk and a few days later came and took the two healthy beasts home to join his one remaining calf.

'You know,' said Sherwin, 'it's lucky we are a load of scaly bastards who believe the worst of human beings. Edward is such a decent chap, he could not really believe that anyone could do such a thing and so he didn't stand his ground when that farmer said it could not be so. We know better! I think this calls for a sherry,' and out came the bottle. While he, John and I were sipping there came a phone call, funnily enough from the farmer.

After listening intently for a few minutes and saying almost nothing, Sherwin put the phone down and said, 'That's a rum go. The farmer has decided to take no action, but sent the lad to a child psychiatrist here in Addenbrooke's Hospital. What happened was that the lad saw the article in the *Farmers Weekly* and was aggrieved that he, who looked after the calves, did not get his photo in the magazine and decided to get his own back on the farmer. He did that in a big way. Poor deranged child.' Sadly human activity is too often the cause of discomfort, disease or death in animals.

The 'thin sow syndrome' is well known to farmers. One of the problems with breeding sows is that they put on too much weight while they are feeding their baby pigs and so once they are weaned it is difficult to get them to conceive. To avoid this problem and not cause a problem in the nutrition of the young pigs is a fine balancing act. If the sow is infected with worms, then the problem becomes more complicated. We were confronted with just such a problem with the client of one of our Cambridge practices John Grieve (yet another Edinburgh graduate, although some years after me). The first samples to arrive were faeces from half a dozen 'thin' sows. We were unable to find any worm eggs in the samples and so John persuaded the farmer John Grout to bring in two of his thinnest pigs. I took the history myself and it seemed that Mr Grout was doing everything by the book and that there was no shortage of food. We put the sows to sleep and I examined the carcases.

They showed some mild bed-sores over the joints but no signs of mange or other external parasites that can cause a rapid loss of weight. Once we got inside the carcase there were all the classic signs of emaciation/starvation: there was not a scrap of fat in the body not even round the kidneys or intestines and between the muscle bundles there was a yellowish oedema fluid that occurs when the blood plasma is deficient in protein. The stomach was devoid of contents and in the intestines all that was seen was some dried mucus and bile, that fluid produced by the liver which helps with the digestion of fat among other things. There seemed to be no lesions or abnormalities in any of the organs – liver, lung, heart, kidneys. Nothing.

Here was a real problem, why were the sows starving in the midst of plenty? We made bacterial cultures from the organs and took samples for Cyril to cut his sections. Nothing. We isolated nothing, the sections from the various tissues, apart from showing the effects of starvation, gave us no indication of the cause of the problem. Nothing.

John Grieve came into the office and we sat down and thrashed out the matter but our deliberations got us nowhere, we kept coming back to the fact that sows were starving in the midst of plenty. John had examined the record of food purchased for the farm and it had shown no decrease on former years, in fact if anything there had been an increase in food consumption over the past year. It was agreed that John would set up a meeting on the farm with himself, myself and the food company.

I carried out my usual investigation, asking questions about the farm policy, the numbers of animals in the various age groups, how the individual groups were managed and of course I concentrated on the breeding and feeding of the sows. Mr Grout was a good enthusiastic farmer who purchased only the best-quality food. The chap from the mill had carried out his own evaluation of the food consumption of the sow food over the previous six months and shown that it was sufficient for 230 sows: Mr Grout's aim was to keep the number of sows to 200, so that he had enough accommodation without having to overcrowd his pigs. At no time in the past six months had the numbers gone above 210 and because of the problems he had sent several off to the abattoir before they became too thin to sell so he was running about 190 on the day of the visit. We examined every building on the farm, all the pens and finally the food store where the sacks of meal were stacked. Everything was in apple-pie order and all was clean and tidy. It was a real puzzle that had all of us beat! We all agreed that we continue our investigations and I would try and sum up our findings in a report.

When writing my report the Sherlock Holmes dictum that I have mentioned before came into my mind: this was the 'impossible' factor. I discussed the case with Sherwin and John and said, 'I've come to the conclusion that the food is being bought but that the sows are not receiving it, and that means only one thing: the pigman is not feeding it to the pigs but using it for his own ends.' Again I thought of the Holmes saying, 'When you have eliminated the impossible, whatever remains, however *improbable*, must be the truth.' We were confronted again by that unpalatable truth.

'You will have to handle this carefully if you don't want to end up in court on the wrong end of a libel allegation, and so can I suggest you run your recommendations past me before you send them out?' Sherwin said.

'You bet,' I said and went and worked on the report. I can remember to this day the exact wording of my report which was: 'I have come to the conclusion that there is no disease problem on this farm and the only explanation I can offer is that rats are getting at the food.'

The shit hit the fan. A couple of days later I had the farmer on the phone saying that he was going to sue me for every penny I had.

'How do you make that out?' I said.

'You've been very careful with your wording but we all know what you are saying, that either the pigman or I are selling the food.'

'I do not remember writing that,' I said

'Don't come the smart Alec with me, you're for the high jump and no mistake: I will not allow you to malign my staff.'

'If you have no better solution to the problem than mine,' I emphasised, 'I think that this conversation will go nowhere.'

'Don't think you have heard the last of this, my lawyer will be in contact,' and with that he slammed down the phone.

Later that day I had a phone call from John Grieve. 'I'm in the same boat; he called me all the names under the sun for bringing you, "idiots" was his word, in. He has also dispensed with my services and is going to ask Alec Scott to take over the farm, and so with your agreement I will send Alec your report.'

'I stand by my report one hundred percent, and both John and Sherwin have read it and concurred with the contents before I sent it out. You may do what you like with the report: it was written for you. It was an honest report based on my experience and what I found in the lab and on the farm.'

No more was heard for a couple of days until Alec pitched up in the lab on his way back from visiting the farm.

'I think things are starting to improve on the farm: according to Mr Grout the animals do not seem to be getting any thinner, but I have no idea what the problem is. I am sure something is going to happen there because the atmosphere on the farm was dire and it seems that the farmer and the pigman are not talking. There have definitely been words there. One thing is for certain, I am going to charge him a bomb for the visit, as I do not approve of farmers chucking their vet for doing their best for them. He is definitely not a client that I want but I went because I thought the pigs might need some treatment.'

Something did happen: about a fortnight later I had a phone call from John to tell me that he had been reinstated as Mr Grout's vet with an apology.

'Come on,' I said. 'Don't keep me in suspense, what happened?'

'The pigman has done a bunk and flown off to Canada with his wife and family; they just left the house and went. They had sold up all the furniture that belonged to Mr Grout and gone. Apparently, he was knee deep in debt: he owed a great deal of money to the bookies and was trying to pay it off by selling off the food. Had he been a little more careful he might have got away with it, but his debts were mounting rather than decreasing. He would load up the boot of his car with a few sacks of meal each day. He left a note for Grout apologising for the trouble he had caused, and so I suppose there is some good in him.'

I did not receive an apology from the farmer, but then I did not receive a letter from a solicitor either. I often wonder what it is that causes people to gamble: I can understand the odd flutter on a horse, but to put your family at peril and have to flee from the hounds? In my view that pigman needed help every bit as much as Tony who killed the calves.

The next detective tales happened in Kenya and not Cambridge, but they fit in here. Pedigree Friesian calves between two and three months of age were found dead in their pens and there were often signs of haemorrhage from the anus and in some there was a great deal of clotted blood on the bedding. There was a suggestion of rodents having been eating round the anus. The calf was examined and sure enough we found what looked like tooth marks round the anus. After checking for and finding a few ticks under the tail and round the ears, the skin was removed and the animal looked very anaemic. The body lymph nodes were enlarged but this is not un-usual in a young animal in Africa, as it is experiencing ticks for the first time and the saliva of ticks has antigenic properties, to which the glands respond. Sometimes in that saliva the tick transmits animal parasites that can cause disease (in a similar way to the mosquito transmitting the parasite that causes malaria to a human). Three parasites commonly transmitted by ticks in Kenya are *Theileria*, *Anaplasma* and *Babesia*, the parasite that causes redwater; we have that last parasite in parts of Britain where we find ticks, the West Country, Wales, north-west England and almost the whole of Scotland. It is good if the calves become infected with *Anaplasma* and the *Babesia*, because at a young age they develop an immunity without becoming sick.

The abdomen of the dead calf was full of clotting blood but there were no other abnormalities, apart from the pallor, until the examination reached the rectum where there was a large jagged tear which was the cause of the haemorrhage and death. This was before the case of the calves killed by the stockman, and so I did not immediately suspect human involvement. However there was no way that a rodent could get inside a rectum. I discussed the case with a few colleagues but they could offer no suggestions.

A second case was presented with identical lesions and I came to the conclusion that this had to be a malicious attack. I asked the farmer to come in and we discussed the case. I said that I was certain that somebody was inserting a sharpened stick or bamboo cane into the anus and then pushing it in as far as it would go and just waggling it about. The lesions on the anus were the result of unsuccessful attempts to insert the weapon.

'Do you have any enemies or disgruntled staff members around?' I asked.

'Certainly the latter,' he replied. 'I had to sack a couple of the milking staff a week or so ago: they were ripping me off by selling some of my milk to their neighbours. They all get a few pints to take home for their own family but this had developed into a real "family" and half of the village were buying my milk from Njogu. They were not happy with their dismissals and said they would get a witch doctor to put a curse on my animals.'

'I doubt that they would get a man to do it, there is too much risk of his being seen on the farm, but does he have a small son?'

'They all have small sons, medium sons and large sons, in fact too many sons and daughters!'

'I suspect that one of the workers put his son up to doing it and explained how to do it. Your practice of tying the calves would make access a simple problem. You must set somebody to hide in a place where he can see what is going on but not be seen, and keep watch. It will only happen during the day because any visitor would be noticed at night and the wandering dogs tend to discourage human predators.'

And so for two days the head cowman lay silently in a pile of straw watching, and his patience was rewarded. Njogu's son tip-toed into the kraal bearing a short stick tapered to a point; making sure that no one was looking, he silently approached a calf and was about to insert his stick when with a great leap the cowman was out of the straw and grabbed the small boy who screamed in terror thinking that he had been taken by one of his gods.

The local tribal police were called. The farmer, Njogu, and the head cowman all seated themselves in a circle. The boy was put into the middle of the circle and told how his father had shown him what to do and told him to kill all the calves, just one at a time. Next, Njogu told his story and said it was not his fault because he had been told that he could take milk for his family and then he was put out for doing just that. He thought that it was grossly unfair that he had lost his work and the farmer owed him money but despite all this he never asked his son to hurt the calves: it must have been the boy's idea because he was cross for not getting his milk before he went to school. The tribal police took the father away to the local police station to go before the magistrate. He was sentenced to six months in the King Georgie Hoteli, as prison was still called years after independence. Another case solved.

The last case in the series also occurred in Kenya and involved a man going to jail. Those of a sensitive nature had better skip to the end of the chapter because this is rather unsavoury. A European employed by a European farmer as a stockman was causing his wife some trouble and she approached his employer as she thought her husband was committing unnatural acts with some of the animals and she did not know what to do.

'He has to be stopped,' she said. 'He's a good man but we are having marital problems and financial worries and he certainly is behaving strangely in many ways. Will you please keep a sharp watch and if you see him misbehaving please go to the police.'

A few days later the farmer saw the man indecently assaulting, I think that was the term, a nanny goat. He phoned the police and asked them to get there quickly: strangely enough they did – perhaps because it was a mzungu misbehaving – and they arrived just as the man had completed his act. He was arrested and the goat was taken as evidence. A local vet was summoned and he took a sample of the fluid from the goat's vagina and sent it to us. Had we been in Britain there were many tests that could have been done: however, we demonstrated semen in the fluid but were unable to determine the species from which it came. With DNA testing the species would present no problem and would probably have identified that the

201

farm worker was responsible. None of this was available to us and we could just report that there was semen present in the vagina. Had the man decided to fight he might have won his case but he did not. He was so ashamed and pleaded guilty, and so I did not have to give evidence in court. Because of the nature of the case I would have found this most distasteful.

Because he pleaded guilty he was given the lenient sentence of twelve months in jail, which is where he passed his twenty-fifth wedding anniversary. He was a model prisoner and received regular visits from the Anglican chaplain. His wife stood by him, the farmer gave him his job back, and I understand he was completely reformed character. So some good came from this sorry episode.

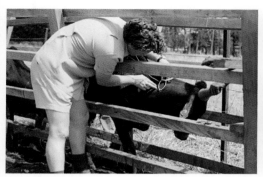

Working in the field in Kenya with cattle.

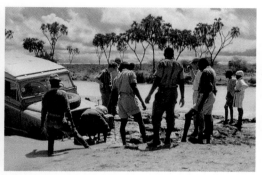

Problems working in the field in Kenya.

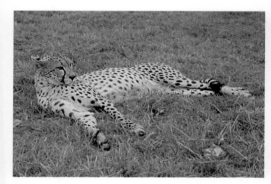

The first patient from the Nairobi Animal Orphanage the day after being treated for severe hookworm infestation.

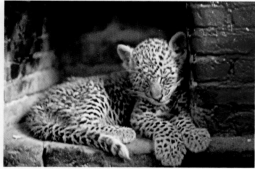

The outbreak of feline enteritis in the orphanage: this young leopard loved the warmth of the fireplace (we had a log fire every night).

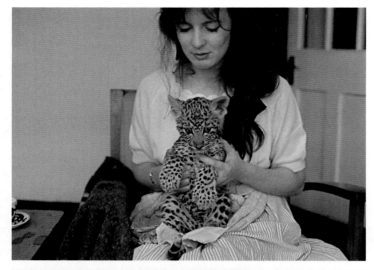

Maxine holding the leopard up so that I could feed it with a spoon.

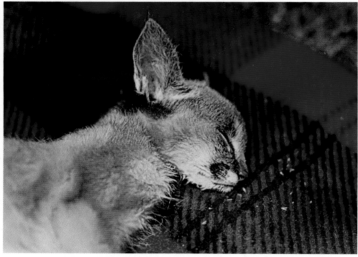

The only wild cat that we were able to save from feline enteritis. *Left*: while sick; *Below*: after recovery.

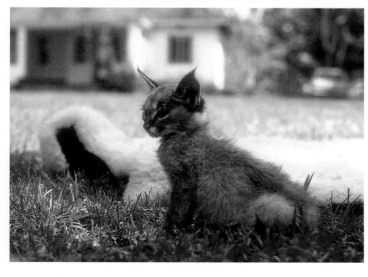

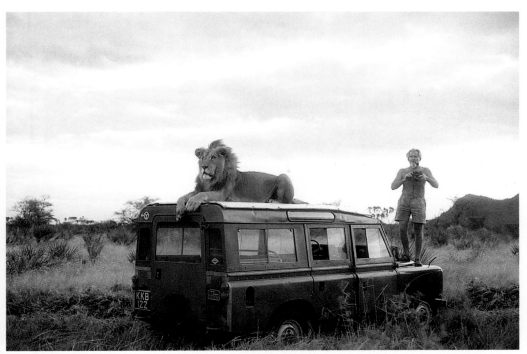

Above: George Adamson looking for the rest of the pride while Ugas keeps him company.

Left: George Adamson and Girl in the camp.

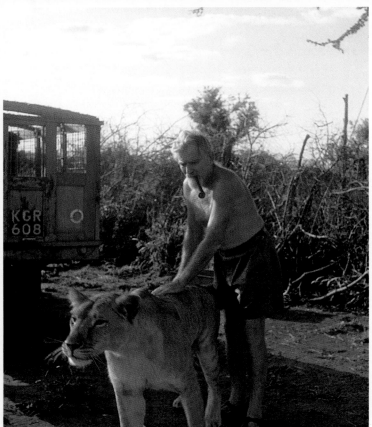

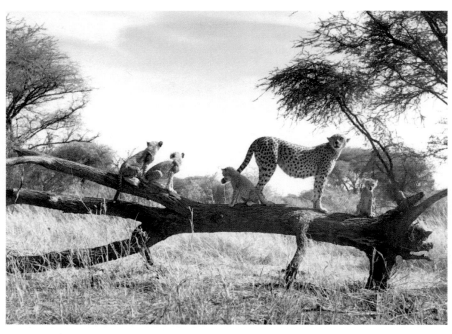

Above:
Pippa and cubs before Dume broke his leg.

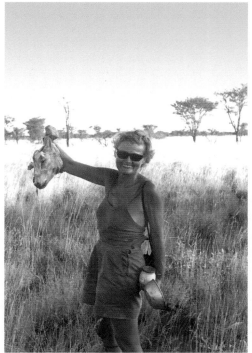

Left:
Joy about to feed her newly released cheetah, Pippa.

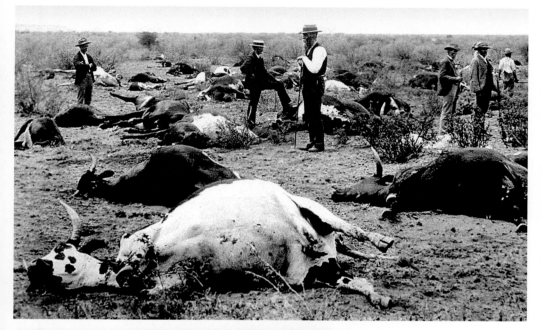

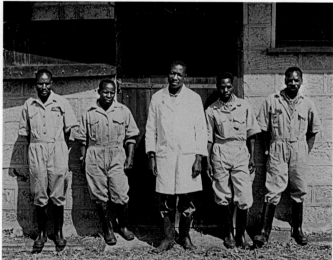

Above: The great Rinderpest epidemic in South Africa in 1896.
© VRI. Onderstepoort, Republic of South Africa

Left: Contagious bovine pleuropneumonia: the team at EAVRO who handled the cattle.

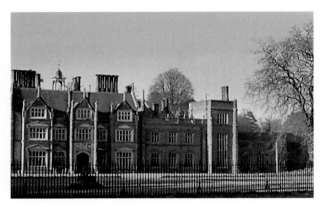

During our stay in Norfolk we rented the east wing of Heydon Hall for £4 per week.

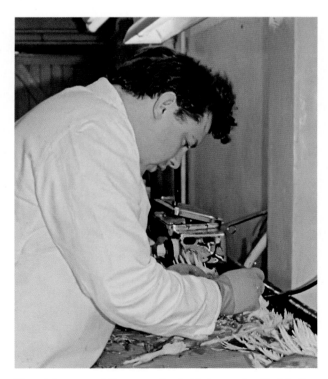

Examining one of the many dead chickens submitted to the Norwich Veterinary Investigation Centre.

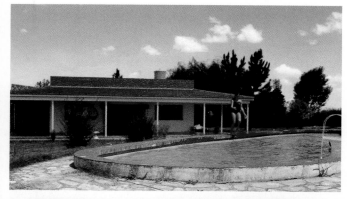

Our house and swimming pool in Cerrillos, north west Argentina.

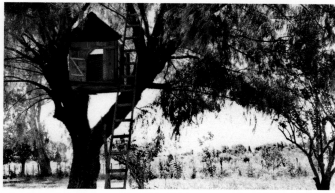

The tree-house in the garden made from a packing case.

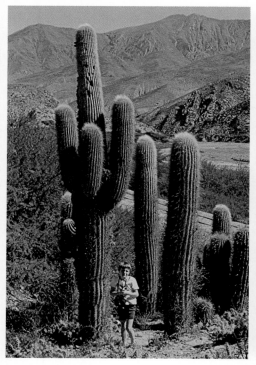

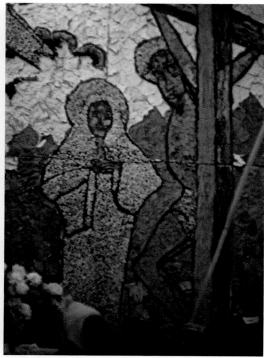

Left: On the border between Argentina and Bolivia. Richard stands by the majestic organ pipe cacti.
Right: Mary at the foot of the cross: a life-sized Tilcara picture made from flower petals.

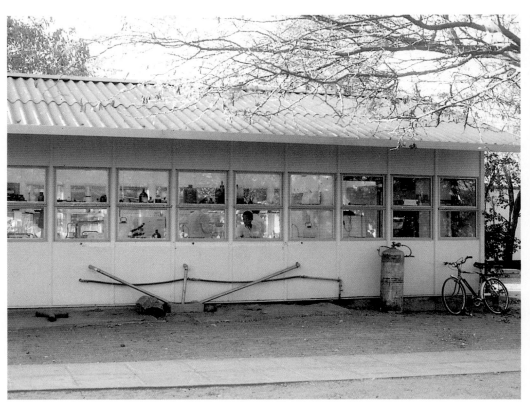

The biochemistry lab building in Gaborone.

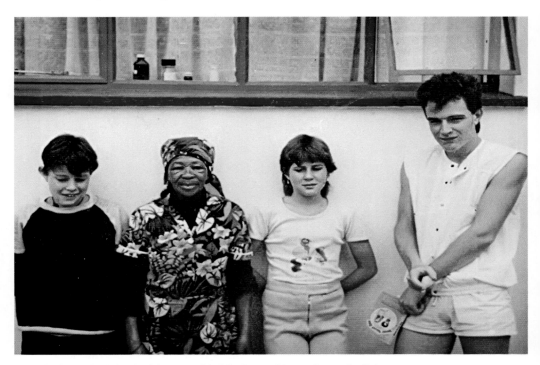

Guy, Claire and Richard with our maid, Dinah, outside our house in Gaborone.

11

Bloody Pig Faeces

'As a rule, when I have heard some slight indication of the course
of events I am able to guide myself by the thousands of other
similar cases which occur to my memory.'

Sir Arthur Conan Doyle, *The Red-Headed League*

Swine dysentery is caused by the spirochete *Treponema hyody-senteriae* which is related to the bacterium that causes syphilis in man – *Treponema pallidum*. For years the disease had been called, incorrectly, vibrionic dysentery because the organism *Vibrio coli* was regularly isolated from clinical cases of the disease, whereas the treponeme is very difficult to isolate or to see in normal smears. It had been around for years but had not caused much in the way of trouble.

This was a different disease and it was killing. The increase in the number of cases mirrored the increase in the number of hybrid pigs being produced and sold in Britain. Pigs had traditionally been bred for pork or bacon because smaller carcases with less fat and big hams were required for the pork butcher, whereas the bacon curers wanted pigs with long backs to produce the best cuts of bacon. The Small and Large White, the Saddlebacks, and a host of other British breeds were developed, as was seen in cattle and sheep. Geneticists in the States had shown that by selective cross-breeding it was possible to produce the pig you wanted in a shorter time with the concomitant decrease in food requirements. These developments were keenly followed by the hybrid pig companies in Britain who supplied what had been closed herds with regular new imports of breeding stock. The traditional system of closed herds whereby a farmer bred his own replacement stock ensured that new diseases were not brought onto a farm. The purchase of hybrid pigs meant the end of closed herds, as you had to buy new stock on a regular basis to keep up with the genetic improvements and these were massive. The regular improvements in production meant that the pig keeping

203

became very profitable and more and more farms began purchasing hybrid pigs just to keep in competition. We do not know whether the hybrid pigs were more susceptible to swine dysentery or whether it was the pigs that were taking the infection to the farm. This will never be known.

Tom Alexander, who worked in the Cambridge Veterinary School, was short with silver hair and beard; a real dynamo, he was one of the leading experts on pig diseases in Britain, the veterinary consultant to the biggest of the hybrid breeding companies and an expert on swine dysentery: he worked with the American Hank Harris in unravelling the story of swine dysentery and as he worked in the vet school, rarely a day went by without some contact between us. He was always prepared to help although he did get cross with us for suggesting that it was the hybrid pigs that were spreading either the susceptibility or the infection. However, the evidence was before his eyes.

Tom showed that if you examined the wall of the large bowel immediately by scraping a little of the lining and mixed it with a dilute salt solution on a warm microscopic slide then you could see these small 'sea serpents' slithering about when you looked down the microscope. Several years later a bacterial growth medium was developed to grow these wrigglies and life became simpler, but it was never simple. Farmers were permitted to add certain antibiotics to the food to 'prevent sub-clinical infections' but they never said of what. These antibiotics were not used in human medicine and so presented no real risk to humans and they certainly increased the growth rate of the pigs. I have never really approved of this practice as it was a really a drug for treating bad management of the animals. It also made the job of identifying pigs affected with swine dysentery all the more difficult as they stopped the growth of the bug without killing it.

The clinical disease was easy to see in untreated pigs. Most infections causing diarrhoea in the pig do so by infecting the small bowel, but this one actually destroys the lining of the large bowel and so the pig would pass pasty faeces in which there were small spots of blood and mucus. If the pig was really sick the whole lining of the large bowel would be destroyed, the dung contained more blood than food material and the pig would soon be dead. Once we had the techniques, it was easy to confirm the diagnosis in such cases. Often the pigs had been treated or had been eating medicated food and that was a different story.

All diarrhoeas cost the farmer money because the pig quite literally passes expensive undigested food without receiving any nutrition. However, most bowel conditions affect the unweaned pig which is still drinking milk from its mother. Dysentery was different; it affected weaned pigs which had already cost the farmer a great deal of food. As the disease began to take a grip on the national herd, we were seeing it more and more frequently in the lab; more and more medicated food was being sold and the signs of disease were suppressed. However, all sorts of alternative pictures began to emerge. A farmer would report a sudden drop of fertility in his herd or a massive increase in neonatal diarrhoea in the baby pigs. Food consumption would increase and productivity fall.

Something had to be done, but what? There was only one effective treatment, dimetridazole which was closely related to the drug metridazole that is widely used in humans in the treatment of gastric ulcers and in women for treatment of vaginal infections. The manufacturers had shown that pigs affected with swine dysentery made a complete recovery after treatment and that the bowel was completely sterilised. This started us thinking, if the drug is almost one hundred percent effective in killing the bug, and the organism is very fragile and unable to live for long outside the pig's body, an eradication plan could be feasible. As we saw with *Streptococcus agalactiae* mastitis in cattle, if the organism has to live in the body it should be possible to eliminate the infection from the herd.

There were many small fattening units in the fens, usually run by a smallholder, who might have ten or more acres of ground which they used to supplement the income from a permanent job by growing fruit, vegetables or flowers. If they had a shed or two they could buy weaned pigs from a breeder and take them up to slaughter weight and then sell them to the abattoir, bacon curers or local butchers. Despite all our attempts to persuade them to buy on contract from a farmer they knew, and so avoid the risk of bringing in disease, they continued to get them 'a bit cheaper' in the market. My mother had a saying which is 'the most expensive is usually the cheapest', and when I was informed by a farmer that he had an eye for a good pig and a bargain, I would ask if he could see the spirochetes in its bowel. They would laugh and shrug it off with, 'I'll be proved right, see if I don't.' Most of these men would pay out huge sums of money in treatment but still managed to make a profit.

The essence of the plan was to put the whole herd, sick and healthy, under an umbrella of dimetridazole treatment. After about three days when we assumed that all faeces passed by the pigs no longer carried the bacterium, the clean-up campaign began. It was a simple enough plan but difficult in the execution. In essence all the dung that was on the farm at the start of the campaign had to be removed before the end, and all the buildings and equipment thoroughly cleaned. This is basically what is done in an outbreak of foot and mouth disease; the difference was that the animals were not to be killed. The first task was to empty and sterilise the midden: this was usually not too difficult a task because there was always a bit of ground far from the pigs where the dung could be heaped and within a couple of weeks it would no longer be a threat. It is of course a wonderful fertiliser for the soil. The key to the success was that there had to be an empty pen, which was the first to be cleaned and sterilised. Pigs were moved into this pen and their pen was cleaned and sterilised in turn, and so on until every pen was pristine clean. The tractors and trailers, wheel-barrows and food trolleys suffered the same fate. We had a plan, now all we needed was a farmer prepared to put it into practice. We had carried out an analysis of the costs of the disease to the farmer in terms of lost production, delays in getting pigs to the market and the ever-increasing costs of treatment. On the other side of the equation there was the cost of the drug, the labour required for the clean-up and the hire of a steam steriliser. We contacted the maker of the drug and asked if they could provide the drug for free to the pioneers in the expectation of big sales if our plan worked: they readily agreed. There were several specialist pig practices in the fens so we put our ideas to them and they were universally enthusiastic. Something had to be done to bring this scourge under control.

Joe Burgess and his father Charlie had swapped houses and Joe had acquired his father's smallholding, which fattened pigs in groups of 100. However, the buildings were never allowed to rest and there were always the tail end Charlies remaining after the bulk had gone for sale which were there when the new ones arrived. Joe and Charlie before him had had a chronic problem with dysentery going back for several years and the medication was making a serious hole in their profits. John Norton, in the Long Stanton practice, was very keen to proceed and so we met on Joe's smallholding. From the start I could see that there could be a problem as there were only two pens with fifty pigs in each; what were they going to do with the pigs while they cleaned out the pen? It was Joe who came up with the solution.

'My dad's got a big truck which, at a pinch will hold a pen-full.'

We provided the drug and explained how it should be administered in the drinking water: they suggested starting on the Saturday which meant that they could start the clean-up on Tuesday. John undertook to supervise the clean-up and keep me informed of progress. On the Friday the report came that all was clean but I could not resist the temptation of going and having a look. They had certainly done a great job. I recommended that they continued the medication until Sunday and then stop it completely. And then we would wait.

A week went past and our hopes began to rise; by two weeks we knew we had succeeded. Joe was over the moon and had already taken steps to find a supplier of weaned pigs from a herd that was free from dysentery. To the best of my knowledge he remained free.

We undertook similar campaigns on the herds of several more fen fattening units. Having agreed to undertake the campaign, the farmers usually did it with a great deal of enthusiasm and our success rate was good, with three successes out of four. We always investigated the causes of failure but they were never apparent: there had to have been some lingering source of infection and it is difficult to be certain that everything has been cleaned. When we experienced a breakdown we asked for the affected pig to come into the lab for examination so that we could provide the drug manufacturer with a sample of the organism to test whether resistance had developed; it never had.

The time had come to put the eradication plan into action on a breeding unit and the Godmanchester practice had a client with a serious dysentery problem. The practice always advertised in the Veterinary Record for veterinary assistants who were Evangelical Christians, and were the only practice that I ever visited that had a Holy Bible in their library. It was next to a book on VAT calculations! Bill Thurlow and I went out to Mr Ellison, of Church Farm. I was pleased that we had the experience of the fattening units behind us, because this was a farm with 300 sows (big for the time), and was not a custom built pig farm but a converted dairy farm with a large collection of buildings scattered round the farmhouse. The only building designed for pigs was the fattening house which was capable of holding 2500 pigs. I did my customary investigation of the management and feeding of the pigs, we walked round the entire complex of buildings and I took copious notes. Over a cup of tea we sat round and discussed what was going to be done.

'Well, Mr Windsor, how many of these campaigns have you carried out?'

'In breeding units, none, but we have had success in three of the four fattening units we have done so far.'

'At least you're honest.'

'There is no point in being otherwise: the object of the exercise is to help you to control swine dysentery. Somebody has to be the first, and truth to tell I would prefer to start with a smaller and simpler unit but you do have a massive problem. '

'You do not have to tell me that, I am spending £300 a week on medication alone.'

'And to that you can add the loss of productivity which must be costing you at least £500 a week. I think our best line of attack is for me to produce and cost a plan for eradication and to work out for you my calculation of your current costs and losses.'

'That seems to be a fair arrangement to me and if your calculations make sense to me, I'll do it, despite your lack of experience,' he said with a twinkle in his eye.

And so we departed.

'He'll do it,' said Bill. 'He tries to be up to date, he is very conscientious and he is concerned about the welfare aspects of this disease; he does not like to see sick pigs on the farm and he is spending a fortune on drugs.'

I spent several days wrestling with this report: I wanted him to have a go but at the same time I wanted him to know what it was going to cost; to start with, the clean-up could not be done in a couple of days; it would take a week at least and that meant it would be cheaper to buy a steam pressure washer than to hire it which would add £3000 (at 1970s prices) to the costs. It was finally complete and I gave it to Sherwin and John to tear to pieces.

'There is nothing like starting at the top,' was Sherwin's comment.

'Too big,' said John, 'it will never work with so many complications.'

'Those complications may be the secret of its success,' said Sherwin. 'All those different buildings might make it easier to get them empty for cleaning and it will enable you to insist that all yards be cleaned and sterilised on a daily basis. I would also make then clean their gowns and boots with the steriliser after leaving each house and again at the end of the day.'

Having taken on board their detailed comments I finalised the report and sent it off to Bill.

About 10 days later I had a phone call from Bill to say that Ellison was going ahead, but wanted to wait till the end of the month when he had about 200 bacon pigs going to the abattoir.

'That will reduce his drug bill,' I said. 'Which makes a great deal of sense and it will make cleaning easier because he will have lots of nice empty pens. Do you want me to come out again before you start?'

'I don't think so. Your plan is perfectly clear and the detail is all there.'

'In that case give me a call when they are about half way through the cleaning process and I will come out and check that they are doing it all correctly, but I would like you to visit the farm on a daily basis when they are underway.'

'Don't worry. I have had my instructions from Ellison that he wants me on the farm at two pm each day that they are cleaning: that is his way of booking my services for the campaign.'

'Let us hope for all our sakes that it works: I have to say I have my worries. It is a huge commitment in time and money on an unproven theory.'

'Don't worry, Roger, nobody will blame you if it does not come off, but I have a hunch we are on to a winner.'

I was grateful that someone had confidence in our success!

The eradication campaign got underway and I received daily reports from Bill about the progress. Mr Ellison had recruited some lads from the village and the dung heap was moved by tractor to the far end of the farm; this had taken almost two whole days but the midden was now spotless, and from there they had moved on to clean all the paths and open spaces. It was decided that these spaces would be cleaned with the steam pressure washer at the end of each day. The fattening house was the next item on the agenda and it was done row by row. The removal of the fat pigs to the abattoir meant that there was a whole row empty, which simplified the procedure. Mr Ellison stage-managed the whole work and according to Bill he was a new man and getting more and more cheerful as each pen was cleaned. He inspected each pen as it was done and if he was not satisfied the men had to do it again. When the fattening house had been cleaned I decided that it was time for my visit. I was favourably impressed by their efforts and thought that if hard work was a guarantee of success then we should win. I complimented them on the results and left feeling a lot more comfortable than I had since we had embarked on this venture.

209

About a week later I had a call from Bill to tell me that the work was done and would I come and give the seal of approval. I arranged with John to cover my 'duty' and went that afternoon: they had all the farm vehicles lined up, as if on parade. Tractors, Land Rovers, wheelbarrows, food trolleys, forks, shovels and at the end of the line the steam pressure washer which had also been cleaned. Feeling like visiting royalty I walked along the line inspecting them all: the vehicles looked as if they were new. At the end if the line were all the workers, including Mr Ellison, in their pristine boots, plastic overalls and rubber gloves. He proudly walked me round the farm, pen by pen and even into the food store which had been emptied and cleaned. Mr Ellison had left nothing to chance, it is the only farm I have ever visited without a cobweb to be seen. They had done a wonderful job.

And now for the moment of truth: it was time to stop the drug. A brave man would have stopped the drug in one fell swoop, but I suggested that we did it by stages. No more dimetridazole for the fattening house. If there were no signs of disease then the next to stop would be the weaner pigs, and the gilts (young female pigs kept for breeding). After a further week it was to be stopped for the dry sows and the sows in the farrowing house and the boars. Step by step we went, with the tension mounting. Two weeks after the final cessation of medication we considered we had won. Mr Ellison and Bill were both delighted. I did a final analysis of the eradication campaign with the detailed costings and Mr Ellison insisted that I remove the cost of the steam steriliser from the balance sheet.

'If I had known how much time and trouble that machine would have saved me I would have bought one years ago.'

Even with the inclusion of the steriliser costs, it worked out that the eradication campaign would pay for itself in three months with the savings on drugs and the increase in the productivity.

I made a final visit with Bill to the farm a few weeks after the completion of the campaign just to have a final look round. In the car coming back to the surgery he was telling me that one of their assistants was thinking of volunteering to work on a Vet Aid project in Mozambique and he asked if I would have a word with her about living in Africa. Living in Mozambique is a far cry from Kenya and working as a volunteer means much less money than working for the British government. However, I said that I would be delighted to have a chat with her.

'I knew you would and so I have arranged for her to be in the surgery now, I hope you don't mind!'

'Delighted,' was all that I said.

Jill was thrilled at the prospect of going off to Africa and eagerly picked my brains for an hour or more. She said how lucky she was because the practice would be supporting her and had guaranteed her a job when she returned. I guess that that is what being a Christian practice means. I gave Jill a warning: 'Do not expect to make rapid progress: it will take time for the local people to accept and trust you. Being a volunteer has its drawbacks.' And I told her the story of Warren Ferris, one of President Kennedy's Peace Corps volunteers, who was a Harvard agricultural graduate. He was sent to work in Ol Kalou in the heart of Kikuyuland. The Peace Corps philosophy, which was to be followed by most volunteer associations, was that the volunteer lived in the community in which he or she worked and had to live a similar life style: pushbikes or a motorbike but certainly no car or truck. Warren became a regular visitor to our house and was always complaining that he could never get anybody to do what he asked them: they just continued with their age old methods.

'Ask them why they are not taking any notice of you, you might find that they've tried your methods before without success,' I said.

'I'll try that,' he promised.

It was about a month later when Warren was back in town and I asked him if he had got an answer.

'Sure, I got an answer and it was some humdinger! I was told straight out that I was no good. I was a bit hurt by this and I asked, "What makes you say I am no good?". Damned if they didn't reply, "If you were any good you would not live in a mud hut like us, you would live in a big brick house like the other mzungus, and you would not have that rickety old motorbike that is always going wrong, but have a smart car!" Do you think I should write to Johnson [Kennedy had been assassinated by then] and tell him he's got it all wrong?'

'No, just stick it out and I am sure they will listen to you in the end.'

And I think that they did and Warren stayed in Ol Kalou for the whole of his time as a volunteer and came to be accepted. But Warren was lucky; he came from a wealthy east coast family and they financed his jaunts to the bright lights of Nairobi. Jill was not so lucky, no rich family and anyway there were precious few bright lights in Mozambique in those days.

On the way home my head was full of Africa, and the wonderful times that we had had. I was glad that I had had a paid job and in those days volunteers had to be unmarried. No, we worked hard but we had the time and money to enjoy ourselves. I am a great traditional jazz fan and, although a classically trained musician, Maxine put up with it for my sake. When Louis Armstrong and his All Stars came to Britain I went to Earls Court and after a wonderful evening I knew I had to go and meet this man and so I went to the stage door. After about twenty minutes the group of us were shown into his dressing room. I was amazed at how small he was in his white dressing gown with a towel wrapped round his head. He was charm and grace personified and I have that signed programme to this day. Louis was coming to Nairobi and would be playing in the New Stanley Hotel. I got up a party and about a dozen of us went off to dine and hear the cabaret. Among our party was Don deTray, an American vet working on the rinderpest campaign. Louis and his band arrived on stage (a low cabaret dais really) to tumultuous applause and started to play. Don turned to me and said, 'Do you know that I used to play with Louis when I was a student in Chicago? I was always broke and playing second cornet to Louis paid a lot of bills.'

'You must go and say hello to him,' I said. After much exhortation from all the party, Don finally went up to the stage. Louis took one look at this unexpected figure climbing up onto the stage. 'Duuuuuunnnnnnnn!' he exclaimed, flung his arms out and embraced Don and dragged him off to the dressing room. They returned with Don bearing his second cornet and they played together for the rest of the evening: Don was not in practice and his lip was not up to playing much at a time but it got better the longer the evening went on. It was a wonderful evening. Louis Armstrong died while we were in Kenya and the *East African Standard* gave him a marvellous editorial obituary which ended with those memorable words 'Blackbird, Bye Bye.'

There were other memorable evenings in the New Stanley Hotel but our first visit was traumatic. Rosslyn Park Rugby Club were touring Kenya and on the Saturday afternoon we went to see them trounce the Impala Club. In the bar after the game we met up with an old friend who was with the touring party. John Davies introduced us to his sister Annie who worked in Nairobi and after a few beers it was decided that we would meet up at eight in the New Stanley for dinner. The problem was that Maxine and I had about ksh 35 (about £1.75), not enough to dine in style even in those far-off days. It was not that we had no money but it was in the bank as one carried no more cash than one needed; credit cards were still several years in the future and restaurants would not accept cheques. We did a tour of the estate at Kabete knocking up friends and trying to beg, borrow or steal their money. We were only partially successful and set off for the New Stanley. We arrived deliberately late so that I did not have to buy a round of drinks; we ate the cheapest dishes on the menu and imbibed the wine modestly. It was a great evening amid a host of people we had not met before. But you can imagine our chagrin when as the end of the evening Morgan Schroeder who was the boss of the Grant Advertising Agency, called for the bill and asked for it to be charged to the company account. Happy memories of Africa filled my head as I drove into the car park at the lab and turned my thoughts again to swine dysentery.

It was obvious that we had a system of eradication that did work. What was needed was a body of evidence so that we could publish, and it was decided that John and I could devote a good proportion of our time to this enterprise. And this is where dear old John showed his worst side: He was great at doing things once he got started, but trying to get him to do anything quickly was another matter. I also tore my hair out trying to persuade him to write up his work. The work was done and I had hoped that an article in the *Veterinary Record* would stimulate the profession into using our technique – and it was *our* technique, not mine and so I was unwilling to publish it without him. By the time the work was published it had been widely used by numerous other workers, who published before us. It did not really matter but at the time it was infuriating. I thought, I am going to keep the next discovery to myself!

12

Vaccine Failure

'Detection is, or ought to be, an exact science and should be treated in the same cold and unemotional manner.'

Sir Arthur Conan Doyle, *The Sign of Four*

I loved working with the students as they kept us very much on our toes. There was an additional perk, that even part-time university teachers had to have a Cambridge degree. You could only teach part time for three years and so, if they wished you to continue, you were given a Master of Arts degree and so, in 1976, John and I duly presented ourselves to the Vice Chancellor of the university, Rose Murray, knelt, touched hands and were awarded our degrees.

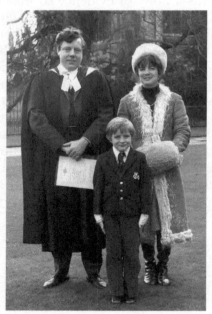

Maxine and Richard with Roger when he received his MA from the University of Cambridge.

214

Some people can be very thick and totally unable to see what is staring them in the face. Sherwin's dictum was you only see what you know (I think that he had borrowed it from one of those Greek philosophers). While I was the principal culprit, Sherwin and John were also guilty. This was certainly true of a string of cases with which we were presented. Weaned pigs of a similar age to those dying of dysentery were showing nervous signs: fits, trembling, unable to stand and scrabbling when lying on their side, showing tetanic spasms of the limbs, high fever and they usually died: some pigs treated with antibiotics did recover and if they had not been too seriously affected then they made a full recovery.

Post mortem examination showed the classic signs of a septicaemia, which occurs when bacteria and/or their toxins are being carried round the body in the blood stream: these signs include congestion throughout the carcase identified by the blood vessels all appearing to be full of blood, strands of fibrin like strips of candy floss were attached to the organs in the abdomen and thorax. When the skull was opened there was a severe inflammation of the meninges, which was seen as a purple colouration over the whole surface caused by the meninges being full of blood. The brain was removed for Cyril's attention and cultures were set up from various tissues including meninges and brain. We failed to isolate any significant bacteria from any of the tissues although we kept isolating faecal streptococci from all the sites. The faeces of normal pigs are hooching with streptococci and it is not easy to stop contamination in the post mortem room when there are many animals to be examined.

Histological examination confirmed that the pigs were dying from meningitis. After several weeks and at least twenty post mortem examinations of which I was responsible for ten or twelve, the penny started to drop. I asked Cyril to stain the brain smears with Gram's Stain and when he did, we found that the meninges were packed with Gram Positive streptococci. These 'faecal' streptococci were the cause of the problem. We had been isolating them for several weeks and throwing them away: you see what you know! We started to look carefully at these bacteria and we sought the services of Dr Stuart Elliott, Britain's leading expert on streptococci, a medical doctor, fellow of Corpus Christi, Cambridge and a personal friend of Rebecca Lancefield, the great American scientist who pioneered the classification of the huge streptococcal genus that is a major cause of meningitis in humans.

Back in the fifties Ivor Field working in the Cambridge Veterinary Investigation Centre isolated a streptococcus from outbreaks of meningitis in unweaned pigs which was shown to be a member of Lancefield's Group S (really a sub group within D, which are the classic faecal organisms). He and Stuart Elliott called it *Streptococcus suis* type 1, which, while an important cause of loss, never reached epidemic proportions. Stuart Elliott showed that our bacterium belonged to Lancefield's Group R and so we called this organism *Streptococcus suis* type 2. We found out this bacterium had been identified causing meningitis in weaned pigs in Holland, but this was the first isolate in Britain and we needed to prove that it was the real cause of disease.

We contacted the Home Office Inspector, who checked on our behaviour under the Animal Experimentation Regulations, to ask whether we could attempt to infect a few pigs with the organism, and received the go-ahead. We obtained three weaned pigs from a farm known to be free from the infection and settled them into a pen in our animal house. They were bedded on deep straw to ensure that they were comfortable and a couple of days later we took a blood sample from a vein of each of the pigs and sprayed a suspension of the organisms that Peter had prepared into each nostril. Rectal temperatures were taken on a daily basis and plotted on graph paper. After a week temperatures of two of the pigs began to rise, then they started to show the signs of fever, and soon after the signs of meningitis were seen: we had our evidence and the pigs were put to sleep. Post mortem examinations confirmed that we had produced the same disease as we were seeing in the field outbreaks. As the police would say, we had enough evidence to convict *Streptococcus suis* type 2 of causing the meningitis. Stuart Elliott and I published this work in a scientific journal, and the flood gates opened. Within a few weeks of that publication, there were reports of the infection from Aberdeen to Truro and Bangor to Norwich, in fact wherever in Britain pigs were kept. It seems that we were not the only ones who had seen these faecal streptococci on the culture plate and decided that they were unimportant contaminants.

Meningitis caused by *Streptococcus suis* type 2 rapidly rose through the ranks to become, after swine dysentery, the second most important cause of loss to the British pig farmer. But what were we to do about it? As Sherwin never tired of saying, 'we were not in business to make diagnoses, but to solve problems'. We knew that if the pigs were treated with antibiotics early enough, and before the onset of the nervous signs then the prognosis was good and most pigs recovered without any long-term effects, but once nervous signs appeared they never made a full recovery. The problem for us was that we knew nothing about how the disease behaved, and whether all pigs were harbouring the infection and some specific event set off the disease or whether if a pig became infected with the organism it became diseased.

There were so many variables and not enough knowledge. We needed to get out on the farms and find out what was happening. This was how I met Polly, a fourth year student, and engaged to a clergyman. When a Cambridge student studies veterinary medicine they start by studying for two years for the Natural Science Tripos part one: this is a very flexible course and the vet students were advised to include anatomy and physiology and other courses for the tripos. For part two of the tripos the students can, within reason, study what they like and Polly chose theology: she was teased unmercifully about this option and the general view was that it was a 'belt and braces job', so that if her treatment failed she could apply to a higher authority. Polly was a small, dark-haired, vivacious young woman with a wicked grin and a great sense of humour: she was also the best student I ever had working with me; apart from her knowledge and ability to learn she had the rare skill, in one so young, of being able to make sound judgements and her technical ability was already streets ahead of mine!

On one farm Polly was one of two students and I demonstrated to them the technique of taking blood samples from the anterior vena cava vessel of pigs. For this you put the pigs onto their backs and insert your needle into the pig where the neck becomes the chest. In pigs up to 50 lb it is a fairly simple technique because the pigs are easy to restrain, and I put the vacutainer needle into the pig, then punctured the rubber cap of the vacutainer tube and the blood was sucked into the tube. There were eighteen pigs to be bled; I did the first one and Polly did sixteen while poor old Sam struggled to get one.

I phoned round the major pig practices in the area and said that we were trying to get information on the new meningitis and so we would like to visit as many farms as possible where we had confirmed the disease. They were a good bunch of practitioners; the response was magnificent and we were run off our feet. Sera and throat swabs,

217

we decided, were what was needed and we decided to take these samples from five percent of the weaned pigs on the farm. Stuart Elliot had a consultancy post in the Public Health Laboratory and he undertook to examine the sera for antibodies to *Streptococcus suis* type 2. Over that summer I spent three afternoons a week visiting farms with the problem, collecting histories and taking samples and Polly was a regular helper. Usually there were one or two more students with us. Meanwhile back in the lab Peter had developed a good system for examining the samples while keeping the amount of work under control.

We had remarkably little to show for all the work that we did. Most pigs on the affected farms had antibodies to the organism in their blood, whereas sera from unaffected farms showed no such antibody but not all pigs on the infected farms carried the organism in their throats. We were no nearer working out a plan for controlling the infection.

There was no doubt that the disease was much more common on the farms that purchased hybrid pigs but by this time the majority of farmers were buying such pigs. We had not, however, identified the disease in a closed herd. A parallel in the field of human medicine came to mind: Sherwin had done his National Service (two years in the army before going to vet school) and was keenly aware of the problem that confronted the army when billeting large numbers of young men together under stressful conditions. Respiratory diseases were rife; possibly the stress lowers the resistance of the soldiers. Meningitis outbreaks in university halls of residence were a constant worry to the authorities. Weaned pigs being herded into trucks, then driven for long distances, and ending up in new accommodation and mixing with pigs from other farms could certainly be likened to the experience of conscripts or students. It seemed more and more possible that the infection was being spread by pigs taking the organism onto a farm.

And so a control method was beginning to evolve. It consisted of setting up isolation premises on a farm away from the main buildings and keeping the incoming pigs in this unit in isolation for a fortnight at the minimum and a month if it was possible. These pigs were to be treated as if they were infected and be fed after the main herd work was finished. Separate boots and gowns were to be worn before entering the quarantine and they were to be scrubbed and disinfected after every use. The incoming pigs were to receive a proper course of treatment for the infection. To start with we took throat swabs from the pigs before they joined the main herd, but since we never isolated the organism this was discontinued. We knew that we had 'made it' when Dan Archer's pig herd (of 'The Archers' radio soap) was diagnosed with *Streptococcus suis* type 2 meningitis and control measures were discussed on the radio.

A further refinement of the quarantine method was made: a couple of healthy pigs from the main herd were put in with the quarantine pigs but were not treated. If there was sub-clinical or hidden disease in these pigs then they would probably transmit it to the untreated farm pigs. We used an identical method for swine dysentery control and with modifications it could be used for any disease in any species of animal. Farmers, like the rest of society, grow lazy when everything is going well, and vigilance slips. Disease control costs money and in these unprofitable farming times with margins squeezed on all sides, who can blame them? We would make a diagnosis of a disease on a farm for which there were excellent vaccines available and then say to the farmer, 'Why don't you vaccinate against this disease?'

To which came the inevitable reply, 'I vaccinated for years, but we've never had the disease, so we stopped.' They ignore the fact that it was the vaccination that had controlled the disease!

'And now you have the disease and that one dead beast has cost you more than you would have paid for several years of vaccine.'

Vaccines were very much on our minds with regard to *Streptococcus suis* type 2; meningo-coccal meningitis in young people is always a worrying problem and the pharmaceutical companies were working desperately to produce a vaccine. With that in mind I phoned an old friend from Kenya days who was now Head of Veterinary Research at Wellcome/Coopers at their Berkhamsted Laboratory, and made an appointment to see him. Armed with all our results I drove down to Berkhamsted and went directly to his house for lunch. Paul Capstick was a member of that generation of Glasgow vets who made a huge contribution to the development of veterinary medicine. He had been director of the Foot and Mouth Laboratory in Embakasi in Kenya and was later to direct the Centre for Insect Physiology and Ecology also in Kenya, but he was currently living in a beautiful eighteenth-century thatched cottage near the laboratory.

Over lunch we talked of Kenya and the friends we had in common, and left work subjects until we were seated in comfortable armchairs in his gargantuan office. I told him about our work with meningitis in the laboratory and on the farms, and of our interest in producing a vaccine for which we thought that there would be good commercial possibilities.

'Do you know the cost and complexity of developing a vaccine these days?' I knew that he was sore about the changes that had occurred in a post thalidomide world. 'For any sort of vaccine for animals we are looking at a minimum of five million pounds and that is only if it works out from the start.'

'Is there no way you could call it an experimental vaccine or something?' I said.

'You have given me an idea; we could produce autogenous killed vaccines for each farm and that would get us away from the regulations. If that worked and we obtained good results then we could think again about making a big investment.'

This would involve them in much more work but much less expense since no form of licence was required for an autogenous vaccine, because the vaccine is made with the strain of the organism isolated from that particular farm. They would make a separate vaccine for each farm. The discussion continued about the protocols of the vaccine; what age, what dosage size, how many shots of vaccine per animal and how we would evaluate the results. We finally produced a detailed plan and I set off home.

Again a call was made to the practices to select a dozen or so farms who would be prepared to take part in a vaccine trial, and soon a list was drawn up; pigs with meningitis were sent in for us to isolate *Streptococcus suis* type 2 and send it to Berkhamsted with a request for the number of doses required. Again the vet students were called in to help with the vaccinations and we had volunteers aplenty. The practising vet was required to visit the farm once a week, the farmer had to keep detailed records and all dead animals were to be sent to us for examination. The first vaccine was given when the pigs were weaned. This presented some problems because the old fashioned practice of weaning at eight weeks was dying, being replaced by weaning at five weeks and some farmers had actually brought it down to three. The reason for this was profit: the earlier a sow was weaned the sooner she could be put to the boar to produce another litter. We decided to vaccinate at weaning, irrespective of age. It was lucky that for some time farmers had been running their sows in batches so that they could be served, farrow and weaned in a group which reduced their work: it certainly reduced ours!

Half of each litter was to be vaccinated and since it is not the general practice to identify individual pigs, a mark was to be tattooed in the left ear of each vaccinated pig. We went out and selected pigs for vaccination by a very basic method of randomisation. The pigs in each litter were paired off, we had a marked card and a blank card, and the farmer chose one card: if he chose the marked card then the pig was vaccinated and its pair left unvaccinated. Two weeks later we returned to the farm and vaccinated them again. No untoward reactions to the vaccine were seen, and so it became a matter of getting on with something else while waiting for the results to come in.

On some farms we had complete protection of the vaccinated pigs, while some of their unvaccinated companions became sick: on other farms the results were not so good and we saw the disease in some vaccinated animals. On those farms where the protection was not absolute there were always more unvaccinated pigs affected than vaccinated. A statistical analysis indicated that the vaccine delivered a significant level of protection but I have always distrusted statistical analyses: if you need to carry out a mathematical calculation to determine whether a vaccine has worked or not, then in my book it has not worked. Despite this I felt that we had shown that a vaccine could be possible and that playing around with the different methods of production, of inactivation and of delivery, it was possible that a good efficient vaccine could be produced. Paul Capstick was happy to wait for an official ministry request to look at the possibility of a commercial vaccine. A detailed report of the trial and an analysis of the results was drawn up and sent to the powers in Tolworth.

What a rebuff we received. What on earth were we thinking of, wanting support when there was not a shred of evidence that the vaccine worked? How they could ignore the farms where we had a hundred percent protection, I do not know. However, that was the end of the *Streptococcus suis* type 2 vaccine. A vaccine was never made and now never will be. I believe that it is the indiscriminate use of antibiotics that has resulted in the plethora of new strains of *Streptococcus suis* infecting pigs today. However, there has been a collapse of profitability of the pig industry in Britain, brought on by a welter of European legislation that only seems to be obeyed in Britain.

At a final meeting with Paul Capstick I told him that I was sorry that we had not achieved our goal and that I felt sad because I was certain that a good vaccine could have been produced. There were certain unanswered questions, such as what would have happened had we used the strain that gave complete protection on a farm where we had only had poor protection?

'It is all water under the bridge for me,' said Paul. 'You would have been dealing with a new Head of Research, as I have resigned.'

'What?'

'The British veterinary pharmaceutical industry is finished; today everything is controlled by the accountants and bean counters, and a solid return of seven million pounds a year in profits is not considered good enough: better sell off the business or close it down and use the capital for something more profitable and to hell with the animals that need the drugs or vaccines. Sir Henry Wellcome would be turning in his grave if he knew what these boys are doing to the company that he loved. Anyway in ten years' time there will be no major British player in the veterinary drug field. The market is too small and there is not enough money to be made.

'And so I am off back to Kenya to run the International Centre for Insect Physiology and Ecology, back to running an institute that can identify a problem and try and resolve it for the benefit of mankind rather than look at the bottom line and decide that it is not big enough.'

'All I can do is to thank you and wish you well in your new venture,' was all I could say in reply.

I thought back to how that institute came to be set up. There is an International Society for the Study of Insect Physiology and Ecology, and I can never think of this organisation without thinking of Victorian vicars roaming the countryside with their butterfly nets. The Natural Science Department Museum in Cambridge has countless thousands of insects collected on their rambles round rural Cambridgeshire. The International Society was firmly established in my mind as a bunch of ancient boffins rushing round the globe looking at insects and the problems they caused. When I was working at the East African Veterinary Research Institute in Muguga we had a visit from the members of this august society on a field trip to Kenya. I had never before, nor have I since, seen such an illustrious collection of Nobel Prize winners gathered together in one room and they were like small schoolboys being allowed out on a field trip. They were just bubbling with an infectious enthusiasm for everything around them. They spent the whole day in our laboratories delving into everything. Their main reason for visiting us was to see the work of the FAO team in producing a vaccine against East Coast fever which was transmitted by ticks and was the biggest killer of cattle in Kenya.

They enjoyed themselves so much that they arranged a dinner for the laboratory staff with them in the Muguga Club, which must rate as the most surreal evening of my life. We sat at tables of four and at my table I was the only one not to have won a Nobel Prize. Two of them were joshing the third (who was responsible for the contraceptive pill) about what he was doing with his prize money: it transpired that he had bought a vineyard in California and was going to market the wine as Smips, which stood for Steroids Made It Possible. The jests flew around and the whole dining room was alive with good humour and mirth.

After dinner we adjourned to the dance hall where there was a small dais and chairs arranged to make an audience. We took our seats and Dr Chan, a Nobel winner for his work on the chemistry of the pill, entertained us to a great variety of brilliantly executed conjuring tricks, mostly involving cards and coins. It was some evening.

As a result of this field trip they set up their Centre at Chiromo on the university campus, where Paul was going as director. My only previous contact with Chiromo was when working in the Diagnosis Section at the Veterinary Research Laboratory at Kabete. I was sitting at my desk when there was knock on the door, which opened to reveal a small dark-haired man with a small moustache and large black boots who was dressed in a dark-blue heavy serge three-piece suit complete with gold watch-chain.

'Is zis zee Department of Chemistry?' he enquired.

'I am afraid not, but come in out of the sun and sit down.' I offered him a cup of tea which he accepted. I explained that the Department of Chemistry was in Chiromo in the centre of the city. 'But do not worry I will explain to your driver how to find it.' Over the cup of tea I found out who my visitor was: another Nobel Laureate who did so much for mankind. He was Sir Ernst B. Chain who, along with Fleming and Florey, gave us penicillin; the start of the antibiotic era that revolutionised the treatment of infections in man and animals. He was in Nairobi to give a lecture on the development of synthetic penicillins.

'Would it be possible for me to attend?' I asked.

'Of course, zee lecture is open to all, pliz come. It is tomorrow at zree pm in zee Chemistry Department.'

He finished his tea and set off to the correct place, but I was thrilled to have met him and had a chance to talk awhile. Several of us from the Vet Lab went to his talk which was a masterpiece of content and delivery. He described how they had isolated the nucleus of the penicillin molecule because it was felt that side chains could be added to the nucleus and in this way antibiotics could be tailor-made to specific infections; such has proved to be the case with a whole range of synthetic penicillins now available.

It was not only the streptococcal vaccine that failed, so did our attempts to keep the Veterinary Investigation Service out of the clutches of the Field Service. Tony Stevens sold us down the river for his own promotion. Tony had come up through the ranks of the Veterinary Investigation Service and had even worked in the hallowed precincts of the Cambridge Centre. However, he was not interested in the Service, only in getting to the top. And like all converts he became worse in his attitude than his Field Service colleagues. It was made clear to us that if we wanted to run a Centre then we had to do our time in the 'Salt Mines', as the headquarters of the Field Service at Tolworth was known. At my promotion interview, Tony laid it on the line to me that if I did not go to Tolworth, then I would never be promoted. I went to Tolworth and loathed almost every minute of it: Divisional Veterinary Officers in the Salt Mines were the lowest of the low, particularly where Sandy Lowe was concerned and he was now in charge of the Veterinary Investigation Service. We did not wish to move house and so I became a weekly commuter to Surrey; I purchased a boat and lived on the Thames at Richmond. The only good thing that came out of this was that I was able to go to the National Theatre and the Barbican Theatre to see the Royal Shakespeare Company two or three times a week.

I was put into the TB and Brucella Section and my boss was Harry Evans from the Valleys. A delightful man but politically naïve, and it could be said that he alone is responsible for the mess that the British cattle industry is now in with regard to tuberculosis. The role of badgers in the life story of bovine TB was just being unfolded by Tony Little at Weybridge and John Gallagher in the Gloucester Centre. They showed that the badger lacked the necessary immune system to deal with TB and so the animal died a rather unpleasant death. It was obvious to several of us at Tolworth that something had to be done about controlling the disease in both cattle and badgers for the well-being of both. Despite the badger being a rather unpleasant and vicious, if beautiful, animal, thanks to Kenneth Graham's *Wind in the Willows* he gets a very good press as a lovely cuddly soft toy. I asked to see Harry and explained that it was essential that the policy of the Ministry should be to control the disease in both species to ensure that both species could lead healthy lives without infecting each other.

'Roger, boyo, we are the Ministry of Agriculture, Fisheries and Food, we are not here to look after all the wildlife.'

How typical of the Field Service mentality, as with that statement he destroyed the cattle industry in Britain. When he said it, there remained only two foci of TB in Britain, Cornwall and Gloucestershire – forty years on and thanks to the 'Badger Lobby' and the cessation of culling badgers, together with a succession of Ministers of Agriculture who have known nothing about farming and cared less, there is not a county in Wales and western England that is not now infected, and the disease is creeping back into Scotland, at a huge cost to British farmers and the taxpayer. If only the Field Service had realised that it was a *service*! When badgers were first culled, the whole sett was killed using a gaseous poison which was highly effective. Culling of badgers has now been reinstated, but the badgers are shot at night: a policy that is doomed to fail. I want to see healthy populations of cattle and badgers living together: to achieve this a proper method must be employed to kill all the badgers in setts where there are diseased animals.

My presence in the section was considered too disruptive by Howard Rees, Harry's boss and another man who was vying for the top job (he made it) and did not want some upstart DVO spoiling his chances. I was moved into the Notifiable Disease Section, anything to get me out of Rees's hair. Here I was put in charge of the Protein Processing Order and coordinating the Monthly Report of the Veterinary Investigation Service. It was, of course the change in the law on the processing of animal proteins that resulted in the bovine spongiform encephalopathy (BSE) outbreak that also played its part in destroying our livestock industry.

For years we had had a policy on the treatment of waste food products, but the companies that carried out the rendering of this

225

waste material into animal feed wanted a change in the law because they felt that they could not compete with their European counterparts. As it stood the law required that waste foods should be heated twice and then extracted with an organic solvent to remove the fat, which was then used in the tallow industry for making candles. Why the law required this was anyone's guess: like so many of the regulations concerning animals they are not based on facts and evidence but on the opinion of a few desk wallahs sitting in Head Office. However, in this case, by some means, they had got it right and they had kept us free from BSE. Not any longer. The processors had their way and, again on the strength of no evidence at all, the regulations were changed: only one cooking and no compulsory fat extraction, and BSE was let loose among our animals. I had stated in my report to the brass (the Regional Veterinary Officer) that no changes in the regulations should be made without a proper reason: I even quoted their reply to our detailed work on TB in pigs requesting that the regulations be changed but again I was only a humble DVO. Again my arguments were rejected.

It seemed that my life at Tolworth was to be one long losing battle with the brass. I enlisted the aid of Tom Alexander, the Cambridge pig disease expert, to try and persuade them that it was not necessary to slaughter pigs with swine vesicular disease, since it was a self-limiting and an unimportant disease of pigs. However, pigs with SVD were slaughtered because the disease looked like foot and mouth disease. They could not see that this was a false philosophy: why not slaughter pigs with any foot lesions because they look like SVD? Tom came down from Cambridge but I was not allowed to be privy to the discussions because this was a Cambridge expert talking to a Deputy Chief Veterinary Officer, the number two in the land. Roger Blamire a man of considerable power, if limited ability, opened his discussions with Tom with the memorable expression: 'Now Tom, don't try and blind me with science.' Not surprisingly, SVD remained a disease punishable by death.

We still had our financial worries and our son Richard was giving cause for concern. He was extremely bright and the local village school could not cope with clever children. He was near the top of the class without doing any work and he was bored. He took out his frustrations on his mother with bouts of extremely bad behaviour. He needed to go to a school that would make him work and so make him happy. We could not afford private education.

I returned home from work one Friday evening to find an un-opened telegram waiting for me. It was from the Food and Agri-cultural Organisation in Rome, offering me the post of Veterinary Microbiologist in Salta, north-west Argentina; we had to get the atlas out to find out where it was. This was the answer to our prayers, I would get away from the Salt Mines and Richard could go to a school where he would be made to work. Maxine and I dis-cussed the implications of this move; once we had started on the treadmill of private education, we had to provide it for all three and this meant working overseas until the children's education was complete – still some twelve to fifteen years in the future. Our parents were getting older and my parents already had one of their three children living out of the country: Maxine's father and my mother died before we returned to live in Britain. We loved our house and did not want to give it up but the Hinds offered to look after the renting out. We decided to accept the offer. But how had it come about?

The answer was not long in coming. Some years previously we had had a delightful Australian, Robin Condon, working in the labora-tory as part of his Master's Degree Course at the Centre for Tropical Veterinary Medicine in Edinburgh. He had returned to Australia and had been recruited by a friend of his to work as the microbiologist on the FAO project in Salta. He and his wife Rosemary had gone off to Argentina but his wife was extremely unhappy there and so he had resigned his post and returned home, but not before recommending me to the Project Manager. The mystery was explained.

I sent a telegram to Rome, accepting their offer. Once I had a contract and a firm date for travel, I informed my bosses that I was leaving: my six months' stay in Tolworth made me the shortest stay prisoner to date. My record was soon broken as other people found the work so uncongenial, not to mention demeaning. There was a huge sigh of relief at Tolworth and I was transferred with immediate effect to the Central Veterinary Laboratory at Weybridge, so that I could 'brush up my laboratory skills before leaving for South America'. It was good to be back in a scientific environment again and I was based in the Bacteriology Section but received tutorials from staff in Serology, Brucellosis, Breeding Diseases, Virology, Rabies, Epidemiology, and from Duggie Wilson himself. It was good to be back in an environment where people treated you for who you were and what you knew, rather than your rank.

The Ministry were very generous in several ways: first because I had moved to the CVL I was again, having changed posting, entitled to be paid a daily subsistence rate, and second I was asked if I wished to be placed on unpaid leave of absence which enabled me to maintain my place in the pecking order. I accepted both with thanks.

The weekends were busy as we had to pack up the house and organise stuff to go to Argentina, stuff to go into store and stuff to remain in the house. Our Willingham friends rallied round and the local clockmaker volunteered to look after our grandfather clock and promised to have it in peak condition when we needed it again. Other friends took items of furniture too precious to be put into store, such as button-backed Victorian chairs and sofas, or antique mirrors. We also had to find a school for Richard. An old Kenya friend was now headmaster of a boy's school in Cheshire, but as we had no family in that part of the world (they were congregated in London or East Anglia) he advised us not to send Richard to his school but suggested we contact Ian Angus, headmaster of Orwell Park School just outside Ipswich. What wonderful advice it was: Ian is the best educator that I have ever met, who believed that every boy excelled at something and that it was the duty of the school to find out what that 'something' was, because 'The moment the boy realises he can do something better than the others, his confidence increases by leaps and bounds and everything else that he does improves. Education is about building confidence in the boy.' He was another small man who was perfectly happy in his size, and made a feature of it by standing on a beer crate to address his audience at speech day. Since this was not the time of year for admissions, Richard was given a series of written papers and was then interviewed by Ian and his wife. He was accepted. Boarding education for Richard gave him a sound education and prepared him well for university, but he did not enjoy being away from home.

We were now all set to go. I was to go first and find a house and generally get set up, and Maxine would follow with the children once the school holidays began. A new phase in our life was beginning and I was to receive further training in a new continent in the art and science of veterinary detection, and the problems of project management.

13

How Not to Run a Project

'Game for a morning drive?'
Sir Arthur Conan Doyle, *The Man with the Twisted Lip*

I have had many fine teachers throughout my life but I had to go to Argentina to find one who would give me a stark lesson in how NOT to do something. It was not possible to fly direct from Britain to Buenos Aires, one either had to change planes in Caracas, Bogota or Rio de Janeiro in South America, or fly from a European city, Paris, Frankfurt or Madrid. I chose Paris as it enabled me to visit my sister and then fly overnight to Buenos Aires.

Usually when appointed to work for the Food and Agriculture Organisation you are instructed to go to Rome for briefing; but for some reason they were so keen to get me to Salta that they dispensed with this phase of the protocol, which meant that I arrived in Argentina with no knowledge of how the system worked, how I was going to be paid or indeed what I was going to be paid. They sent me a ticket and I borrowed money from the bank to tide me over until the salary began to come in. All the United Nations Agencies are controlled within a country by the United Nations Development Program (UNDP) office in the country. I had heard from them that if there was no one to meet me (and there was no one to meet me) then I should take a taxi to the hotel where a room had been booked for me. Ezeiza Airport, like so many capital city airports, is miles from the city itself. I was instructed to get a receipt for the taxi journey and claim the money back.

A delightful taxi driver drove me to the hotel, chatting away all the while, but I could hardly understand a word he said as I had been told that it was not necessary to speak Spanish for the job and so FAO would not pay for lessons before I was recruited. I had done my best to learn from a book and cassettes. But learning a language without having anyone to practice with is like learning to swim from

229

a manual with no pool. We arrived at the hotel and I was told that the cost was thirty five thousand pesos and so I handed the driver a note for fifty thousand, which he returned to me – saying that this was only five thousand. I looked at the note and sure enough it was five thousand pesos. I took out my wallet and handed him another note for fifty thousand, and again he returned a note of five thousand. By then the peso had dropped and I realised that he was palming the note. So one hundred thousand pesos lighter I held on to the note of fifty thousand while he counted the change and then we exchanged notes. Welcome to South America!

It was June, approaching mid-winter and Argentina was ruled by the clock, consequently the hotel had no restaurant; that only operated during the summer months. I was in need of a sleep after my sleepless night on the plane. By 7 pm I was up and showered and feeling better able to face the city. Dinner was the next item on my agenda and I was given directions to a nearby restaurant which turned out to be one of the best in the country and enormous. At least 100 tables each set for four people. This was Buenos Aires, the capital of the most important country in South America (or so the Argentines thought) and I walked into their best restaurant at 7.30 to find a single diner – the Argentines do not dine until 10 pm. I was escorted to my table and positioned with my back to the sole other diner: neither of us could see the other. The menu was brought and in my halting Spanish I ordered dinner. After I had completed my order I heard a voice behind me, 'Would you care to join me, or do you prefer to eat alone?'

This was my first meeting with Dr Richard Sykes, who worked in a senior capacity for ICI (that once great British company); he was in Argentina to, as he put it, 'buy energy for ICI'. He was looking at possible coal or oil purchases for the company. We had a delicious meal and Richard was excellent company, he knew a great deal about the country. We met up a few times in Buenos Aires and he later came and stayed with us in Salta; we became firm friends.

Breakfast next morning was at a little café round the corner from the hotel where you stood at a counter and ate excellent croissants stuffed with ham and cheese while drinking superb coffee. I had to spend several days in Buenos Aires at the UNDP office, sorting out salary payments which had to be paid into a bank in New York. It was fun opening a New York bank account from Buenos Aires, luckily there was a branch of an American Bank based inside the UN headquarters in New York. I was also instructed that upon arrival in Salta I was to open a bank account with an Argentine bank so that they could pay money into it directly. I was paid all sorts of allowances and finally given a ticket to Salta.

At that time inflation in Argentina was running at eight percent per month, which in the end was to cause the closure of the project. The government of the country were tightly controlling the value of the Argentine peso and so each month the cost to FAO in dollar terms was rocketing. To ensure that its staff round the world all have equal purchasing power with their salary, each international employee is given a 'Post Adjustment Allowance' which is recalculated each year. In Argentina it was recalculated each month! My post adjustment increased from $1800 per month to just over $4000 in two years. Fifty percent of your basic salary and all the Post Adjustment had to be paid into your local account. This in turn led to a great scam on the part of the UNDP staff: they received our salaries and post adjustment in bulk from the UN head office in New York and it was their job to forward it to our banks. Each month the money arrived later and later: what they were obviously doing was investing our cash for a week or two or three before sending it on to us, and pocketing the interest. There were ten FAO staff in Salta receiving at least $5000 each per month – eight percent of $50,000 every month was a nice little earner. Because the mail service in Argentina was so unreliable we were allowed to use the UN Diplomatic bag. We were certain that the Buenos Aires office were opening our mail, because things were going astray from envelopes. This was confirmed when my *Guardian* arrived with the crossword partly completed.

One night during my stay in the capital I was taken out to dinner by Bob Houben, a Dutchman who was an auditor for Philips, the Dutch electronics giant. Bob and his wife Marit were a godsend to us. We had met him in Willingham when he visited the Philips plant in Cambridge. Willingham friends knew that he was based in Buenos Aires and thought that it might be useful for us to meet. Marit was in Holland and so Bob took me to dinner in a gaucho restaurant where the menu consists of beef, beef and more beef; you will probably have seen pictures of whole bovine carcases split and being grilled. Bob suggested that he order and I agreed. We started with some chorizos, those wonderful spicy sausages at which the Spaniards excel. I was amazed that Bob had only ordered one portion between the two of us and only one skewer of the brochette. I need not have worried. There must have been a kilo of chorizo into which we made but slight inroads. The brochette when it arrived was more than three feet long. On it there were six cubes of prime beef each about six inches in all directions. Between the cubes of meat were miniscule slivers of onion and pepper. What a feast! I have never eaten such succulent, flavourful beef. I managed only one and a half of the cubes even though they were liberally washed down with first-class Argentine red wine. It was some introduction to Argentine cuisine.

My arrival in Salta was a very different affair to that in Buenos Aires. The project manager David Broadbent and his wife were both at the airport to greet me. I was whisked off to the hotel and told to leave my suitcase there, as we were off to the Broadbents' house for the remainder of the day. They were wonderful hosts and very kind and generous to me. We were not allowed to discuss the project until we got into the office the following morning but we talked of our respective careers. David was actually English and had qualified at the Royal Veterinary College in London but had spent most of his working life in Australia where he was a Veterinary Field Officer, with no laboratory background, before joining FAO. Anita was his second wife, and his son from his first marriage was in Salta but going through a difficult time and causing the Broadbents many problems.

They lived in a lovely little house in the centre of the city and I was made very welcome. Both of them were fanatical classical music lovers and I thought that it would be wonderful for Maxine to have friends who were so interested in music; I am eternally grateful to them for introducing me to the Bruch Violin Concerto which I had never heard before and it remains, to this day, one of my favourite pieces of music. It is difficult to reconcile what happened after Maxine's arrival; once she arrived I never visited their house again and it was only with great difficulty that we were able to persuade them to come and see us.

The project was one of two set up by FAO to assist one of the poorer regions of Argentina. It was thought that the high lands of Salta, Jujuy, Tacna and others of the north-west mountain provinces could be used for the production of steers to be fattened on the lush pampas of the south and east of the country. Our project was to look at the animal health implications of this activity while the second project, run by the Australian Ted Campion, was to investigate the best methods of animal husbandry for the area. Argentina boasted a wonderful regional network of research institutes throughout the whole country – Instituto Nacional de Tecnología Agro-pecuaria (INTA) whose central laboratory was at Castellar, set in a huge farm just outside Buenos Aires. The Salta research institute was based in Cerrillos, a small town about ten miles from the city and I suspect it had been set up on an old estancia, or estate with a colonial style house at its centre. The laboratories were set around the house.

David had collected together a distinguished team of 'experts' of which I was much the most junior, to investigate the diseases of the area. There was John Bingley, an Australian biochemist who was particularly interested in mineral deficiency diseases. The Israeli Ayah Hadani was the director of the Tel Aviv Animal Health Laboratory and a distinguished veterinary protozoologist (he was a particular expert in the protozoan blood parasite *Anaplasma marginale* that was prevalent in Africa and the Middle East). David Le Riche, who came from Jersey by way of Kenya and had a Norwegian wife, specialised in worm parasites in cattle and had worked for research institutes and pharmaceutical companies. And I was there to identify the microbes that caused disease in the area and to set up a diagnostic laboratory. David the project manager had no special scientific skills and this was the basic cause of all the problems that beset the project. Instead of accepting the fact and realising that he had an exceptional team that could produce results, he set out to divide and so rule. He was frightened that if we became a team he would be unable to control events, and so we never discussed policy as a team but were seen one by one in his office so that we could not gang up on him. As a policy it was a disaster and when the Argentines were brought into the equation it was even worse. He would discuss with me what we should do, and then with my counterpart Reuben Gonzalez, a large, jovial bear of a man and known by all as Flaco (skinny!), who would be called in and his opinion asked: he would not see us together.

The Argentines were a very talented bunch: the head of the project Gerado Habich, was studying at the Veterinary Epidemiology and Economics Research Unit (VEERU) in Reading at the time of my arrival, and so I only met him on a few occasions when he was back in Salta. In the interim Ernesto Spath was the acting local director; a trainee protozoologist, he was of German origin and had studied at La Plata Veterinary School, about 100 miles from Buenos Aires, as had most of the Argentines including Reuben who was of Italian origin. Graciela Kühne, also of German origin, was a very able parasitologist, working with David. Graciela was murdered some years later by government agents but we were never able to find out why, although there were rumours that she was supplying chemicals from the project for the drug laboratories. Whatever the truth, she was a delightful woman and by her death the country lost a very able scientist.

There were only a few laboratory technicians – Argentine professionals do not like competition from the para-professionals, most of whom were very well trained. Bacteriology boasted Luis who had a good line in chat and knew where you could get everything. As is so often the case with FAO projects, there was a band of young Dutch people, known as Associate Experts who were really there to be trained. Two in particular stick in my mind: Mik Winnen, because he later came to work with me in Gaborone, Botswana, and Ron Dwinger with whom I shared a cubby hole as an office, and who later passed through my life in various guises and now works at the International Atomic Energy Veterinary Centre in Vienna. FAO also provided training places for young Argentines and there were a bevy of them, including one young married couple of veterinarians, Ignacio and his wife Isabela, who joined us in the diagnostic laboratory.

With such a young, enthusiastic bunch we should have achieved great things: instead we achieved almost nothing, because there was no team. This was particularly noticeable during the coffee break in the morning when the Argentines stood in one group speaking in Spanish and the expatriates stood huddled together speaking in English. I learnt that lesson well and later when I ran a laboratory in Peru the speaking of English was forbidden in the presence of Peruvians. This social division was highlighted because many of the young Argentines could not speak English and many of them resented us because they felt that we were talking about them. The senior Argentines also resented our presence because we were paid much more than them, and they felt that if they had just been given the money that we were able to spend on the project they could have achieved the same results: they might have achieved more.

The school holidays were fast approaching and I had to find somewhere to live. Flats in Salta started at $750 a month and a small house cost upwards of $1500 per month. I wanted a garden where the children could play and I found a wonderful country house a couple of miles beyond Cerrillos on the road to Rosario. All Argentines aspire to live in Buenos Aires and all those who live outside the capital like to live in the provincial capital; only peasants live in the country. All the farm managers on the ranches and dairy farms lived in the city of Salta and travelled out to work each day. Even the foremen did not live on the farm but in nearby small towns such as Cerrillos. When I expressed a desire to live in the country I was thought to be mad. Rich Salteños do love to own a country house to go to at the weekends and the road to Rosario was just such a place. The owner of the house that interested me was a doctor who had recently separated from his wife and so he had no use for the house in the short term, and an income of $500 in dollars a month, paid in dollars, would be a useful supplement in those inflationary times. The house was in a good state of decoration: it had three bedrooms, a large sitting room, a huge hall that easily doubled as a dining room and play room for the children. The kitchen was fitted out with modern units with beautiful green alabaster work surfaces, typically South American, superb on style but poor on practicality because if you spilt lemon juice or vinegar it dissolved the worktop! Around two sides of the house was a covered veranda which meant that the children could play outside during the rainy season. During evenings in the rainy season the toads, which were about nine inches high and lived in the down drainpipes, came out to play and to serenade us: they made a delightful noise.

The garden was almost four acres with an orchard and a swimming pool, both of which had been sadly neglected; the grass was about five feet high and the paint was peeling off the pool. There were also swings for the children. With David's help I brought in some labourers to clear the garden and within three days it was done, but before I knew what was going on they had set light to the whole thing: this was the traditional way to get the plants to grow again. We had a wonderful blaze in the garden but were left with the aftermath of the fire – ash and charcoal and the rains were not due for a couple of months. The house was furnished but we needed plates and pots to tide us over until our freight arrived.

Maxine and the family arrived and we all stayed in the hotel for a few nights to allow them to adjust: this was a real problem because we could not get dinner until 10 pm by which time the children were famished and exhausted. Maxine did a round of the wives and found her way round town. We agreed to move in to the house at the weekend when I could borrow a project car. There was no problem getting to and from the laboratory because there was a bus for the junior staff that went past the house and I was able to use that – much to the astonishment of the senior Argentines who would not have dreamed of travelling on a bus with a load of smelly campesinos. I have never stood on my dignity and it got me to work until the car arrived, and in fact for the whole time I was there because it enabled Maxine to have the car.

Maxine was horrified when she saw the state of the garden.

'How am I going to keep the children clean and get their clothes free from soot?'

She was even more horrified on the Monday morning when the water was cut off. The city of Salta's water supply came from the Rosario dam/reservoir and once each year part of the supply was cut off so that the processing plant could be cleaned. We lived on the wrong side of the road! Although we lived in a country house we lived on the east side of the road along with the campesinos – with the exception of our house all the country houses were to the west of the road which had a different supply that was not affected. Representations were made to the local engineer, who was sympathetic but could do nothing. It would be a fortnight before the water supply was returned. It seemed ironic to me that the supply was turned off to houses where people lived but all the empty houses had a regular supply throughout the whole time. South America again.

'I told you that you should live in the city' was the general view of my colleagues. However a temporary supply of dustbins and bowls were driven home on a daily basis. The children got filthy, their clothes were filthy, but by now we had a maid who cleaned it all on a daily basis. Even when the water returned we still had problems until the rain came down and washed all the ash and soot into the soil. But the gardeners were right, with the rain the plants came to life and we found rose beds that brought forth wonderful flowers, We tried to grow vegetables but they were all eaten by the wild guinea pigs that were everywhere. There was an irrigation system that ran through the garden twice a week and within weeks we had a lovely garden with lawns (if that is the correct word for wild grass beds) – however, the beds threw up beautiful small orchids every time that it rained. There were magnificent mulberries, huge, ancient eucalyptus trees, a great fig tree and some small but excellent plum trees as well.

236

We cleaned and painted the pool and then tried to fill it. We were only receiving water on alternate days and we calculated that it would take a month to fill. A visit to Sr Gomez, the water engineer, was called for; he arranged for water bowsers to fill the pool. But only having water on alternate days was a problem as there was only a small tank on the roof. The owner of the house agreed to put a large storage tank in the ground with a pump to fill the roof tank. Problem solved. However, we never knew how much water there was in the upper tank.

Andrew James, a computer expert, solved that for us. Andrew had been sent out by VEERU in Reading to assist us in developing a computer disease recording system for the project; this was my second glimpse into the world that would take over our lives. Andrew worked with David Broadbent, but not the rest of the project, on developing this system that went on to become PANA-CEA a really useful programme for the analysis of disease at the farm level, as opposed to VIDA which was a method of analysing disease records at the national level. When he was in Salta he enjoyed coming out to the house ostensibly for a swim but in reality to play with the children; he was missing his own. The James Patent Water Meter was his first improvement to the Windsor house. A wine bottle was half filled with water, a length of fishing line was then fixed in place by the cork which was jammed into the neck and sealed with the wax from a candle. The bottle was floated in the roof tank and the fishing line was hung over the side of the tank and down the wall of the house. A four-foot length of broomstick was tied horizontally onto the end of the fishing line and the taps turned on until the tank was empty. A thick black line was painted on to the wall below the broomstick, and the tank was filled till water poured from the top. The bottle had risen and the broomstick had fallen, and so a second line was painted on the wall. Our water meter was complete.

Andrew's second improvement was to the pool. There was no filtration system and no means of 'hoovering' the grot off the bottom. During a trip to Buenos Aires I had visited Argentina's only swimming pool accessory shop to find out about filters and 'hoovers', and pills for keeping the water sterile. Everything was imported from the States and I had to sit down when told the price: a small filtration system would cost about $30,000 – we would have to swim in dirty water. Andrew suggested that we make our own filter from a forty-four-gallon drum which we filled with graded layers of gravel and sand, finishing with ten kilos of filtration sand from the pool shop. Here Sr Carlos Massé came to the fore. An architect by profession he found it more lucrative to run a hardware shop and it was a palace of delights; to this day we still keep the sharp 'Massé knives' (Brazilian made by Tramontina) in the kitchen although they are now more than thirty years old. Carlos organised all the welding for the inlet pipes and the 'hoover' and got the vacuum tubing for us. The total outlay for the filter and 'hoover' was $500 or it would have been had I not purchased the filtration sand, that ten kilos cost a further $500; well it was imported. Andrew cunningly modified the pipes to the water tank pump so that we could use the same pump for cleaning the pool. We stopped buying the pills too: since they cost twenty dollars each and lasted a week. Instead we purchased bottles of a low-grade chlorine bleach which cost about fifty cents, and we used two or three a week – but you did not go in the pool for a couple of hours after treatment. Now that we had a pool we were the focus of attention for the project staff. It no longer seemed such a mad idea to live in the country, particularly when we were paying a $1000 a month less in rent.

By now our luggage had arrived and life was more comfortable. This was when the first of our medical disasters occurred. I was dismantling one of the large crates in which the luggage had arrived and Guy, ever the craftsman, was following the work intently. The top of the box was about to fall and so I told him to stand back, which he did. The top did not fall and so he went to inspect it, just as it did fall and smacked right across his left knee. I lifted the box to see the damage and watched as his knee swelled like a football being inflated. I carried him into the house and put him on his bed; he was being very brave and trying not to cry. I went into Cerrillos to get the doctor. Luckily we knew the address of a general physician whose father was a paediatrician (you find out these details at an early stage in a new town!) and even more luckily I had the use of a project car for that weekend. I found Dr Rodriguez and he was delighted to attend the son of an Englishman. He looked at Guy's leg, gently felt around the swelling and then pronounced that nothing was broken – there was nothing to worry about and nothing that a little pawpaw would not cure. We looked at him in surprise.

'Tienen papaya?' he asked. We always had pawpaw in the house as it was an excellent breakfast fruit. 'Traigala, y un cuchillo,' he instructed and Maxine brought the pawpaw and a knife. He

238

proceeded to cut the pawpaw into strips and put them on Guy's knee.

'En dos dias, cien por ciento.'

I drove him home but he would accept no fee: it was an honour to treat a British child (this was before Las Malvinas, the Falklands War). Guy made a complete recovery and suffered no long-term effects from the blow.

I flew down to Buenos Aires to meet the people in the main laboratory of INTA at Castellar, and the team working on human brucellosis in Hospital F.J. Muñoz, Upsallata, Buenos Aires, and to collect my car and drive it back to Salta, a thousand or more miles and a two-day drive. Like the roads in central Nigeria, the terrain in the pampas is exceedingly boring: flat, green and uninteresting. Mile after mile of fence posts and barbed wire with the occasional oven bird nest on top of the post to break up the monotony. These fascinating birds build a closed nest of mud that is so complex that predators are unable to get in. There were skunks aplenty and you could smell them as you passed them. The farms were so large that the farmhouses were few and far between, and many a farm had developed into a small village with church, police post and school. There were police blocks at each inter-state border, where you were stopped, your documents examined and possibly the car would be searched – the police needed something to break their monotony, but they were always courteous and polite to foreigners and not looking for 'dashee'. Eventually the foothills of the Andes were reached; the scenery became more congenial and the villages closer together. The night was spent in Tucumán, the birthplace of Argentine independence from Spain and an interesting city with many fine old buildings. The back of the journey was broken as Tucumán was two thirds of the way home. After an excellent steak (there was little choice in restaurants) with some good local wine, it was time for an early bed to be fresh for the journey the following day.

Once I had my car and was no longer dependent upon David for use of a project vehicle we could begin to settle down. The first necessity was a school for Guy and we were in luck; in Cerrillos there was a small school for the children of American missionaries. These protestants had a forlorn time in a strongly Catholic country, but there were enough children for a small boarding school and it was our good fortune that it was sited in Cerrillos. Julio Castro his wife and dedicated band of missionaries ran an excellent school and were persuaded to take Guy. Maxine repaid their kindness by helping with the music teaching. A 'jardin' was found for Claire but this was in Salta and so Maxine had to make the trip each day. Claire loved the company of the little girls and language was no barrier as she soon was fluent in Spanish.

We had decided to use one of the boxes that our luggage had come in as a tree house. There was a magnificent eucalyptus tree by the pool which had the perfect structure for securing a tree house. The house was reconstructed from a packing case, but how to get it up in the tree? Here the le Riche and Campion families came into their own; David and Dikke had a daughter and three sons, the youngest of whom was slightly older than Richard, and the Campions also had an adult son, who was visiting them for the Christmas holidays. First the support struts were nailed to the tree so that the box could be securely fixed. A rope was slung over a bough and fixed to the house. With David up in the tree we hauled on the rope and up she went. David manoeuvred the house onto the supports while we took the weight. He then put in the first securing nails before the young lads were allowed up to complete the job. This took some time and refreshments were required, and so the rope was put into use again to raise and lower David's boot with a thermos of coffee or a box of mince pies. We had been unable to purchase a rope ladder and so Maxine had made one out of broomsticks cut to a suitable length by me and carefully fixed to two lengths of nylon rope. We had brought with us the *Readers' Digest Do-It-Yourself Manual* which gave detailed instructions on the making of a rope ladder. The rope was then firmly attached to the doorway of the house. Once up, the children could raise the ladder and be unreachable. I had some concern because the house was some twenty feet off the ground but the children never had a problem.

It was now time to concentrate on the purpose of my journey to South America, developing a veterinary investigation centre for the north-west of Argentina. With no support from my boss and no interest from my counterpart this was tricky. Reuben, while not opposed to the concept of the laboratory, was really only interested in mastitis and spent all his time and most of our resources to this end. There were many dairy herds in the north west of the country and all of them were dire. Most farm owners lived in Buenos Aires, the managers all lived in Salta or other big cities in the region, and basically the peones were left to their own devices. As a consequence, the husbandry was appalling, the hygiene worse, and the milk unless sterilised was unsafe to drink. Pasteurisation was inadequate to control the contamination.

A single example will suffice as explanation. We would visit a farm to sample the cows at the morning milking; this often meant that we had to leave home at 3 am for the two-hour or more drive to a farm to be there when milking commenced at 5 am. It was still dark. On this particular farm I thought it odd that the dairy had a black ceiling, but made no comment. As milking progressed and the samples stacked up, dawn broke, the sun came up and the temperature rose; I noticed the ceiling starting to move. It was the flies beginning to wake up in the warmth: soon they were buzzing round our heads. This was where a basic human foodstuff was produced, no wonder it had to be sterilised before it could be consumed.

To give Reuben his due he tried hard to convince the farmers that by improving the husbandry and hygiene, they would make much more money. Without the presence of the owner or manager, his talk fell on deaf ears. The samples were taken back to the laboratory where they were processed in much the same way as in Cambridge, although few cell counts were made because this was in the days before electronic counters were commonly used, the laboratory did not have one, and all counts had to be done by hand. Once the cultures had been streaked out on the agar plates they were stacked up in modified milk churns. Inlet and outlet taps had been welded into the lids of the churns so that we could increase the level of carbon dioxide in the atmosphere which improved the conditions for bacterial growth. We had a large walk-in incubator with the temperature controlled at 37° C. The following day the plates were examined and they were usually alive with environmental bacteria – *Escherischia coli*, *Klebsiella*, *Aeromonas*, *Pseudomonas* – together with the more usual causes of mastitis, the *Staphylococcus* and *Streptococcus*. Each farm represented a mountain of work and to what end? After half a dozen of these filthy farms I asked Reuben what was the point of doing all this work when I could give him the results without doing anything? We were no closer to identifying the causes of mastitis, all we were doing was demonstrating what bacteria were present and we did not know which animals had mastitis.

An exception to the rule of farmers not living on their farms was Sr Marinaro, and his dairy farm was next door to the INTA estate. He was an enthusiastic, rather than good, farmer but he did try and put into practice what he was told to do. It was obvious that he had a major mastitis problem and I finally persuaded Reuben that one of the causes of the problem was the milking machine. Luckily I had brought with me the equipment that Robin Mackintosh had taught me to use, so it was decided that we would have a major investigation into Sr Marinaro's problems and invite Argentina's top mastitis man Dr Alfredo Rodriguez from INTA Castellar to join us. As we had already carried out a herd sampling it was not necessary to visit the farm at the crack of dawn, but we assembled on the farm at 9 am and started with a discussion in the farm office before proceeding to an evaluation of the machine. Dr Rodriguez obviously knew his stuff and was also impressed with the quality of the testing equipment. By midday we had determined the major problems and poor Sr Marinaro was in for an expensive time replacing the pump, much of the rubber tubing on the machine and all the vacuum cup liners; keeping cattle can be an expensive business. We did not eliminate Sr Marinaro's mastitis problem but were able to reduce it considerably,

When the owner was present they invariably provided hospitality and Sr Marinaro was no exception. After we had finished and cleaned up we were invited to lunch in his garden, where a cook was hard at work turning a sucking pig on a spit. The animal must have weighed about sixty pounds and was mounted on a contraption that I had never seen before; below the pig which was lying on a metal grid was a massive bed of charcoal glowing red, but above the pig was a sort of corrugated iron roof, upon which sat another bed of glowing charcoal. It was obvious that the pig was almost ready to be eaten. We sat in the shade of an enormous paraiso tree – so called because when in flower it is supposed to smell of paradise – drank beer and discussed politics, or at least the Argentines did; I kept out of it. All were bitterly opposed to the military junta that ruled the country, but all were agreed that the policies of the civilian Minister for the Economy, the Old Etonian José Martinez de Hoz, were working.

I went into a sort of reverie thinking about the country: the only country on the planet to extend from the tropics to the Antarctic, with a plethora of different climatic zones and farm lands. In this fabulous country they could grow everything from oats and rye to mangoes and coffee; they produced the best beef in the world and certainly some wonderful peaches and apples, some very drinkable wines and they could grow any cereal. There was mineral wealth in

242

the Andes and fish in the sea – the coast line was more than 2000 miles in length and they were populated by an intelligent and industrious people. And yet in a period of sixty years, successive governments had brought the nation to the verge of bankruptcy.

My thoughts were interrupted by the call to the table – set under another paraiso tree. We started with chorizos before turning to the main course, the sweet succulent flesh of the roast pig: it was superb, served simply with salad and bread and accompanied by the local St Galadriel red wine. I ate two gigot chops and felt stuffed; I was not and still am not accustomed to eating a large lunch. Sr Marinaro, Drs Gonzalez and Rodriguez together with the cook ate the rest of the pig. It never ceased to amaze me how the Argentines could consume such huge quantities of meat and remain so slim. It also surprised me that in a country with such huge social divisions no one thought it odd when the cook joined us at the table. The day on the farm was an interesting insight into the life of the rural Argentine middle classes.

Not all farms had milking machines, there were still many that milked by hand, yet they had as many problems as those with machines, a further indication that the root of the problem lay in the husbandry and hygiene. I remember taking samples on one such farm. I stood and watched the milker, sitting on his stool, hunched over the bucket and wheezing into it. Every so often he would give a soft gentle cough. He has TB, I thought, and so it proved. We informed the manager that we thought that one of his staff was ill and what we thought was the problem, The farm manager was a conscientious man and so instead of sacking the worker, he sent him to the local clinic, where it was confirmed that he had an 'open' case of TB – indicating that he was actually breathing out the organism. And straight into the milk, I thought! I remembered the saying of Professor Gordon Ferguson at the Dick – that the major role of the veterinary profession was to ensure that people could safely drink raw milk. Again I thought that veterinary medicine is often as much about people as it is about animals.

A major problem in the laboratory was the complete disparity in the staff ratios: we had five vets: Reuben, Ignacio, Isabela, Mik and myself, and to assist us there was Luis, our single lab technician. There was one secretary/typist to type reports but she had to serve the whole project. There was an old boy to clean the post mortem room and several willing women to wash up and sterilise the equipment; in those days we used glass plates for our cultures, not disposable ones, and so these had to be washed and sterilised. Over the years I have worked out that the most efficient staffing ratio for a laboratory is to have two or three laboratory technicians, one administrator/receptionist/typist, and one washer-upper to each vet, and two post mortem attendants for the whole unit. In Salta the vets were used as laboratory technicians (and not very good ones at that) and even as cleaners in the post-mortem room. This was common throughout Argentine life: the professionals did not like delegating work to para-professionals: nurses were almost non-existent in their hospitals and lawyers had no clerks.

Just as a detective requires clients to provide him with work, so for a laboratory to operate properly it requires practising veterinary surgeons working in the field to send in specimens. When the FAO project in Salta commenced there was not a single vet undertaking large (farm) animal practice. As time went by more and more vets arrived in the neighbourhood and offered their services to the farming community: most subsidised their work by selling drugs to the farmers. Perhaps the one benefit that the project bestowed upon the community was that we left behind a number of thriving veterinary practices.

The vet who made the greatest impression on me was Ernesto Podtz, a Porteño (born in Buenos Aires) of Belgian origins. This man would have made his mark wherever he worked: he was able, thoughtful and hard-working. He closed his practice in Buenos Aires and moved his family to Salta because he thought that where there was such a bunch of international 'experts' he would be able to learn a great deal. He did not, however, give up his biggest client, and each year at the onset of winter he would set off for the pampas. In a little over a month he would carry out more than 40,000 rectal examinations for pregnancy diagnosis. This work earned Ernesto more than $60,000, enough to give him a good living without doing any more work, but that was not the man. I asked him how he could carry out more than 1,000 examinations a day. The system had been carefully developed over the years to ensure great efficiency. There were two crushes side by side, for holding the cattle and many helpers. One read the ear number of the cow and the farmer wrote it down. One man lifted the tail and Ernesto inserted his arm and decided whether or not the cow was pregnant. If she was not pregnant she was separated from the mob and sent for slaughter. As

Ernesto did one animal the team in the parallel crush were preparing their animal. Ernesto used each arm alternately, and the team worked hard. At the end of the day was the time for the 'asado', the transverse cut of the beef ribs, cooked on the plancha (often an old disc harrow) with plenty of coarse salt and consumed with crusty bread, a green salad and great quaffs of wine; one of the truly great dishes of the world and a fitting end to a hard day's work.

'Why does the farmer pay you huge sums of money to identify barren cows?'

'It is simple really – because he makes money out of it!'

'But how?' I was showing my ignorance of the Argentine agricultural economy.

'It is simple really. With the onset of our winter, however mild, the grass stops growing, or at least it slows down. These breeding units are stocked to maximum capacity for the full growth of grass. Every barren cow takes food from the ones in calf. With too many barren cows, the young calves suffer. Better to turn the unproductive ones into corned beef. The farmer has a great check on my skill, because pregnant cows get downgraded in the slaughterhouse and so he loses even more money. I have no worries, my accuracy is almost a hundred percent. It is not difficult work: hard, but not difficult, Some of the cows are almost nine months pregnant and you can feel the calf as soon as you put your hand in. The farmers want the cows to calve at the end of the winter when there are fewer flies about and the young grass is there for the calves.'

A simple lesson in farming economics that was not applicable to Britain but which served me well when I went to work in Botswana. The value of these herds was enormous – 40,000 cows even if they were only worth $1000 a head, still works out at an investment of $40 million!

Ernesto appreciated the value of a diagnostic laboratory and so he regularly brought us samples for evaluation. He understood that it was cheaper to check a representative sample of faeces for worm eggs than to treat the whole herd for worms. He sent us milk samples for mastitis, blood slides for protozoan parasites, calf faeces to identify the causes of diarrhoea. And when his treatments failed he would send in the dead animal for post mortem examination to find out why he had failed. He came round to our house one evening to ask if I would be interested in a farm visit the following morning.

'Are you up to an hour on a horse?' he asked

245

'I can try,' was my reply; I had not spent that amount of time on a horse since I was a student, when we returned ponies belonging to the anatomy lecturer, Jimmy Speed, to his home in Fife at the end of the trekking season.

Early the next morning Ernesto collected me from home and after a brief visit to the laboratory to collect sampling equipment and sample containers, and to explain what I was doing, we were off up into the hills. We drove for about half an hour into the rolling farm land and pulled up at a gate where a group of men were waiting with a bunch of horses. After brief introductions, Ernesto said, 'Give him the quiet one!' and explained that I had not ridden for some time.

The pace was quite leisurely and after a few moments of dread I began to enjoy myself. We all had to be able to ride at the Dick Vet; an afternoon a week was set aside for us to ride in the indoor school and when we were competent, out in the countryside. I am not a horseman, and never really overcame my fear of falling off these large animals. At the pace we were going now there was little danger of that.

On the way to the farm Ernesto had explained that the farmer (absent of course) had about 500 cows of mixed breeds, some indigenous and some crossed with Angus or Hereford, two breeds very popular in Argentina because they produced so well under the conditions. The farm produced yearlings which were sold down to the pampas for fattening. Exactly what our project was all about. Recently cows had gone off their feet, become drowsy and after a few days they died. The alarm bells were ringing. Before I dismounted from my horse, I knew what was wrong with the cow: she was suffering from rabies.

I do not know what it is about rabies, but there is no mistaking an animal with the 'dumb' form of the disease, there is something about their eyes and their whole demeanour that shouts 'RABIES'. I had never before seen rabies in a live cow, but I just knew what the problem was. It was the same with the dog in Vom, I just knew the diagnosis by looking.

'We should not kill her here to carry out the examination: it would be much better if you could bring her to the laboratory because we will need to remove the brain to confirm the diagnosis.'

The owner replied that that would present no problem, there was a main entrance to the farm for vehicles. We had used a back entrance to the farm because the animal was near to the road – if you can call a 45-minute horse ride near. It was arranged that the cow would be brought from the farm the following morning.

Dumb rabies in cattle in South America is normally spread by vampire bats; cattle (and other ruminants) are usually what we call 'dead end' hosts for the virus because it does not normally spread from a diseased cow. Unlike dogs they do not go round biting each other, or people, which is the normal way that the virus is spread. Vampire bats are almost unique in that they can be infected with the rabies virus but not suffer from the disease; most other infected animals die.

'Do you have vampire bats on the ranch?' I asked.

'We have always had vampire bats on this ranch,' came the reply, 'but we have never seen this disease before: I have been manager here for more than 10 years and these are the first animals that I have seen like this.'

It seemed to me that the bat colony had recently become infected but the problem was how to control the disease in the cattle? At the time there was no adequate vaccine for use in cattle, it was still a few years away. It would not be possible to eliminate the bats. I was stumped. A partial solution would be to move the cows as far from the hills as possible, or graze these pastures with the young and consequently less valuable animals. This was considered to be a practical proposition.

We were offered lunch but the ranch house was a further hour's ride away and so we politely declined and made our way back to the road. A lone guide accompanied us. The cow was duly delivered to the laboratory the following day, it was killed with an injection of barbiturate (you cannot use a humane killer if you want to examine the brain), the brain removed and sent to the public health laboratory for examination (only they were allowed to diagnose rabies). Rabies was confirmed.

What were we to do with the carcase? The laboratory had a post mortem room but no means of disposing of the carcases once the work was completed. The material was either buried or more commonly put out in the field for scavengers. This was not a very efficient way of stopping the spread of infection! My experience in Kenya proved useful: we had no incinerator there, but a 'long drop', which formed the basis of most toilets in rural Kenya. A hole is dug in the ground to a depth of three or four metres and in the case of the laboratory system a concrete platform is made round the top so that a lockable lid could be fitted. Modifications to this basic system had been made over the years and now the practice was to line the walls with concrete sewer pipes of one metre diameter to prevent the walls caving in. The principle was simple: the carcases were decomposed by bacteria and in the process all the pathogens were destroyed. The only drawback to this system was that care had to be taken to prevent the contamination of water courses. In all the time I have had use of this system I never knew one that filled to the top, and providing the concrete platform was kept clean there were no flies and we never had problems with odours. For once I had total support from David and construction soon began. The Argentines thought we were mad, but once it was functioning their opinion soon changed. Nevertheless for several weeks I checked at the end of each day to make sure the padlock was securely in place and that the slab had been completely cleaned.

'Could you possibly look after the children in the lab this afternoon? I have a hair appointment and will then do some shopping in Salta.'

'I am in the laboratory all day today and so just drop them off on your way into town.'

I was in the post mortem room when Maxine arrived with the children. There was a hatch from the laboratory into the PM room and Maxine popped her head through the window to say that she had brought the children.

'By the way, on the side of the road I saw a small dachshund dog that had been knocked down: I picked it up. Please have a look at it when you have time – Jenny is looking for a dachshund as hers has just been run over.'

Jenny was the wife of Ted Campion, the project manager of the FAO Husbandry Project. The Campions were Australian and we had become firm friends. Ted ran his project in a completely different way to David, but then he was a competent scientist and he gave me more help and advice than I received from my boss.

I shouted to the kids to behave themselves and that I would shortly be with them: Guy popped his head through the hatch and asked if he could come in and watch what was going on. Things were a bit mucky in the PM room at the time and I suggested that he watch through the hatch. He soon got bored and returned to play with Claire and the dog.

When I had cleaned up and divested myself of boots and gown I walked into the lab and saw with horror that my two children aged five and six were sitting on the floor cuddling and caressing a rabid dog. I tried not to panic as I did not want to frighten the children but I had to get them away from the dog and get them cleaned of its saliva. I took a towel off the hook put it on the floor and said, 'I think that we should put the dog down and make him comfortable. Then we had better get you clean and tidy before Mummy returns.' I led them to the sink and gently washed their hands and faces with running water, trying not to rub at all. I picked up towel and dog and took them into the PM room.

By the time Maxine returned the vets had all trickled back into the laboratory and been appraised of the situation. It was too late that afternoon to do anything and if we called the public health laboratory they would want us to bring the dog to them alive. I did not want to wait for the dog to die as I knew it had rabies.

Maxine was furious with herself for putting the children at risk. 'But there it was walking across the side of the road and seemed to be staggering, I just couldn't leave it.'

'Of course you couldn't; it was just a pity that the children were in the car and all they wanted to do was help the poor little dog. Don't worry darling, things will be fine.'

'I wish I could be so sure.'

'All that will happen is that we will all have to be vaccinated. I do not know what they use here but it will be a WHO-approved vaccine and I can tell you it will be more than one shot.'

The dog was still alive the next morning and my first job was to put it to sleep and remove the brain. I took the brain to the public health laboratory and within a couple of hours the diagnosis was confirmed. I then discussed what should be done with Maxine and the children and was informed that the whole family would have to be vaccinated – I was not to be spared despite having had the vaccine in Kenya.

'We use a vaccine made from the brains of unweaned mice for treatment of people; this is superior to the old Pasteur Vaccine that was made from the nervous tissue of adult rabbits. Because the mice are immature the nervous tissue has little myelin round it [this acts like the plastic insulation sheath on an electric cable]. It is this myelin that causes the unfortunate reactions that some people have to the Pasteur Vaccine. You must go to the general hospital and be vaccinated.'

And so for the next fortnight Maxine made a daily trip with the children to receive the basic vaccination course. I was only required to have the booster course. The children were angels and received their daily injection without complaint. Perhaps the sweets they were given after the injection played their part. The major problem was not the injections but the fact that during the course of treatment we were not allowed to eat meat. I did not understand the rationale behind this but felt we should obey the instructions. This really irked my carnivorous children and I cannot say I enjoyed the enforced fish and vegetarian diet although Maxine did her best. This was our second medical misfortune but worse was to come.

14

Journeys for Work and Pleasure

'You have attempted to tinge it with romanticism.'
Sir Arthur Conan Doyle, *The Sign of Four*

One of the more agreeable tasks of the veterinary detectives is to attend international conferences; it is also useful to be seen at these meetings in order to further one's career. My work with strepto-coccal meningitis in pigs had attracted a great deal of attention and I was invited by The International Pig Veterinary Society to deliver a paper on the topic to their international symposium in Copenhagen. The ticket was only from London and so I had to find the funds to get me to London. The Wellcome Foundation was kind enough to offer me a small grant towards expenses. I had to leave home while Maxine and the children were still undergoing their rabies vaccination.

The cheapest way of getting from Salta was to fly by Aerolineas Argentinas to La Paz in Bolivia, flights which only took place on Sundays. I had to spend half a day there before catching the Lloyd-Boliviano plane to Miami, and after a further long delay on to London by the British Airways daytime flight. However the same route could not be used for the return flights because the days did not fit and the BA promotional price did not operate for the journey. Luckily there was a direct flight from Miami to Jujuy (about 100 miles from Salta) twice a week operated by Aerolineas Argentinas and Mr Laker was offering flights to Miami for £100. The problem with Mr Laker was that you could not guarantee a flight unless you were prepared to queue up at the Victoria ticket office when the flight you wanted was opened – this did not happen until the previous flights were fully booked. My father volunteered for this duty, but there was further snag; to get a ticket you had to show your passport with its American visa. Luckily I had my UN Laissez-Passer which would allow me to travel within Europe so my father

251

could keep my passport. The Internet and credit cards have made life so much simpler!

The conference was a great success and my paper was well accepted. It is not the formal parts of conferences that are the most beneficial – it is the discussions in small groups over a beer or two where the ideas on approaches to research or investigation are thrashed out, new techniques discussed, new suggestions for collaboration are made, new links are forged and new friends made, that make conferences worthwhile. Copenhagen was no exception. The organisers had put me into a delightful hotel close to the Royal Palace with a bunch of old friends. Not surprisingly there were no Argentine vets present; the pig industry was almost non-existent then, and most vets could not be bothered with pig and pig keepers. It was only vets like Ernesto who were prepared to investigate their problems.

There were some outstanding papers on diseases of major importance and on developments in husbandry and breeding. One of the problems for me with the modern methods of pig husbandry is that in the quest for profits the well-being of the pig is often forgotten. Modern techniques are more about the comfort of the pigman than the comfort of the pig. This conference was a watershed, when the tide turned and major changes in attitude towards welfare occurred; this resulted in the banning of sow stalls, where the animal is tied up for twenty-four hours a day unable to move around. The reason for doing this was that the sow was less likely to trample or lie on her piglets.

We visited several very smart pig breeding units where disease security was paramount. We had to don plastic overboots, and a plastic coat, gloves and hat. The staff on these units all spoke perfect English and were very enthusiastic about their methods and their success. I was very pleased to have been part of this conference and looked forward to putting some of the new ideas into practice, even in Argentina. It was time to return. I got to London to find that my father had been able to get a ticket for the flight that I needed. A family lunch was held and then it was time to get to Gatwick Airport, my first visit to that place. I checked in and went into the departure lounge, and what a tip it was; tables in the café had not been cleared and there were mountains of dirty crockery on every table. There was rubbish everywhere, and to cap it all there came an announcement that the Laker flight to Miami was delayed by six hours. This meant that I would miss my connection to Jujuy.

We finally arrived in Miami at four in the morning and, with no connecting flight, I had to go through immigration. The form asked if I was carrying any animal or plant products. I certainly was: it was impossible to buy bacon in Argentina and I had several pounds of vacuum packed bacon in my suitcase. The form asked if I had visited any farms while out of the country. I certainly had. I duly noted the fact on the form. The customs officer was a short dumpy Latina, who eyed my form with dismay.

'You gotta meat products in that case?'

'Yes ma'am.' It pays to be courteous to people in authority, especially at 4 am.

'You say you bin on a farm.'

'Yes ma'am.'

'In that case I gotta call Aggie.'

At that time in the morning it took me a while to realise what she meant, but a few minutes later a tall gangly man in a khaki uniform came out of an office rubbing the sleep out of his eyes and straightening his cap. In a deep southern drawl he said, 'What's all this about you importing meat?'

I explained to him that I was a veterinary surgeon and had been to a pig veterinary conference in Denmark, that I was on my way home to Argentina, that we could not get bacon in Argentina and that I was taking vacuum packed bacon for the family. Had my plane not been delayed six hours I would by now have been winging my way home.

'And you've put here that you have been on a farm.'

'That is correct. Participants at the conference visited several farms where the disease security was very high: we all had to don protective clothing from top to bottom.' I thought it politic not to mention that disease security in Denmark was much better than in the States and that there are no diseases in Denmark that are not present in the States.

He took his peaked cap off and scratched his head. Pause ...

'Do you know anyone in Miami?'

'No, not a soul,' I said, quite truthfully as it happened.

Pause ... and he scratched his head again.

'I'm gonna trust you,' he said. Pause...

I waited.

'I'm gonna let you keep that bacon, but you must promise me y'all not gonna open the packets in the States.'

253

I shook my head. Pause...

'I hope your kids enjoy it when you get home.'

'Thank you very much.'

'Now,' he said. 'I don't want you to think I'm being difficult, but if Jesus H Christ walked in thru those doors, and he had been on a farm,' pause ... 'I'd have his boots off him. '

And that concluded our discussions. I went out into the airport, found the Laker desk, and to my surprise was informed that they would pay my hotel bill until I caught my connection. I was given a voucher for the airport motel next door which was excellent and which I have used regularly each time I have had to stop over in Miami.

Once my ticket had been sorted out I had a couple of days to sample the delights of downtown Miami. I even spent some time on the beach and bought a television (prices in Argentina were prohibitive). I had informed the New York office of the UN of my problems and somehow they managed to get word to Maxine (how, I never found out) of what had happened, and when and to where I was returning. She was in the airport in Jujuy to meet me and it was great to see her. She had had her own problems while I had been away.

When Carlos Masse heard that I had gone away he insisted that she take his pistol to defend herself, because we had had a break-in the week before I left. Gas cylinders, bicycles and our tape recorder had been stolen. All but the tape recorder were recovered from Sr Ramon, a rogue who was almost our next door neighbour. She had tried to remonstrate with Carlos that she had no idea how to use a pistol and had never fired one in her life. But there was no arguing with him. One night Maxine heard the noise of would-be intruders outside the house. Not wanting to wake the children she took the loaded pistol, went into the sitting room with the lights off, and stood there until she heard the noise of someone slipping in a dog's mess and swearing, whereupon she shouted that she had a gun, but that she did not want to fire it because of waking the children. The intruder was also informed that it might make a hole in the window! Silence ensued and she eventually went back to bed. It had been a nasty moment for her alone with two small children in a house out in the country with no telephone. I am not sure about the value of the gun, as I believe that possession of a firearm puts you at greater risk. On the previous occasion the thief had got in through the door which was not well secured whereas all the windows were fitted with ornate wrought iron burglar bars

A new disease, or at least new to me, was being seen in young broiler chickens, where the feathers developed poorly and the abdomen swelled up with fluid. Apart from the keeping of backyard hens, the poultry industry was new to Argentina and a few entrepreneurs had imported breeding stock from the USA. When we opened the birds the abdomen was full of gelatinous fluid and all the tissues were waterlogged. The lungs were full of fluid and it seemed that the birds had drowned in their own exudates. A salient feature in all the birds was the marked enlargement of the heart. It seemed to us that the birds were suffering from a type of altitude sickness and that the growth of heart and lungs was not keeping pace with the rapid growth of the muscles. The geneticists have a lot to answer for: in Britain they had produced birds whose muscles outgrew the ability of the skeleton to support them. Lack of oxygen, as occurs at altitude, could also result in cardiac enlargement and failure. Some of the water in the Andes has a moderately increased sodium level and this is well known to cause a rise in blood pressure.

We would have to visit the farm to find out what was going on in order to sort it out. The farm was in La Quiaca on the border with Bolivia, and to get there would require overnight accommodation. Easter was fast approaching and so it seemed a good idea to combine business with tourism. The town of Tilcara on the road to La Quiaca had a traditional Easter festival and the citizens made pictures for each station of the cross out of flower petals and other parts of the plant.

We drove up on Thursday so that we could take part in the candlelit procession to welcome Good Friday. It has always seemed to me that one of the great differences between the Catholic and Protestant churches is that the Catholics pay more attention to the crucifixion and the Protestants give greater prominence to the resurrection. And this is particularly true in South America where churches are full of statues and paintings of horrific scenes. The first procession was on Thursday night and it was repeated again on Good Friday. The main crucifix from the church was erected on a huge cart which was pulled round the stations of the cross by the faithful who vied to be selected for this important task. The town band led the way, followed by the priests and altar boys in their robes and even the local nuns were allowed out. The procession stopped at each station of the cross where one of the priests said not a few words and then a hymn was sung and then off we went to the next one. Each of the floral depictions was a true work of art and dedication. My favourite was that of the crucifixion itself about five feet by three feet, with a distraught Mary standing at the foot of the cross and on her face a single tear made from a tiny pale-blue petal. It says a great deal for the evening that the children were not bored.

Over the weekend we explored the town and the environs and the children loved the swimming pool in the hotel. Guy finally found the confidence to dive into the water. After that there was no stopping him.

On Monday we were off to La Quiaca and the chickens with waterbelly. It was a real frontier town, 11,500 feet above sea level, with seemingly no law and order: we were allowed into Bolivia with only a curt instruction to make sure we came back. It was like crossing the centuries going into Villazón: the women were just as you see in the pictures, wearing voluminous skirts and bowler hats. The streets were of dirt and the whole place reeked of deprivation and poverty in comparison with their rich, modern neighbour. There is little doubt that the Argentines spent a great deal of money in La Quiaca to ensure that it looked as different as possible from its primitive Bolivian counterpart, from its prim Plaza de Armas to its wonderful church with its alabaster windows. Just outside the town we could see the real South America, with the trains of pack llamas bearing illicit goods between the two countries high up in the hills and far from the roads so that the police, who were restricted to motor vehicles, were unable to apprehend them. I never understood why they did not use horses for the chase, but perhaps they were too well paid by the smugglers.

We found the farm of Sr Rochas, if such it could be described; it was more of an animal factory. The buildings were specially designed for the job, but not for the altitude, and they were poorly insulated so, at 11,000 feet, it could get very cold at night. Everything was being done by the book; day-old chicks were flown in from a hatchery in Buenos Aires, the chicks were held in a restricted area which was increased as they grew, warmed by a heating lamp and fed a commercial starter mash with adequate drinkers. Losses were almost nil until the chicks were four to five weeks of age when they started to swell up and die. Several batches had been successfully reared, but the problems had started with the onset of winter. The birds still came from the original source but the food company had been changed, because their rations were said to produce faster growth and bigger profits: greater losses I thought.

We sat in the office and the maté pot was produced, filled with the leaves that looked like grass and a good helping of sugar added. The pot was filled from the kettle and the beautiful silver filter straw was put in place. As was customary, the host drank the first filling to make sure that all was well. The pot was refilled and I drank. I had acquired a taste for maté, which would have happened more quickly had they not used so much sugar. We discussed the options: obviously the strain of bird was adequate for the conditions because several successful batches had been produced. However, it seemed to me he was living on the edge with the potential for things to go seriously wrong at any moment. It was essential to reduce all risk factors where it was economically possible. Insulating the roofs of the sheds would reduce the heat loss in the winter months and make for a more stable environment for the birds. Sr Rochas must forgo larger profits, which would be counterbalanced by reduced losses, and go back to the original feed supplier. A further possibility was to feed the meal with water as a mash which slows the bird's intake and hence the growth. It was possible for Sr Rochas to obtain cheap supplies of distilled water which he could mix with the water from the well. Now that Sr Rochas understood the problem he could play around with the nutrition, balancing growth rate against disease. We left a satisfied client and began our return journey.

I never ceased to marvel at the plant life in the Andes, there were cacti everywhere, tall ones, short ones, round ones and woolly ones. I had been brought up with cacti as my father was an avid grower and collector. He would have loved the area around Humahuaca where the countryside is a miniature forest made up of thousands of these spiny plants. Guy noticed some bearing seed pods and so we stopped the car and picked the pods to give the seeds to my father – who, of course, got them to grow.

It was too far to get back to Salta that night and so we stayed on the hacienda of Sr Ricardo Leach and his wife at Los Lapachos near the city of Jujuy. Los Lapachos was in fact the farm but it had developed into a community of more than a thousand people all living on the land of Ricardo: police, priests, teachers, a doctor and shopkeepers. Ricardo was the Honorary British Consul in north-western Argentina and had an office in Jujuy. He was of British descent and was later interned during the Falklands War. He farmed almost a quarter of a million hectares of reasonably productive land and I had helped him when he had problems of mastitis in his dairy herd. He thought that I was a lousy vet to have working for him.

'I grow tobacco and sugar and produce milk and you consume none of them; you are definitely not a good salesman for me.'

The family had been established in Argentina for several generations and Ricardo loved Argentina dearly but other members of his family were leaving as the economic climate of the country worsened. They were most hospitable; I suspect that if you live out in the sticks, visitors are a welcome relief. It was a good place to stay because they had a guest wing to their villa that could comfortably sleep twenty people.

Early in our stay in Argentina we had met the Misdorps, Andrew and Sheila, with their tearaway sons Carl and Frans: they were from Rhodesia. Andrew, who was a tobacco farmer, had lost a leg in a motorbike accident, and had been working on a tobacco estate in the east of the country towards the Mozambique border when his farmhouse was attacked by Zimbabwe rebels and his artificial leg badly damaged by gunfire. Working on the assumption that it might be the good leg next time, Andrew decided that it was time to move. His employer was looking to establish a ranch in north-west Argentina and asked Andrew to manage it. They managed to get their money out of the country by turning their assets into gold and jewels which were hidden inside his artificial leg. The whole family are there to this day despite the break-up of the marriage. Both boys are married to local girls. Carl and Frans were the same ages as Richard and Guy and were totally wild.

Our third medical problem started with Carl and Frans being off colour. Sheila noted their urine was a dark brown colour and so took a sample and brought it to our house in a bottle and a paper bag: the bottle had leaked but we thought no more of it. I took the bottle to the laboratory and the results indicated that young Carl was suffering from hepatitis. In young children it is not normally a serious disease and they rapidly throw off the infection without serious damage to the liver. Some weeks later Guy and Claire went yellow and passed dark urine but seemed to be only a little off colour and otherwise fine.

A major holiday had been planned, to drive across Paraguay into

258

Brazil to visit the Iguazu Falls, one of the great sights of the world. The party consisted of the five Windsors, Ted and Jenny Campion together with Ted's parents, and Aya Hadani, his wife Ilana and son (another tearaway) Ronny. The plan was to drive across the Chaco (that great northern forest of hard, hard wood, where temperatures can reach 50° C) to Clorinda on the border with Paraguay and spend the first night in a hotel. We would then cross into Paraguay and go directly to Asunción where the Campions had friends who had put their house at our disposal as they were back in Australia. We were to spend some days there before driving on to the Paraguay/Brazil border.

The plan had been to drive in convoy but Aya drove his Renault 4 at no more than forty miles an hour, and had we gone at that speed the children would have rioted. So we drove to a nice place and stopped and waited … and waited; when we saw the little blue Renault on the horizon we set off again. The Windsors and Campions alternated in waiting and we were the first to arrive in Clorinda in mid-afternoon.

I said to Maxine, 'Do you think it is getting dark?'

'There is something going on,' she replied. 'Do stop the car. I am sure that something is happening!'

We parked the car and Maxine looked around through the binoculars and up at the sun, and noticed a segment missing. It was the start of a total eclipse of the sun, the first I had ever seen. For a few minutes it was like night, until the moon moved from its blocking position as the sun and moon continued on their way.

The Campions mistakenly tried to check into a brothel, before finding a 'family' hotel that could take us all. We waited at the entrance of the town for the Hadanis, who had caught us up by the time Ted returned to lead us to the hotel. That night the lurgy struck; we never found out what it was, but I think that it was a Salmonella or a Shigella. One by one we were all affected with a high fever and severe gastric pains while some had diarrhoea and vomiting as well. Despite feeling decidedly unwell, I drove on to Asunción. On arrival the senior Campions and the Windsors were allocated rooms with beds because Joe and Maxine were the most severely affected. The children slept in sleeping bags in the car. We spent several days exploring Asunción while the infirm slept. The disease was awful while it lasted but luckily the duration was short.

In the nineteenth century Paraguay had a president Francisco Solano López, who during a visit to Paris fell for an Irish prostitute and took her back to Paraguay. He never married her but she acted as his wife throughout his presidency and bore his children. López had a fixation that he was Napoleon – the Paraguay flag is similar to that of the French, with the stripes horizontal rather than vertical. He started the 'Chaco War' to gain territory that he thought rightfully belonged to Paraguay, and fought pitched battles against the Argentines, Bolivians and Brazilians, all at the same time. He lost. In addition he lost almost twenty percent of the male population, a disaster from which Paraguay, more than a hundred years later, is still recovering. In memory of those dead, López built a copy of Les Invalides, with a tomb of the unknown warrior, guarded night and day by guardsmen in their traditional uniform and with an eternal flame burning.

It was fascinating to see the houses of parliament looking like a well-decorated birthday cake, with bullet holes in the walls. All around were the most beautiful government buildings, but walk behind them and there by the river were the most desperate slums with children in rags and without shoes, playing on the river bank. The Paraguay river in Asunción is more than half a mile wide despite being more than two thousand miles from the sea, and is navigable by ships of up to 10,000 tons. It was fascinating watching conscripts unload sacks of cement from a barge, walking a gang-plank barely six inches wide that was bouncing up and down as they crossed over – but we never saw one fall in.

With the party more or less back to full health we drove on to Puerto Stroessner (now, after the fall of the dictator Stroessner, renamed Puerto del Este) the border with Brazil. What a town. It was a paradise of contraband; there were more cases of whisky than I have ever seen in a Scottish town. Every shop in the long straight high street had cases of whisky stacked from floor to ceiling and it was possible to buy almost any brand. When I returned twenty years later nothing had changed but the name of the town. Paraguay must be the contraband capital of the world. It was said at that time you could buy a very cheap Mercedes: you gave the order for model, the year and the colour and you would receive it within a week. The only problem was that you could not take it outside Paraguay as it had been stolen from either Argentina or Brazil!

The journey was without incident – not so the entry into Brazil. We passed Paraguayan immigration without a hitch and drove across to the Brazilian side where we received a very frosty reception. Despite our diplomatic number plates and UN Laissez-Passers we were greeted with blank indifference. We were handed immigration forms by the white officials at about 2 pm. We explained to one officer that we were sorry, although we spoke Spanish, none of us spoke Portuguese and could he assist us as the forms were only written in Portuguese?

'No.' And he turned his back on us.

I do not know how many times we completed the forms but the officers took one look at them and tore them in half muttering that they were all wrong. It is one thing to listen to Portuguese conversation which has a close relationship with Spanish and to understand the language. It is quite another to try and read it. We had difficulty in restraining Aya from thumping one officer in particular. It was approaching five o'clock and growing dark when the shift changed: all the white immigration officers left to be replaced by black ones. Within ten minutes we were through, the staff could not have been more helpful. We found a hotel which was closed for the winter but because of the size of the party they opened for us. Maxine stayed with the children in the car so that we did not have to pay for them. The hotel restaurant was also closed, but they offered to cook some steaks and serve them with a salad, which they did. Wonderful fillet steak, served with a sublime salad.

I have seen several of the world's great waterfalls but none compares with Iguazu. From the Brazilian and Argentine sides they are two different falls. We started in Brazil and climbed down and down the side of the fall, watching the water crash down below us. At the bottom there is a platform built out into the falls and for a few cruzeiros you can hire a brilliant yellow plastic mac and sou'wester and stand just a few inches from the raging torrent where it smashes into the rocks. We retraced our steps and climbed right to the very top, where again there is a platform built out over the falls from which the whole depth of the fall can be seen. It is not a direct fall – about half way down there is a sort of step which the purists say detracts from its beauty but in my view it adds to its majesty.

During the siesta hour Aya, his son Ronny, my two boys and I went across on the ferry to discuss with the Argentine authorities the regulations concerning the import of household goods from Brazil, where the prices were very much lower. Aya wanted to buy a TV. It was perfectly straightforward, the official informed us. There would be no problem about our bringing anything with us, provided we had the requisite authority from the Ministry of Foreign Affairs in

Buenos Aires: Aya was stymied as he had no such letter of authority and no means of getting one. It was not possible to purchase return tickets on the ferry and I had bought the tickets to cross to Argentina. When Aya bought the tickets back to Brazil we found out why! I had paid in crucieros the equivalent of about a dollar for the two adults and three children. The return trip in pesos cost more than ten dollars. Same boat, same crew and same distance, but each country kept its own take: Aya was incensed; even my offering to split the costs did not calm him down.

The following day we drove down to the union of the Iguazu and the Paraguay rivers, where the boundaries of Argentina, Brazil and Paraguay meet. We crossed into Argentina, found a hotel and went exploring the falls from a totally different viewpoint. The falls are not a single body of water, but the river which is about a mile wide in a rough horseshoe breaks up into numerous individual falls, each with a name. Brazil has the single greatest body of water but all the other falls are in Argentina and it is possible to walk right into the middle over a series of bridges. The centre falls – La Gargantua del Diablo (the Throat of the Devil) – is the most dramatic as the water pours down three sides of a square into a witches' cauldron with 'steam' emanating as if from a magic potion; it seemed most magical. Guy's Spanish teacher Sra Graciela had asked Guy to bring her some water from the falls and he chose this moment to remind us that we had yet to collect any. The only receptacle we had for collecting liquids was the lens cap of Maxine's camera, and so on hands and knees I collected the precious liquid which had to be carefully guarded until we could find a proper container to take it back to Salta, where Sra Graciela was both delighted and, I think surprised, to receive her sample from the falls.

The return journey was completely through Argentina: we drove through the state of Misiones to Corrientes in Entre Dos Rios, where we spent the night. It was a time of high political tension in the country. The hotelier was very suspicious of this large group of foreigners staying under his roof and phoned the police, and so in the middle of the night we were all woken and had to present our papers and documents for the cars to a group of helmeted and armed soldiers. All was in order: the soldiers apologised profusely for disturbing such distinguished guests and we resumed our sleep.

The ponies were delighted to see us after our ten days away. Somewhere along the line we had acquired two ponies: the first I had treated for a nasty cut on the lower foreleg. I bought it home to treat because it needed regular bandaging. When it was fit I was about to take it back home when the owner asked if I would like it for the children: his last daughter had gone off to university and no longer had any use for it. The second came from Guy's school who did not have enough grazing for it. I rode it from Cerrillos and a very pleasant ride it was. However when I tried to turn it to cross the road to enter our garden, it would not go, something had spooked it. It was not going to cross the road. I went back down the road and tried trotting up and making a swift turn but it was having none of it and stopped dead. I dismounted and tried to lead it across with no success, even tugging on the reins. By now the family had seen what was going on and I was receiving a great deal of gratuitous advice. Had I a sack I would have put it over its head before leading it. The children brought handfuls of lucerne (alfalfa) hay to tempt it. In desperation Maxine brought the car up behind it and gently nudged it forward while I led it and the children waved hay. Once it had entered the garden the spell was broken and the pony completely relaxed. The garden was almost big enough to provide a couple of ponies with grazing and we supplemented their grass with purchased alfalfa hay and a small quantity of concentrate. It was an ideal place for the children to learn to ride because once they were fairly secure on the pony they could be allowed to ride up and down a lane behind the house which was not used by motor traffic.

Not far from us was a riding school which hired out skinny nags for a modest fee. The first time we visited the stables which was at the bottom of a long, straight, downhill drive, Richard was the first to mount and set off up the track: he was given strict instructions NOT to cross the main road at the top but to wait there for us. He cantered up the hill despite this being his first time on a horse. He turned and galloped down the lane and when he saw us watching dropped the reins and stood up in the stirrups and waved with both hands. It must have been in his blood as his grandfather had been in a cavalry regiment and took part in the last cavalry charge of the British army at the end of the First World War. The remainder of that riding trip is long gone from my memory, expunged by Richard careering down the track totally oblivious to his fate. Maxine never really enjoyed the riding and so we did not go too often as I could not look after three on horseback by myself. Carlos had a son Horacio who was the same age as Richard, and both loved to gallop up and down the lane at top speed, shouting encouragement to each other.

Down the road towards Cerrillos was a fruit farmer who grew the most wonderful peaches and apples. He also was a dealer in pigs and kept a few breeding sows. When one of his sows aborted, Sr Salvador brought the aborted piglets and placentas to the house. I suggested that it would be better to take them to the laboratory so that we could carry out a proper examination.

I had never seen anything like it and nor had my Argentine colleagues. The placentas appeared full of fluid (rather like the abdomens of the broilers with waterbelly), but the striking lesions were in the organs of the aborted piglets, where everywhere there were dark brown abscesses like lumps of chocolate distributed through their small bodies. We were all certain that we were dealing with a bacterial infection, but what? Smears were made from the abscesses onto glass slides and they were stained with the Gram Stain; tiny pink rods were seen. The penny dropped and we asked for smears to be stained with the modified Ziehl-Neelsen which I described earlier. *Brucella*, unlike the mycobacteria that cause TB, is not truly acid-fast but it is resistant to decolourisation with weak acids – and sure enough the beastie causing the mayhem was a *Brucella*. Once we had cultured it, we were able to confirm its identity as *Br. suis*. Out came the books, which informed us that the organism was commonly found in domesticated and wild pigs in South America, although none of my colleagues had seen the disease before nor heard of it causing problems. It also occurs in northern North America and Russia where it causes disease in moose, caribou, reindeer, Arctic foxes and wolves. Unlike its close relative, *Br. abortus*, that causes abortions in cattle all over the world, *Br. suis* can be transmitted venereally in the semen. *Br. abortus* is not transmitted this way: to become infected the cow has to ingest the organism which is why infected placentas are such a problem in cattle. Also unlike *Br. abortus* there is no vaccine for control. There is also no economically viable treatment.

Once we had a confirmed diagnosis Reuben, Ignacio and I set off for Sr Salvador's farm. There were only a dozen sows and about seventy-five fattening pigs. To us the best course of treatment was to stop purchasing pigs for the present, slaughter the fattening pigs as they were ready, to allow the remaining sows to farrow (three more aborted), sell the young pigs once they were weaned and send the sows to the abattoir. When the place was free from pigs then a good clean up and disinfection was to be undertaken which Ignacio or I would supervise. They could then begin again.

The night that we carried out the examinations a large box of the most wonderful peaches was delivered to the house. A few days after we visited the farm, at about eleven o'clock at night there was a knock on our bedroom window. Maxine got up and opened the door, and a beaming Sr Salvador carried a dressed suckling pig into the house. He was obviously pleased with our work and the results. We gave a party: Carlos and his wife Zulma helped Maxine with cooking.

This was not the first *Brucella* species found to be causing a problem in Salta. When Robin Condron was working there he had carried out a large serological survey of cattle, sheep and goats. He had found that *Br. abortus* was not a problem in cattle and *Br. ovis* was not a problem in sheep but that *Br. melitensis* was a serious problem in goats, and since the people were drinking unpasteurised milk there had to be a problem in the human population. It had been a common disease in southern Europe until it was brought under control and it caused serious disease in man – in Europe it was called Malta fever (hence the *mellitensis*, meaning literally 'from Malta'). One of the great roles of the laboratory worker is to liaise with workers in other disciplines, particularly when the disease is zoonotic – one that spreads between animals and man; the aim being to help solve the problems common to both humans and animals.

Discussions had been held with the Public Health Department in Salta, but we were unable to raise any enthusiasm in their staff for a survey among the human population and we had no remit to examine humans. The medics in Salta were not idle, just overrun trying to control Chagga's disease. This is a chronic disease affecting millions of people in rural South and Central America caused by *Trypanosoma cruzi*, which is a cousin of the organism that causes sleeping sickness in humans and animals in Africa. The organism is spread by a bug (a type of beetle called 'vinchuca' in Argentina) that lives in crevices in walls and ceilings in the houses. These bugs come out at night and suck blood from their sleeping human victim and because they prefer the skin of the face they are often called 'kissing bugs'. When the bugs drink the blood they take in the parasite from an infected human and later pass it out in their faeces which they deposit on the skin of their victim. Once infected, the patient is probably affected for life and the infection results in chronic heart problems. The resources of the Public Health Department were seemingly all taken up by trying to control this disease by eliminating the vinchuca from the houses. It seemed to me to be a pity to prevent a man from dying of Chagga's disease only for him to die of brucellosis.

But we had our own health problems to worry about. I was feeling wretched, and in the middle of the night Maxine woke me to go and look at Guy.

'I'll see him in the morning,' I said and turned over. Maxine spent the rest of the night watching him and roused me early in the morning. Despite still feeling wretched I went and looked. I was horrified: he looked like a mummy, all shrivelled from dehydration. I put my clothes on in a rush and raced down to Cerrillos for Dr Rodriguez: he brought his own car and as always he was the epitome of calmness and comfort.

'I think it would be advisable to take him to the hospital, because he needs to be rehydrated as quickly as possible. Please go to the pharmacy in the hospital and buy the following items and I will meet you in the ward.' He scribbled down the list and left. Luckily Maria our maid was there and she took charge of Richard and Claire while I carried Guy to the car and put him in his mother's arms. He had para-typhoid, confirmed by laboratory examination. Because there were no nurses, Dr Rodriguez had to come to the hospital and put the drip in place. One of us had to attend to him at all times. I did the first shift while Maxine went home to sort out the house and children. Guy and I both slept. I was not a very good nurse. Maxine returned after lunch and I went back to attend to the rest of the family.

Claire was having a wonderful time in the pool with the young American missionaries and Richard and Horacio were thundering up and down the lane on the ponies, when suddenly there came a loud shout of alarm from Richard. John the young missionary was the first to get to him: the girth strap had broken and Richard and saddle had landed in the dirt. John tenderly carried Richard into his bedroom and put him on his back. We thought that he was probably more shocked and winded than hurt and I decided to wait before troubling Dr Rodriguez. It was not long before he was back on his feet but very shaken. I think that he was relieved that he had not fallen off the horse in front of Horacio.

The day was still not over, as I had to attend a Project party for some visiting dignitaries at the Broadbents' house. I called in the hospital and found Guy sitting up in bed and looking very chirpy: his skin had returned to normal. It was agreed that he could go home later that evening. I got to the party and socialised for about an hour, drinking one small whisky, and decided that it was time to collect Maxine and Guy and get home while I could still drive. Everyone had been most sympathetic about Guy and all were delighted that he was on the mend.

We got home and even before I went to bed I knew the worst: having seen the colour of my urine, I knew I had hepatitis. The doctor came on Monday gave me a shot of B vitamins and told me to do nothing until I felt better. For the next fortnight I spent the time with the children doing complicated jigsaw puzzles and teaching Claire to read. I remembered Maxine's father's dictum: when you have hepatitis you should eat and drink what you want. That is what I did. I ate my birthday cake and drank beer. The cake provided energy and the beer the vitamins. When the news got round that I had hepatitis our friends deserted us. Not a soul came to see us: not even the Misdorps who had introduced the virus into the house. After two weeks I was definitely on the mend but still very feeble.

It was time for Richard to return to school when we noticed that some of our carefully stashed dollars were missing and we needed dollars to pay Richard's school fees; these would be taken back to Britain after being sewn by Maxine into his clothes: Granny then removed them and paid the school. The reason for this rigmarole was that half my salary and all the 'post adjustment' had to be paid in Argentina although it was paid in dollars. The cost of sending money out of the country was prohibitive and you had to get official permission which might take forever. We assumed Maria had taken the money and since we never saw her again, there was little doubt who took it! She was also clever enough not to take too many, thinking correctly that if it was only 100 dollars or so we would not bother to go to the police. She was right of course but we wondered how she found them.

The family drove to the airport which was not far away being on our side of the city of Salta. As Richard went through the departure gate Maxine burst into tears, something she never does and so I knew we were in for trouble. As I dabbed away her tears I saw that her eyes were yellow. She had hepatitis, and she totally collapsed

267

there and then at the airport; she had been stopping herself from becoming ill so as not to spoil Richard's last days of holiday.

I would have to drive home and I was not sure that I was up to the task. We set off and I had difficulty in focusing my eyes. I found that if I closed the left eye I could see well enough, and I was not planning to make the journey in record time. We realised that this might be the last time for some time that we would get out of the house, and so we stopped in Cerrillos to stock up on basic foodstuffs plus things for the house and chocolate for the children.

We put Maxine straight to bed and the children amused themselves while dinner was prepared. We did not know of Maria's defection until Monday when she did not turn up for work. At least that saved us from a row. The missionaries sensed our plight when Guy did not turn up for school and came to see what they could do. When they heard that our maid had gone they sent Angela. They came and collected Guy for school and brought him home at the end of the day, and they sent regular meals to be heated up for the family. They were a true godsend. Dr and Sra Castro may God bless you. Before Angela took over the duties I did the washing each day in the bath as I took my shower – I 'trod' the dirty washing and the soapsuds like winemakers treading grapes. They were rinsed by the same process, as it was too much effort to bend over and do it by hand. Assisted by Claire we got the washing on the line: it was not ironed.

Maxine was really ill, and there was talk of her going into hospital which she immediately vetoed. She developed massive haemorrhages under the skin of her back as if I had been whipping her, and for several days she was unable to do anything for herself – and she had a rotten nurse, although he did his best in the circumstances. The vitamin K injections soon stopped the haemorrhages but she took a long time to recover. She never did recover her ability to drink, and now a glass or possibly two of wine is the most she ever consumes. We both finally recovered and with recovering health we had friends returning, who all had perfectly acceptable reasons for why they had deserted us.

The word was going around that FAO would not renew the project when its term finished at the end of the year. The massive inflation in Argentina coupled to the artificially high value for the peso meant that costs were rocketing, and although the job was far from done there were positive results that the Argentine government could use for future development of the north-west of the country. We would all need to look for new jobs. Ted Campion took me aside and asked me if I would be interested in running the laboratory in Botswana.

'Jack Falconer is looking for someone who will sort out his lab: he has had a bevy of people none of whom he has kept for more than one term. I think that you might be just the man he is looking for. If you are interested let me know, and write him a letter because I will be seeing him in a couple of weeks when I go to a conference in Bethlehem in the Orange Free State in South Africa. By the way did you know why Christ was born in Bethlehem in Israel and not the Free State?'

'No, but you're going to tell me.'

'Right – they couldn't find three wise men and a virgin in the Free State.'

'Thanks Ted, I will let you have a letter for Jack Falconer.'

I felt that I was now ready to take on the task of running a laboratory and Argentina had taught me many things not to do. A laboratory has to be run by a team, with everyone valued for the contribution they make: there must be no artificial discrimination and division of the team into 'them' and 'us'. The cleaners and post mortem attendants have a vital role to play, as in a laboratory 'cleanliness is definitely next to godliness'. Each member of the team must know what is expected of him or her and there must be open meetings where everyone can have their say.

I certainly had ideas for Gaborone. That all important letter to Jack Falconer the Director of Veterinary Services had to be very carefully drafted. It was a fine balance between stating my experience without overselling myself. The letter was finally written and hand-carried to Botswana by Ted. He and several of his Argentine colleagues had attended the conference on animal nutrition and arrived a couple of days before it started, to overcome the journey and the jetlag. They were not very complimentary about the facilities in Bethlehem: dinner in the hotel was sharp at seven in the evening and there was nothing to do in this dismal town. They were reduced to walking up and down the railway platform until it was time for bed. Ted went on to Gaborone after the meeting while his colleagues returned to Salta. Ted had a meeting with Jack Falconer, gave him my letter and before he left Botswana, the DVS told Ted to tell me that the job was mine and he would write to me.

269

We waited and waited and no letter came, until one morning David Broadbent had a telephone call from a secretary at INTA Castellar asking if there was a Dr Windsor in his project as rather a strange letter had arrived. David said that there was and the letter was sent on. The envelope was addressed:

Dr Roger Windsor MRCVS
Casilla de Correo Argentina,
INTA.

It was not so surprising that it had taken so long; what was surprising that it had arrived at all. The letter confirmed Ted's statement that Jack Falconer wished to recruit me to the post of Provincial Veterinary Officer in charge of the Veterinary Diagnostic and Research Laboratories: he wanted me out there as soon as possible and that I should contact the Overseas Development Agency (now the Department for International Development) on my return to Britain. He would put in motion the necessary request from the Botswana government.

Then a complication developed: a telegram arrived from Rome informing me that I had been appointed to the post of Veterinary Microbiologist in Beirut, Lebanon. Maxine and I decided that I should take no action on this until I was in Rome, in case the Botswana job did not come off.

It was the time to write my final report and close down the work: by and large the Argentines were not sad to see us go: Reuben had been converted to the idea that a laboratory should offer more than just mastitis, but he was off to the USA for a scholarship to study for an MA in mastitis. He never returned to Argentina. Many of the other project members obtained scholarships to study for higher degrees, and this was another of the project's successes.

Because of the inflation and the controlled value of the peso, prices in the country were sky high. My Peugeot 504 sold for $22,000, $3000 more than I had paid for it two years previously. The TV that I bought in Miami for $400 sold for $1000. Perhaps the most incredible sale was my Asahi Pentax camera that I had bought 15 years earlier for $100 and sold for $250. We had arrived in Argentina with massive debts; we left the country with the debts paid off and 'a fistful of dollars': everyone paid in cash dollars. It was said that, at the time, there were more hundred-dollar bills circulating in Argentina than in the USA.

Reuben did even better: he bought a car from one of the project members and then when he heard he was off to the States he sold it for $22,000. He was paid the money on the Saturday morning and as the banks were closed he was unable to convert the money into pesos and put the money in his account. On Sunday night the President made the statement that the country was devaluing its currency, in order to give the peso its true value. The rate of exchange went over night from 4000 pesos to the dollar to 40,000. In Argentine terms, Reuben's car had increased in value tenfold. He immediately paid off the mortgage on his house.

We spent Christmas with the Massés and Campions, said goodbye to all our friends and set off via a round trip of the States, collecting Richard in Miami. My first task on arriving back in Britain was to visit ODA and ensure that the Botswana job was real. It was. I could then set off to Rome to deliver my final report, knowing that I did not need to go and work in a war-zone.

Never in my life have I been subjected to such a barrage as that which met my statement that I would not go to work in Beirut.

'Security is no problem, your wife and family can live in Cyprus and each weekend we will provide you with a return flight to Nicosia.'

'I do not want my wife and family to live in a different country, I want to live with them.'

'They will really enjoy Cyprus, it is a lovely country.'

'Fine, if you offer me a job in Cyprus I will certainly be happy to discuss it with my wife.'

Every person that I dealt with from the Animal Health, Country Planning, Finance or Personnel Departments pressured me to accept the job. The reason for this was that the Director General, Edouard Saouma, was Lebanese and they were having difficulty finding anyone prepared to work in Beirut: it seemed that I was their last chance. The final ultimatum was, 'If you do not accept this job you will never work for FAO again.'

My resolution was beginning to weaken and so I phoned Maxine and told her what had been going on.

'Do you really want to work for an organisation that employs such tactics?'

The next day I went into the office and stated categorically that I was not going, **PERIOD**. It was fifteen years before I got another job with them, when they had to come to me to help sort out contagious bovine pleuro-pneumonia problems in southern Tanzania.

It was on the flight from London to Johannesburg that I realised I had finally graduated from Journeyman to Master, and that I was going to be the head of my own laboratory. I now had the opportunity to put into practice what I had been taught by Ian Beattie, Maryk Gitter, Walter Plowright and Sherwin Hall, not to mention a host of other people who had helped with my education.

PART 4
Master, 1981

15

Botswana

'But I could not afford to fail'
Sir Arthur Conan Doyle, *The Devil's Foot*

The long wait was over: I had served my apprenticeship, worked as a journeyman, had a wide experience of disease diagnosis and control, and I was now to have my own laboratory. 'Would I make the grade?' I wondered. 'Could I make a success of my own laboratory?' I said to myself, 'If you put into practice all that your great teachers have taught you, you must succeed.' Whatever happened I was going to have fun.

When the Botswana Airways DC4 Dakota touched down at Gaborone Airport, I had the feeling of coming home. Africa was in my blood. It is said that once infected by Africa you never recover, although Maxine would not agree. The cheerful immigration and customs staff also bade me welcome to their country. The formalities were soon completed and I was in! Mik Mares, the acting head of the laboratory, was there to greet me in his colonial shorts and regulation long socks. He was a tall, bean-pole of a man with a mop of curly greying hair, a freckled complexion, and an engaging smile.

'Welcome to Botswana,' he said extending his hand.

'We have booked you into The Horrible Inn. It's quite close to here which means it's a bit out of town, but it does have a great swimming pool, and a casino, if you are interested. The only other hotel is The President which is right in the centre of town, is noisy and has neither swimming pool nor garden.'

'The Holiday Inn will do me fine.'

'We will leave all discussion of work until tomorrow but Ruth is expecting you for dinner tonight; I will drop you at the hotel and let you get settled in and call for you at six thirty this evening,'

I had arrived. Dinner that evening was a very pleasant affair and Ruth had gone to a great deal of trouble over the production of the

275

meal: smoked salmon was followed by excellent roast of Botswana beef and the final delight was mangos served with mango sorbet, all accompanied by excellent South African wine. Botswana was in a common customs union with South Africa and as a result all South African goods were available in the country. I was invited to join them the following evening for the Capital Players production of 'My Fair Lady' in the strangely named MOTH Hall, which stands for the Most Honourable Order of Tin Hats, the Southern Rhodesian (now Zimbabwean) equivalent of the British Legion. It was a fantastic show in a delightful little theatre and I was amazed that there should be so much talent in so small a town.

The Veterinary Diagnostic Laboratory was in the grounds of the Princess Marina Hospital not far from the centre of the city. It had originally been built to serve the hospital and the Veterinary Department but had been arbitrarily divided into two when the wives of some of the ministers complained that they did not like their pregnancy tests being carried out in a veterinary laboratory. Now, although they were two separate laboratories there was still a great deal of cooperation between them. The laboratories shared four rows of prefabricated asbestos buildings with tin roofs and no insulation, set in a well wooded site, a stone's throw from the hospital itself. Right on the perimeter of the grounds was our small post-mortem room which luckily was not a shared facility!

The staff lined up to greet me. Stan Rogers, the number two in the lab was a big man in every way. Stan could be nothing but an Irishman, and an Ulsterman to boot. Although not a church-going man, Stan was a vitriolic Protestant: in my mind's eye I can see him in a dark suit with a bowler hat and an orange sash marching behind a pipe band. He was a lovely man, kind and generous to a fault. He had been an Athletics Blue at Trinity College Dublin and played for the Veterinary School first XV at rugby. He could not see the irony of the fact that his closest friend in Botswana was Kevin Cullinan, a Dublin-born Catholic who was head of the CID: they were inseparable drinking pals.

Stan was ten years older than me and with much greater experience in Africa than I had. He could have made my life hell, but he didn't. He was my most loyal supporter, defender and friend. He had worked under a succession of bosses, most of whom had done little to develop the laboratory that Elizabeth Hobday had set up so well 15 years before. He wanted the lab to succeed and he knew that I had

had a wide experience of laboratory work. Give Stan a task and he would do it; sometimes accuracy went out of the window, but the job got done. His great passion was fishing and he loved working at Motopi when we were testing the foot and mouth disease vaccines. The testing started on Monday when the animals were challenged; they were then checked daily until Friday when they were killed and examined. Monday and Friday were busy, but Tuesday, Wednesday and Thursday a couple of inspections and the rest of the day was free, in Stan's case to get a boat out on the Motopi river and fish for tilapia (river bream). The resultant catch, sometimes 100 lb or more, was filleted, frozen and brought back to Gaborone to be distributed. Stan never refused the offer of a trip to Motopi. He had bought a house in Strangford so that he could spend his retirement years with a boat out in the bay fishing. Sadly ill health prevented him from practising what he had so loved to do.

The next to be introduced were Mike Fortey and Ken Digby. Mike was the best technical man I ever worked with: he could repair any piece of equipment with the exception of electronic boards. As an example of his ability it is only necessary to tell the story of the atomic absorption spectro-photometer. Mike was desperate to acquire one to speed up the biochemical analyses. The British High Commissioner was persuaded to give us one from his special fund and we were able to buy it from South Africa, because it was of British make and servicing would be easier from our neighbour. The machine was installed and within a week it ceased to function. Mike examined the machine and realised that the magnetic aperture ring was not working: he phoned the agents and told them.

'They never go wrong, but we will be up on Monday.'

On Monday they found that it was the magnetic aperture ring that was faulty and they had not bought a new one with them. They had to send to Johannesburg for it.

Mike had had a dreadful experience shortly before my arrival: he came home from work one afternoon to find that his wife had left him and gone back to Britain with their son. No word, no letter, nothing. Mike's response to all crises was to drink and this was his undoing. He became less and less reliable as time went by. His drinking was the cause of his second marriage breaking up. He was furious with me when I finally obtained for the laboratory a post of Chief Technician and did not appoint him to it, but brought in a man from outside. Some time after I left, Mike had become an alcoholic and the Ministry dispensed with his services. Stan and friends poured him onto a plane bound for London and that was the last we heard of him.

Ken liked a drink or two but never to excess. He was a micro-biologist and if there is such a term as 'green fingers' to be applied to growing bacteria, well Ken had them. Ken was married to Maria whom he had met on an earlier project, when Maria was working as a secretary in the British Embassy in the Yemen. He was a keen sailor and so frequented the yacht club, but socially they tended to keep themselves to themselves. Both Mike and Ken were well liked by their African staff and both were patient and good teachers.

Emmanuel Galeforolwe and Leonard Manthe were the two senior African members of staff and both had talent, but not as much as they thought that they had. Leonard had been awarded a scholarship to study veterinary medicine in the United States. Sadly he failed the second year of the course and had to transfer to a microbiology course, returning with a bachelor's degree. Emmanuel was not thought up to doing a veterinary degree and came to Britain and studied medical laboratory technology at which he succeeded; he finally made it to the post of Chief Technician. There were a host of young Batswana both male and female in training posts and it was immediately obvious that there was a great wealth of talent waiting to be drawn out for the benefit of the country.

The laboratory even boasted its own 'Mma Ramotswe' (from *The No 1 Ladies Detective Agency*) in Magdalene Ngwanang the laboratory secretary, who was of 'traditional build'. Like her fictional counterpart, she was well educated, intelligent, and fiercely loyal to her country and the laboratory. She was responsible for answering the phone, meeting the public, typing the reports (at the time there were not many of them) and filing them. She did this with great efficiency and was always good natured. It is not surprising that she ended up as secretary to the Permanent Secretary in the Ministry of Agriculture.

Having met the staff, toured the buildings, been shown the equipment and given a briefing on the work, I sat down to discuss the future. My first meeting was a one to one with Mik (his name was Robert, but as a baby he was so small that his father had called him Microbe, and Mik had stuck) and he wanted to stick.

'I tell you Roger, I want to stay in the lab. I am too old to go back to field work. I could do all the administration for you.'

That was exactly what I did not want, somebody coming between me and the team I wanted to build. And so this presented me with my first difficult decision. He had been running the laboratory for a year or more and it was obvious that it was working at a fraction of its capacity and ability. Mik had no background in laboratory work and in my opinion he was too old to start. He had come from Malawi where he had succeeded Phil Bannister (who was now in charge of meat inspection at the Lobatse Abattoir) as Permanent Secretary to the Ministry of Agriculture, having had a distinguished career as a veterinary field officer in that country. But I did not want an administrator: I would do my own, and following Sherwin's way I would want all the senior staff to do their own and shoulder their own responsibilities.

I did not exactly dodge the decision, but I said to Mik, 'I really do not want an administrator, I want all the veterinary staff to take a full part in the work of the laboratory. But let's wait a bit and see how things turn out.'

It was time to go to headquarters and meet the Directorate. Mik drove me to the department which was housed in a collection of buildings similar to the laboratory. It transpired that at Independence when the capital was moved from Mafeking to Gaborone, the sites for the ministries were planned out and temporary buildings (sheds made from asbestos concrete, as were most of the government houses) were erected on the sites. Over the years these buildings were knocked down and replaced by fine modern brick buildings. The capital city is still exactly as it was when freedom came to the country and yet it is totally different with all these smart new office buildings. I was ushered into Jack Falconer's office but Mik was left outside.

Jack was a small solid man from the Black Isle in north-east Scotland, and I found out later that the best man at his wedding was Mr Iain Coull, my very first bank manager in Edinburgh: the man who taught me the basics of managing my finances. Jack was genuinely thrilled to see me.

'You do not realise what a mess I have had to put up with for the past ten years. I have had a succession of laboratory heads who knew little and cared less. I have had to get rid of the lot of them, and I am not a difficult man to please. I just want the laboratory to function and give me results. I have every confidence that you will do the job – you came highly recommended by Ted Campion, and he's a man who knows a thing or two. We have a lot of vets out there working in difficult conditions in a harsh climate and they need back up, support and above all RESULTS. We've got foot and mouth under control, we've opened up beef markets for Europe and now we need to increase production so that we can meet our quota. You do a good job and I will give you all the resources you need. If the work increases and you need more staff you will get them. This department is financed by a levy on the meat going through the export abattoir.' He hardly drew breath.

'This is a big country with few towns and even fewer people. It is a hard climate and almost the only thing you can do with the land apart from dig diamonds out of it is to grow cattle.

'First you have to get a house, but we have a good one ready for you, and get yourself sorted out. Get yourself a decent truck and some kit. So I will not push you but what I want you to do first of all is get out and see the country, meet the people who you will be serving and see for yourself what we are up against. I know, I know.'

So far I had not said a word.

'The first problem you are going to have, is what are you going to do with Mik Mares? You should get rid of him.'

I made a gesture of disapproval as I thought, well, it was you who employed him – perhaps you will soon be saying the same about me. I did not like to contradict my new boss, particularly at our first meeting, but I ventured to suggest, 'I have read about Sebele and the Botswana Agricultural College, do you not think that he could help out teaching the new veterinary assistants and livestock officers?'

'You know, Roger, Botswana has a very good and simple system of animal disease control. Every village has its own veterinary assistant who is the farmers' first port of call. These young men, at the present time there are no women, have a year's training at the BAC in recognising the different organs of the body and what normal tissues look like. They are taught how to cut up a carcase and take samples from any tissue that looks abnormal. I would like the laboratory to become more involved with this course. We teach them how to handle animals and give simple treatments like drenches and intramuscular and sub-cutaneous injections. When they are trained we give them a bag of tricks, to enable them to work, together with a small pharmacy of drugs, and they are sent back home. They sell these drugs to the farmer and purchase replacements from us. The small margin of profit on the drugs boosts their income and makes the farmers realise that treatments cost money. When he gets stuck, he contacts his livestock officer who comes out to assist.

'After two years as veterinary assistants, the best ones are selected to return to the BAC to undertake the livestock officers' training course for two years, on full pay. This course is a para-vet course and something like the Tanzanian "Barefoot Vet" scheme. The difference being that with us the livestock officer works in the field under the guidance of a veterinary officer. The LO is responsible for up to a dozen veterinary assistants, and when he is stuck he goes up the line to the District Veterinary Officer.'

I later found out that the system worked incredibly well.

'Do you, Roger – oh and by the way, it is all Christian names here, so please call me Jack – do you know that BAC might just be the solution to our problems? I'll transfer him to Sebele as soon as your feet are under the table, and I'll not mention that it was your idea.' He said this with a twinkle.

That was Jack: straight, honest, blunt but totally ruthless in pursuit of his goals, which were the success of his department and the country he loved. He spent twenty-eight years in Botswana, eighteen of them as Director of Veterinary Services. Long after independence there was no move to oust him and he went on until his retirement age. Woe betide anyone who crossed him by not doing their job. A veterinary officer let him down by not examining animals properly before they boarded the train for the abattoir (the greatest sin in the book, because they did not want the disease in the abattoir). On arrival at Lobatse there were several animals with clinical foot and mouth disease and, when inspected, a good number had chronic lesions in the mouth and feet: the man had not done his job properly, if at all. He was duly summoned to HQ for a dressing down. At the end of this Jack asked him for his resignation as he could not have in his department vets upon whom he could not rely. The livelihoods of too many people depended upon the export trade. The man demurred, he had a wife and family and could not possibly resign. To which Jack's retort was that he should have thought of wife and family before failing to examine the animals properly. The man was adamant, he would not resign. Jack's response was to transfer him to Rakops, the equivalent of the Russian Gulag, which in those days was a four-day journey in an ox cart from Serowe. When he came to the end of his contract, the officer did not ask for a renewal.

The next office to be visited was that of Martin Mannathoko, the

Motswana chosen to succeed Jack and an affable and competent vet. It was made known to Martin that he had been chosen for his ability and not just because he was a Motswana. He was tall and well built with a round smiling face and a dreadful predilection for wearing flared trousers. He was not a true Motswana, being a Kalanga from the north: the Kalangas were descended from the Zulus who left South Africa during the reign of Dingane to settle in Rhodesia and become the Matabele Tribe, which in turn gave rise to the Kalangas.

Martin welcomed me warmly to his country, wished me a pleasant stay and good luck; he also told me how important it was that I succeed.

From there it was off to see the two Deputy Directors, Tom Stewart and Eddy Bradley. Tom was about to retire and this was my only meeting with him, but Eddy was to become a good friend and his wife Jean, also a vet, soon joined the staff of the laboratory. Eddy was in charge of the budgets and he made it clear that if I wanted money, it was to him I should turn and not Jack. As well as departmental business I was given a run down on the social scene: the one cinema, Capital Players, the golf club, music societies and the Gaborone stables: there was a lot to do and it seemed that Maxine and I would not be short of entertainment. Having seen the HQ, viewed the stores and the pharmacy, it was time to return to the lab and talk to all the senior staff to find out what they wanted.

This meeting became the forerunner of what was to be a regular monthly meeting of senior staff in the Cambridge style, but on that day it was Stan and Mik, Ken and Mike, Emmanuel and Leonard, and Magdalene and me. They were there to talk and I was there to listen. Stan set the ball rolling with an overview of the problems; there were few dairy farms in the country but there was a steady trickle of milk samples; the major supplier of samples was the nation's beef herd where parasites were a problem and surprisingly fascioliasis (liver fluke) was of sporadic importance (surprising because the snail, the intermediate host in the life of this parasite, requires a permanent water supply to survive and Botswana was semi-desert). Anthrax and clostridial diseases were seen from time to time and particularly when there were droughts. Tick-borne disease went in cycles and luckily there was no East Coast fever but there was a constant problem with reproductive diseases. Plant poisonings were also seen during the regular droughts. The only sheep of any consequence were down in the far south where it was almost complete desert and the farmers, mostly Cape Coloureds as they were then known, kept Karakul sheep for their Persian lamb pelts. There were plenty of goats in the villages and also a few pigs and hens. The lab provided a biochemistry and haematology service to the only real small animal practice in the town, Falconer and Bradley.

'What?' I nearly fell off my seat. The Director and the Deputy Director of Veterinary Services were running an after-hours fee-paying clinical service, and it was thought to pay very well. It transpired that profit was not the motive but purely that of providing a service to the pet-owning public in the city. They held a clinic every evening from 5 pm until it finished and on Saturday morning after the 9 am surgery, routine surgery was performed – the clinic was held in one of Jack's servants' quarters that had been modified and was well equipped for most eventualities. I had to get the subject back to the laboratory.

'And what is the rabies situation?' I asked.

The general consensus was that it was not too bad with occasional flare ups. Thanks to regular programmes most of the dogs were vaccinated on an annual basis. Vets working privately carried out the vaccination for a fee, and provided a disc for the collar and an internationally valid certificate. All dogs were entitled to free vaccination but not discs or certificates. When they were vaccinated during a campaign they received a splodge of paint on the head and a week to ten days later the veterinary staff went round the towns rounding up unpainted dogs (they were put to sleep out of the public eye). In the villages notices were put up informing people about the shooting campaign. Teams drove round the villages and any unpainted dogs were shot. In this way the disease was kept under control in settled areas. However, out in the bush where the jackal was the main vector, sporadic cases in cattle, goats and donkeys were seen. There were two exceptions to this general picture: western Botswana was completely free from rabies. Despite the disease being present in eastern Namibia, from Ghanzi south the country was free. There were also two sectors of mongoose rabies, one around Lobatse and one around Francistown, and this manifested as clinical cases in cats with occasional cases in humans.

Ken talked about the diagnostic work not being very demanding but the work for the abattoir required large amounts of staff time and vast quantities of media. The laboratory sent a vehicle each morning from Monday to Friday down to the abattoir to collect samples of tongue, corned beef and meat extract together with any material detained on the slaughter line. He would certainly be grateful for more trained hands to carry out the evaluation work as it was not just the animals that were sampled but the benches, knives, walls and water.

Mike was involved with a large scale food supplementation trial in conjunction with the FAO Animal Husbandry Project which was managed by Nick Buck, a graduate of the London veterinary school whom I had first met in Nairobi. The trial was based in Nata, halfway between Francistown and Maun, then the end of the tarmac road. Mike and his team went up each month and took blood samples from all the animals on trial and these were examined for various minerals. The trial was to evaluate the effects of supplementing the diet with bone meal, a by-product from the abattoir and a good source of calcium and particularly phosphorus, in which southern Africa was especially deficient. He had a long list of equipment that he required, of which the atomic absorption spectrophotometer topped the list. He was happy with his junior staff but being the only trained biochemist he had to do all the interpretation. Leonard worked with Ken and spoke for the junior staff: there was something of the union man about him and in such meetings he tended to become a bit pompous. I felt that had he been wearing a jacket he would be gripping the lapels. They wanted me to do something about the field allowances that they did not receive, whereas the same grade staff working out of their area were paid daily allowances for living out in the bush.

'It is much more expensive to live in Gaborone and these people when they are in the bush get meat from the land.'

'It is just not fair Sir,' Emmanuel agreed, but then Emmanuel almost always agreed with what people said: he was a born again Christian and loved everybody.

Mik talked about the systems that he had tried to set up in the lab but which had not been popular and had not been widely followed. It came home to me very forcibly that I must not impose my views: I must be much more subtle and get them to suggest what I wanted them to do. It had been a really friendly meeting and I had learned a great deal, particularly what an excellent bunch of colleagues I had to work with. When the meeting broke up I invited them all to join me in the Holiday Inn for a beer or two. The two Batswana declined but the rest came to the hotel and we drank a few 'Castles'. The chat was widespread, mostly about colleagues and mutual friends. Maria, Ken's wife had worked in the embassy in Asunción and so the talk turned to South America and the looming problems with Argentina. It had been a wonderful first day and I knew that although there were challenges ahead the next few years were going to be fun. I needed a motor car to make myself independent. Mik knew of an old VW Beetle going for £100 from an expatriate who was on his way home. I had placed an order for a small South African made Nissan and asked a firm of Rhodesian motor mechanics to look out for a good second-hand Land Rover for me: I was still flush with the money we had brought back home from Argentina in hundred-dollar bills.

I had viewed the house we were to live in and it was a delight: 'an improved Type 2'. It still only had three bedrooms but one was in a separate guest wing with its own bathroom which was accessed through a door in the sitting room via a delightful tiny closed garden with a wonderful banana palm that bore regular bunches of small sweet bananas. It was the last house in Tawana Close, with our garden abutting one of Gaborone's small parks and immediately opposite the Russian Embassy. The house came furnished with solid government issue furniture. The sitting room furniture was definitely not designed to lounge in and so I went to a newly opened shop 'The Finishing Touch' and bought a bright and jolly comfortable three piece suite which was to be delivered once I had taken possession of the house.

I was taken to meet David Findlay, a Scot and like me an Edinburgh graduate. He had come out to Botswana to work in the administration as a District Officer and at independence he had decided to throw in his lot with Botswana and became a citizen. Through ability, industry and a burning desire to see his adopted country succeed he too had succeeded and rose rapidly through the ranks. He was now at the top of the civil service despite being only slightly older than me: he had made a good choice, such promotion would not have happened in the British Civil Service. He too was eager to see the laboratory performing as it should as the future for beef exports looked rosy and he could see that Botswana might have difficulty in meeting the quota of meat allocated to it by the European Economic Community.

'Get your domestic arrangements sorted out, get the family settled in and get started,' were his instructions.

There were many people wanting me to succeed and prepared to help when it was needed. It was time for the Veterinary Diagnostic and Research Laboratory to show what it could do. Once settled in, I intended to do it. Maxine arrived with the family and, unlike her Argentine experience, she arrived to a lovely house set in a large, neat well-maintained garden with running water, electricity that worked for most of the time, a telephone in the house and the ability to dial England when it was needed. The sea freight arrived in good order and soon she had her piano tuned and was playing again.

This piano set her on a course which she follows to this day. While in Botswana she studied for and obtained the Teaching Diploma of the Associated Board of the Royal Schools of Music and she taught while she was studying. In Gaborone she met an inspirational musician, David Slater, who taught music at Maru-a-Pula School, an independent, co-educational boarding school. David was the main driving force for music in the city and conducted the excellent Gaborone Symphony Orchestra and the Gaborone Singers, a very fine choir. Concerts were a regular feature of the calendar and it was amazing how much musical talent there was among both the indigenous and expatriate communities.

Jack and Christine Purves were musicians from the Oberlin Musical School in Ohio, USA, who had come out to teach in 'high school' and were based in Maun where Jack was the headmaster. They transferred down from Maun as Jack was required to work in the Ministry of Education. Christine had a great rapport with the local people and soon had her own choir running in Gaborone. There were two Swedish sopranos with voices like angels, Anne Olofsson and Ann Kristin Bergland. Ulrich Balke straight from the Hannover Opera Orchestra came to run an SOS Village near Gaborone and had brought his cello with him. Gunhild Neumann-Redlin, who was also from Hannover and a professional violinist, had come to live in Lobatse with her mining engineer husband. There were American clarinettists and horn players, sopranos, tenors and bass singers, an English bassoon player who also taught physics, string players and singers, and there was even a South African lawyer who played the double bass. There were a large number of very talented people who came to Botswana not only to work, but also to play.

David immediately realised Maxine's talent and she was called upon to assist as a rehearsal pianist, from which she soon graduated to performing in concerts and as a soloist with the symphony orchestra. I can remember her playing Beethoven's First Piano Concerto, with the Gaborone Symphony Orchestra in the hall of Thornhill School in mid-summer with the temperature almost 40° C. She had a wide piano stool on which was a 'cool-box' containing ice-packs. When not playing she kept her hands in the box to prevent them over-heating. Both she and the orchestra gave wonderful performances which brought the audience to its feet. With music for Maxine and theatre for me, I soon realised that we were going to enjoy our stay in the country.

Note on terminology in Botswana:
The country is BOTSWANA
A citizen is a MOTSWANA
Several citizens are BATSWANA
The language they speak is SETSWANA.

16

My First Safari

'My practice could get along very well for a day or two,' said Dr Watson.
Sir Arthur Conan Doyle, *The Naval Treaty*

BM Engineering was a small, developing company of motor mechanics and was considered the best in town. It was run by two brothers who had come down from Rhodesia, dismayed by what was going on there, and they had rapidly established a reputation for integrity, reliability and quality. Brian phoned me to say that he had found a five-year-old Land Rover that had been well look after and maintained: it could be mine for £4500 sterling. It became mine, and my Argentine pool dwindled.

'I will make sure that everything is in tip top shape,' said Brian, 'but you will need to carry spares where you will be going.' He also listed for me the tools that I should carry in case things went wrong. There was a wonderful Aladdin's cave of a hardware shop owned by a Yemeni family, and they stocked almost every tool known to man. They supplied me with all that I required and a splendid box to put it in. Brian decided that I needed extra jerry cans for fuel, water containers at the front and a ladder at the rear to make access to the roof-rack easier.

The Botswana government preferred its staff to use their own transport, on the reckoning that people look after their own property better than government property. Consequently they paid a good rate for official mileage with a differential for 'off-road' usage and allowed staff to use a government driver in their own car. The official laboratory driver was Alford, a bright and cheery Kalanga who, I was to find, was an excellent travelling companion; his main role was to drive to Lobatse each day to collect the samples from the abattoir, but going up country meant 'field allowances' which added to the family exchequer. We would be going to Francistown where he came from and so there would be relatives to see and free accommodation.

It was planned to be a round trip, visiting the Veterinary Offices in Mahalapye, Palapye and spending the first night in Selibe Phikwe where there was an excellent hotel that served the copper mine. The next morning would be spent in the Veterinary Office with Russell Leadsom, the DVO, before driving the 100 miles to Francistown. At the time there were two hotels in Francistown, The Grand that wasn't and The Tati that was! The Grand was thought to be the least worst: a problem in both hotels was that if you had a room on the ground floor you had to keep the windows tight shut or the whores climbed in looking for business. A whole day was planned for the Veterinary Office in Francistown which was the departmental headquarters for the north of the country. Then to Nata to see the Sebele research project and on to Maun, where there was a choice of tourist accommodation. I chose Crocodile Camp on the advice of Alan Wellwood the DVO. We would spend a morning in Maun and then drive to Ghanzi with its famous Kalahari Arms Hotel which had a hitching post for your horse outside and swinging saloon double doors to enter. A real 'wild west' hotel.

At the last minute it was decided that we would not drive back across the Kalahari through Kang as the journey could not be done in a day and so we would have had to carry the complete camping gear. Instead it was decided that we should return the way we went. Ken asked if I could take a passenger who wanted to see Ghanzi. He was the Pakistani husband of a Canadian volunteer microbiologist who worked in the medical laboratory. I am glad that I did as he introduced me to the music of John Denver and even gave me some of his tapes when he left the country. Aziz, or Azi as everyone called him, was a good travelling companion and the three of us had a most enjoyable time on the road.

My first trip in my first Land Rover started early in the morning before the sun was too hot, or at least it was supposed to. Brian had not been happy with something in the Land Rover and asked me to call in on my way north. He had decided that I needed a new condenser and it proved more difficult to replace than he thought and so it was after ten when we finally set off.

As Nigeria and the Argentine pampas, so Botswana – the land is flat for mile after mile with only the odd apology for a hill to break up the landscape, but it was much more interesting than either. In Nigeria the bush was all the same; here there were majestic thorn-trees and a great variety of small bushes. Like Argentina the roadside

289

was fenced but there were no oven bird nests on the posts. Instead there a great variety of beef breeds of cattle, some pure but most crosses. There were small pockets of game animals but not many; small antelopes and an occasional majestic kudu with his huge curly horns were seen and towards Selibe Phikwe we saw a small herd of giraffe.

We soon arrived at Mahalapye with its wide dry river. Mahalapye stands where it is because of this 'sand' river – the water runs all year but mostly underground and so does not evaporate. Throughout the town along the river people dig wells and put pipes into the river and pump out the water. From the town there are roads into the desert and the various 'cattle posts'.

Botswana has a strange system of land ownership and usage. In certain parts of the country such as Ghanzi and the Tuli Block and around the principal towns it is possible to buy and sell land, but the vast majority of the land is owned by the tribe and can be allocated to individuals. Once you have been allocated a piece of land you are entitled to sink a borehole and erect buildings around it. No borehole may be drilled within five miles (eight kilometres) of another. This borehole is the 'cattle post', and although a person may buy and sell cattle posts, the land does not belong to him but to the tribe. Any new owner has to be approved. The land may not be fenced, although it is permitted to erect holding yards and crushes where the water is pumped from the ground, but cattle are unlikely to wander more than five miles from their water supply. This has great implications for disease control because cattle will not mix or have contact with cattle belonging to other owners. On fenced properties, farmers are more inclined to use all the land they have and to carry water to outlying parts, and so ironically cattle on fenced farms are more likely to have contact with those belonging to the neighbours. The owner of a cattle post rarely lives there; he employs a local man to run the place but visits it on a regular basis to bring food for the staff, diesel for the pump and supplements for the cattle.

The Batswana think of themselves as cattlemen and every tribesman yearns to have his own cattle post. There is the delightful story about President Sir Seretse Khama; when he was feeling overworked or depressed he would go at the weekend to his cattle post, sit on his Botswana chair made of rough wood with strips of dried cow hide for the seat, and just watch his cattle and presumably wrestle with the problems of state in peace. His peace was disturbed one Saturday afternoon when Kenneth Kaunda, the President of Zambia, arrived in Gaborone for an unplanned visit. There were no mobile phones to recall Sir Seretse, and so Kaunda was taken to him. They sat together on their chairs drinking bush tea with their aides kept at a distance, and what they talked about nobody knows.

It is therefore not surprising that the Botswana government wanted to promote their cattle industry and that Jack Faulkner was so powerful. It was said that he was the only person allowed to attend cabinet meetings in shorts. Many Batswana men owned cattle and all Batswana men wished to. When asked why he was so concerned about the livestock industry when diamonds were producing so much wealth for Botswana, Sir Seretse's famous reply was, 'My people cannot eat diamonds.'

At the time there was no Veterinary Officer in Mahalapye but there was a Senior Livestock Officer in charge of the district and he made us very welcome. We sat outside the office under a large mophane tree and drank Indian tea – I could never get used to the rooibos tea so favoured by the South Africans and Mma Ramotswe. Cattle were trekked to Mahalapye and then entrained for Lobatse. There was a large holding ground by the station where the cattle were held and inspected before being let on to the train. The tongue of every animal had to be carefully inspected for signs of foot and mouth disease; Mr Njui had a bevy of veterinary assistants for this work and any tongue less than perfect was referred to a senior officer to check. Ground conditions are so dry that lameness is not common in the country and when it occurs it is usually caused by overgrowth of the horn which can be remedied by judicial hoof trimming. Any lame animal in the kraal had its feet inspected but this was not a routine.

Mr Njui was happy with his lot and his life in the Veterinary Department; he enjoyed running his district and I found out later that he was highly respected by all, especially by the old Boer farmers who had settled farms round the town. These senior Batswana Livestock Officers were the salt of the earth; Jack trusted them implicitly and they repaid his trust by their devotion to their work, the department and the man.

Unlike Nigeria and Argentina, Botswana had an excellent telephone service to all the major towns, even Ghanzi on the west of the country. When I was in Shakawe in 1995, and heard of Stan's death over the radio, I was able to call from the DVO's office to Maxine, in

Scotland, to inform her of the sad tidings. But it was the radio that interrupted our discussions. At 1.45 pm the Veterinary Department had the use of the radio frequency to speak to the various offices beyond the reach of a telephone. Woe betide any officer who failed to make the daily briefing. The laboratory was later able to join in this discussion and we were able to pass on the results of our examinations. In this way Jack could control the foot and mouth disease vaccination campaigns from his office in Gaborone. The first part of the time was given out to informing people which districts were to speak and in which order; this was done to prevent chaos with twenty or more people on the air. There was nothing for Mahalapye. Jack had instructed all staff that there was to be no mention of foot and mouth disease, instead they had to say 'they thought that Christmas was coming'! When asked why they should use this message, Jack's reply was typical: 'Whenever I ask for money for the department I have to do battle with Ministers of Health, Education and Finance, but I have only to tell them that we have foot and mouth disease then all the money I want is available, just like Christmas.' Jack put out a brief to all northern stations that I was on the road and so they should sort out what they wanted from the laboratory.

At the end of the radio interlude we said our farewells and set off for Palapye, where we were met by another Senior Livestock Officer and more tea was drunk as we discussed the problems of the district and what they wanted from the laboratory. The same complaint was repeated to me at every stop, they wanted the reports the day before they sent the samples! They wanted to know what they were to do before the animals died or recovered. I had always believed that laboratory reports need to be working documents and not historical records. I asked what he did when he had problems that he did not understand or a disease that he had never seen before.

'I phone Dr David [Brown] in Serowe and he will always come down, it is only forty miles from here and he is a very good man.'

Serowe was the ancestral home of the Bamagwato, the biggest and most powerful tribe in Botswana, of which Sir Seretse Khama had been Paramount Chief before his untimely death from pancreatic cancer. His son Ian was too young to be enthroned and a Regent was appointed. I was given a lesson in racial politics in Palapye: I was told that when Seretse Khama became President of Botswana he was Paramount Chief of the Bamagwato and Member of Parliament for

Serowe. He decided that it was a job too many and that he could not do all three adequately, and so the constitution was amended so that the president, although elected by parliament rather than by the popular vote, was not required to remain a member for a particular constituency. He stood down and asked his friend from childhood days, Colin Blackbeard, a trader and son of a trader, to stand for the constituency. Colin pointed out that he was white. This cut no ice with Sir Seretse; Colin was a Motswana, born and raised in Serowe, spoke Setswana as his mother tongue and was known to all as a man who dealt fairly with everyone.

'But the electors are all black.'

'Forget colour and race, they will vote for you as a man.'

Colin stood for parliament and with the support of Sir Seretse he achieved more than ninety percent of the votes cast. I heard the details of this story again at a later date from Colin himself; the Blackbeards lived in the close adjacent to Tawana.

After requesting that if they had any problems they should contact us because the laboratory was there to serve them, and to call in and see us when the staff were in Gaborone, we set off on the last leg of the day's journey. We were later than planned and did not arrive at the Pikwe Hotel until after dark. Alford and Azi made their own arrangements. When I checked in the receptionist gave me a note asking me to phone the home of the District Veterinary Officer. Russell Leadson came straight over and the first thing he did was to apologise for not inviting me to dinner. He and his wife had been in a quandary about what to do, not knowing whether at the end of a long drive I would want to socialise or just have a bath, dinner and bed.

'Think no more about it: it has been a long hot day and I am sure there will be plenty more opportunities for me to meet your wife.'

We fell to talking about the problems of the district. Russell had only recently taken over from Tony Holmes who together with the vet lab was held in high esteem in Selibe Pikwe. Tony had been walking into town on a Saturday morning when he heard a scream and saw the mine manager's wife in her garden being attacked by a dog. He rushed into the garden and got the dog off the woman, who had been bitten in several places. Finding a garden implement he cornered the dog and kept it there: a crowd had gathered and the manager of the mine was sent for, to bring a rifle. The dog was shot, its head was removed and put in a sealed plastic bag and placed in a bucket. Tony phoned Stan at home, because in those days the laboratory did not work on Saturday mornings. Stan agreed to get the lab up and running to check the brain for rabies. Meanwhile the victim was being treated in the Pikwe hospital.

The mine plane was called into use and the dog's head in the bucket was flown down to Gaborone. The mine representative was there to collect the bucket and take it to the laboratory where Stan's team were ready. The brain was removed, smears were made from the Ammon's horn and stained with fluorescent antibody. Within two hours of the brain's arrival a positive diagnosis of rabies was made, which was phoned through to the hospital. Stan was informed that the hospital had no vaccine: the laboratory always kept vaccine in case of accidents in the laboratory. Luckily the plane was still in Gaborone and so the pilot was able to take the vaccine back and within six hours of being bitten the woman had received her first dose of vaccine. She survived! The mine staff were impressed. This is what veterinary investigation is all about. We had another beer and I said I would be in the office at nine the next morning to give him time to get the necessary administration out of the way. There is nothing worse than having visitors first thing in the morning.

The following morning I was able to see Selibe Pikwe for the first time. It was a pretty little town with many trees: the eastern half of the country receives more rain and as a consequence is more densely forested. It had more in common with a small town in England than those towns I had seen so far in Botswana. It was neat and tidy and all the roads were paved. I presumed that was because the mining company had laid out the town and probably paid for the upkeep. However, the veterinary office was government issue; all veterinary offices were the same – one or more lines of rooms with a covered walkway joining them and raised about two feet from the ground to prevent flooding from the rare downpours of torrential rain.

Russell was smartly turned out in shorts and long socks: it is amazing how smart such attire can be, and in that climate it was good to have a bit of a breeze about the knees. We had a useful discussion about the disease problems in his area which extended to the borders with South Africa and Southern Rhodesia (now Zimbabwe) and so he had to deal with problems of smuggling. The Tuli block which was an area of settled farms (probably the most productive in Botswana) was some distance from him and those farmers were often the most demanding, so he spent a great deal of time travelling. He needed the laboratory to come out and help him investigate infertility problems and results were needed quickly when samples were sent. Plant poisonings were of concern particularly in the dry season. He wished to carry out some simple testing in the office because getting samples to Gaborone could take time. I have always been in favour of vets examining blood smears for anthrax and protozoan parasites and examining faecal samples for parasite eggs, only sending samples to us from time to time to check that their results were correct.

Tony Holmes in Francistown also felt that they should have the ability to undertake simple examinations in his office. The journey to Francistown took less than three hours. We picked up Azi in the town; he had come across a bunch of Pakistanis and had had an enjoyable time. We arrived in late afternoon and I settled into the Grand Hotel (unfortunately on the ground floor) but was quickly rescued by Tony who took me home to meet Cynthia and to have a couple of beers on the veranda before an excellent dinner. Tony was an Edinburgh graduate, but some years after me, and was well into his second tour in Botswana and enjoying the experience. There was a post for Principal Veterinary Officer (North) and Tony was hoping to be offered it. He covered a huge area from the Sua Pan in the Kalahari right up to Kasane on the border with Zambia and Southern Rhodesia. There were several large ranches along the Tati river where there were also disused gold mines. From time to time he was asked to visit the Orapa Diamond Mine, which was closer to Serowe, but the mine had constructed a good road to Francistown. The mine was almost self-sufficient in milk, beef, pork, chicken and eggs as they had invested heavily in a farm at the mine. The mine also boasted one of the best restaurants in Botswana: I was later able to confirm this.

When we met in his office Tony voiced his concern that Botswana would be unable to meet the quota we had been given by the EEC. Already getting animals to the abattoir was a major undertaking; cattle were trekked and trucked and finally put on the train to Lobatse; his resources were really stretched trying to cope with the inspections each time a mode of transport was changed or the animals passed a cordon fence.

The cordon fences caused much anguish to the wildlife community, although they did little to interfere with most wild animal movements. In Botswana, foot and mouth disease was associated with contact with buffalo: these animals harboured the South African Types (SAT) of the virus and were a threat whenever cattle and buffalo mixed. There were only buffalo in the north of the country and so the north was the most at risk, although uncontrolled movement could take the infection south and the disease with it. By means of these fences the country was divided into three areas. The northern area known to harbour animals carrying the virus was called the infected area and all cattle were vaccinated twice a year: meat from animals in this area was not exported to Europe. Animals from the south of the country were known to be free from the infection, were never vaccinated and their meat could be exported anywhere. Between these two zones was a buffer zone where animals were not vaccinated and their meat was not exported to Europe but was acceptable to the South Africans. Wherever the fence crossed a road there was a quarantine post with a holding ground. All vehicles passing through were stopped and the number plate recorded; the goods being carried were inspected and it was forbidden for meat to be brought south.

Because vaccinated and unvaccinated animals could not be allowed to mix, sending animals to the one commercial abattoir in Lobatse had to be tightly controlled. This was what was giving Tony a massive headache at the time of my visit. When the abattoir was slaughtering for Europe then cattle from his area had to stay put. When the slaughter finished, the abattoir was opened to all and it was essential to get the northern animals down there before it was time to shut the abattoir again, give it a complete spring clean so that it could be opened again to animals from the south.

There was a European Senior Livestock Officer, Ken Ward in HQ, who basically did the organisation of lorries and trekking parties, but it was Tony's job to get the work carried out and the animals to the abattoir. It was a hard and onerous job but had to be done so that the farmers could be paid for their work. This involvement had really got to Tony, so much so that he had invented a board game rather like Monopoly where the object was to get your cattle first to the abattoir. Among the hazards that I can remember are:

Driver of lorry cannot find the cattle post
Driver gets drunk
Driver finds a girlfriend in a bar and fails to turn up for two days
Lesions of foot and mouth disease found on inspection

He lent the game to me so that I could better understand the problems of livestock farming in Botswana. The children thought that it was a pretty enjoyable game to play, but it was never put into the shops.

I could understand why Jack was so keen for me to go round the country because at each stopping place I was learning something new about the jigsaw puzzle that is the Botswana livestock industry, but it was getting difficult to remember all the names; to us most Batswana names are very difficult to pronounce and even more difficult to remember.

We broke the journey to Maun at Nata, where the Kasane Road to the borders with Zambia and Rhodesia branches off. The Nata project was an FAO project and not a Botswana government one; they did not know we were coming and there were no senior staff on hand to explain what was happening, although there would be other times. At Nata the tarmac ended and it was a dirt road for the rest of the way. We did not stop at Motopi because there were no trials going on at the time, in fact there was only activity for one week a month. The rest of the time the place was in the care of a bunch of staff who looked after the cattle and made sure nothing got in or out. They also looked after the building that was the office, the dining room, the store and laboratory, and the rondavels that provided the accommodation for visiting workers.

Crocodile Camp was a bit off the beaten track and Maun is a maze of unbeaten tracks. The soil is very sandy here from the silt deposited by the Okavango river; as a result it is very fertile and there were extensive fields of vegetables growing near the various tributaries of the river. This river never makes it to the sea but breaks up into a delta and dies in the Kalahari sands and Maun is at the end of the main branch of the delta. At the time there was no main street in Maun just a myriad of shops and pubs and houses with the odd hotel and government office for good measure. But Maun was the fun place to be and Crocodile Camp was where it all happened. The owner Lindsay Birch had been the Head of the Game Department, and on retirement had started this tourist camp. Like Motopi it consisted of a central building that was reception, lounge, bar and dining room, with surrounding rondavels each with a comfortable bed and a private toilet and shower.

Lindsay had one aim as an inn keeper which was to get all newcomers to the camp absolutely paralytic. I must hang my head in

297

shame and admit that he succeeded with me. I do not know how he ever made any money at hotel keeping, because he mostly paid for the booze that got his clients drunk. I had not been warned of the dangers of Crocodile Camp and did not know what I was letting myself in for when after a good dinner I was informed that it was customary for all newcomers to be given a set of traffic lights as an introduction to Maun. They had to be drunk in the order that the lights changed. The red was cherry brandy, the green was Chartreuse and I suspect that the yellow was van der Humm, a South African liqueur. All a bit sweet to my taste. By then the bar was full of habitués who realised there was another sucker in town; half a dozen played Colonel Bogie, in which you shake two dice and the first person to roll a total of seven gets to choose a drink or combination of drinks such as brandy, port and Benedictine which actually tastes rather good, the second who rolls seven, pays for it, and by a strange coincidence it was Lindsay who had to pay. And of course I got the third seven and it is he (always a he, women are too intelligent to play this game) who has to drink it. After the second round, where by strange chance I was the third person to get a seven and so drank a mixture of something quite vitriolic, I suspected that the game was rigged and declined to play further. But it was too late, a combination of about ten different spirits had done their worst. Luckily my rondavel was not too far away. I drank a pint or more of water and collapsed onto my bed wondering why the room was going round and round.

It was with some surprise that I woke the next morning at seven without a trace of a hangover and able to eat a traditional English breakfast. Two nights had been allocated to Maun, one to give a measure of a respite after the long daily journeys, before facing the road to Ghanzi, and also it was not a good idea to complete the journey in the dark for fear of getting lost.

Alan Wellwood had also been at Edinburgh, a contemporary of Tony Holmes and seemingly a confirmed bachelor until he married in his mid-forties. Alan was not your immaculate veterinary officer: his standard outfit was a pair of shorts, a shirt worn outside the shorts and his feet untroubled by socks were encased in a pair of flip flops. When working I never saw him in anything else. His patch was enormous, joining with Francistown and extending on the west to the border with South West Africa (now Namibia) and to the north Shakawe and the Caprivi Strip. In the south his boundary with

Ghanzi was at Sehitwa where the road splits and the Shakawe turning branches off. The whole of the Okavango delta was in his area. To get to some places in the delta was a two-day journey, and during the rainy season some places were inaccessible by road. The Okavango delta was a tourist paradise with its huge numbers of elephant, buffalo, rhino, large and small antelope, giraffe and lion and leopard. There was a great variety of birds and throughout the delta there were safari camps to suit most pockets.

Alan just loved his job and the life in Maun. Apart from foot and mouth disease, his main concern was the tsetse fly and trypanoso-miasis, that wiggly little protozoan parasite that is transmitted by the fly, which sucks blood and transmits sleeping sickness in man, and a serious debilitating disease in cattle and other species of animal. Unlike the mosquito which is a 'silent biter' using its proboscis as a fine needle to suck the blood, the tseste fly is a 'slasher', with mouth parts like scissors that chop a hole and the fly drinks from the pooled blood. At one time almost the whole of Africa and certainly the whole of Botswana was infested with the tsetse fly, but the great rinderpest pandemic of the 1890s killed so many game animals as well as cattle that in marginal areas the fly died out. Only the Okavango region was infested with the fly; not even on the banks of the 'Great, Grey, Green Greasy Limpopo River', which forms the border with South Africa in the east, did it survive. The Botswana government was determined that it would not spread to the Lim-popo, and when you passed through a quarantine post leaving the tsetse area, your car was sprayed with insecticide to kill any flies like the tsetse which are attracted to moving objects.

There are two different species of the trypanosome that cause disease in man but these parasites do not usually infect other species of animal. There are three common species that infect cattle and unfortunately all can infect man, producing identical clinical signs. Alan was not keen to talk about trypanosomiasis because he had arranged for me to meet the Chief Tsetse Control Officer in the afternoon. He was however keen to talk about contagious bovine pleuro-pneumonia which was present across the Namibian border. He was certain that it was only the presence of the South African Defence Force (the army) that stopped the disease crossing into Ngamiland (north-west Botswana). There was a double fence the whole length of the border between South West Africa and Bots-wana and this was patrolled twenty-four hours a day. Herero people live on both sides of the border and up into Angola: the women wear the most wonderful outfits copied from the wives of the German missionaries who came to the land in the nineteenth century with bustles and huge horn-shaped headdresses. Pleuro-pneumonia was kept alive in the herds by the regular illegal movement into and out of Angola which the Defence Force seemed unable to stop.

How prescient were Alan's remarks. After the Independence of Namibia the South African Defence Force was withdrawn; a few days later the fence was cut and cattle were moving back and forth, and it was not long before pleuro-pneumonia was confirmed in Botswana for the first time in more than 60 years.

After lunch Alan took me to meet Jeff Bowles; he was a graduate from the London School and a contemporary of Sherwin. Jeff was enjoying life in Maun, the work was interesting and rewarding and he and his wife enjoyed to the full the social life that Maun offered. He was keen to tell me about the eradication programme for the tsetse fly. Aerial spraying was being employed using 'Samarin' at four grams per hectare. Samarin was being used because it specifically targeted tsetse fly without affecting any other insects. It caused no harm to mammals and the only adverse environmental effect reported was that it affected fish that were stopped from breeding for a season, although their long-term breeding seemed not to be affected. Each season they were spraying a defined block and then they went into the area and painted the trees round the margins, which are used as resting places by the tsetse, with 'Aldrin', an organo-chlorine compound that can only be obtained on special licence. This was to stop tsetse recolonising the area.

At the start of the campaign a headquarters in the delta was selected with adequate road communication to the spray zone. A helicopter was used to get staff in and out from this base camp but the basic supplies were brought by road. I was invited to come up and watch the spraying in progress. A year or so later I went to see the spraying in action. The base camp was only fifteen minutes by helicopter or a twelve-hour drive in a truck. It was my first ascent in a helicopter and we had a German pilot who was a complete maniac. He made sure that we had strapped ourselves in and donned our headsets; he left the door open to give us a better view of the game – it seemed a strange idea to me, but those who had flown with him before thought it normal – and off we went. Before long we saw elephants in the swamps and with a whoop of joy he dropped down to give us a good view. Before I knew where we were, the helicopter was on its side and we were staring through the open door at an elephant about twenty feet below us. I thought that if the seatbelt broke, I would be sitting on its back; I was petrified and remained so throughout the rest of the flight. However we arrived safely at our destination. No beer was drunk before dinner, which was a warming stew as it can get cold in the night out in the swamps and after dinner we dressed warmly and set off in a line of trucks to the spot where we would link up with the planes.

Spraying was at night so that the spray did not evaporate; it also had to be a still night to prevent spray drift. On a chart six to eight target points were marked for the spraying to commence. At the appointed time the truck would be on the site with a massive searchlight mounted on the back and the beam would be shone in the sky. The plane would fly directly over the beam on a pre-determined course and would commence spraying. The pilot would fly for ten miles, stop spraying and return to look for the searchlight in its new position and flying the same course he would spray for another ten miles. The ground crew were in radio contact with the pilot. The spraying would be repeated until the evening's work was done, the plane would return to base in Maun and the ground team would return to camp for a well-earned couple of beers. The next day the sprayed area would be examined to see that there had been no untoward effects. Each year the area occupied by the tsetse fly grew smaller and it was hoped that the insect might be finally eradicated. It was extremely hard work during the campaign but there was a great team spirit in the camp and there was no shortage of volunteers prepared to live for several weeks in the bush.

Of course this work was not without its detractors: the open-toed sandal brigade as they were called thought it quite wrong to disturb the balance of nature but these people had never lost a child from sleeping sickness or seen the flesh drop off their prize animals.

'If you've nothing better to do, why not come home at the end of the day and have a swim?'

'I can think of nothing better to do,' I replied.

'Just come when you are ready.'

Jeff had the reputation of a guest never swimming a length of his pool before there was a can of cold 'Castle' waiting, and sure enough as I completed the first length, there was that tin sitting on the side. I declined an invitation to stay for a pot-luck dinner because after the predations of the previous night I needed to get to bed early and sober. I made the excuse that I had to write up my notes. After dinner at Crocodile Camp I went into the bar but there was no repetition of the previous night – I had earned my spurs

Alford and Azi arrived at Crocodile Camp spot on eight in the morning just as I finished my breakfast: I had settled up the previous evening and my bag was packed. We were on the road once more and what a strange road it was. It was like a maze in heavy sand. Different drivers had different tactics for driving on this sandy bush road. This was not a proper road, despite it being the main road to a major settlement. The cattle were trekked along the Francistown route to Lobatse but the road from Maun to Ghanzi was one of Botswana's major arteries: sometimes the road branched into five or more tracks, but Alford assured me they all joined up again. After Sehitwa we lost the really heavy sand, the road more resembled a road and we were able to increase our speed. By mid-afternoon we were in Ghanzi, the one-saloon town.

This hotel had accommodation for all and to suit all pockets; we all stayed together although Alford did not eat with us but sought the food he liked at a price his subsistence would allow. The hotel owner regaled me with stories of a previous Veterinary Officer, Tony Williams, of great size and great drinking habits. He could consume a case of twenty-four cans in an evening and still remain sober. When he carried out private work on the local farms, he never asked for cash but charged in cases of 'Castle'.

The food in the hotel was pretty good considering how far Ghanzi was from any other town. There was only one regular flight to Ghanzi a week and that was the Barclay's Bank plane on a Wednesday which arrived at 11 am and left again at 3 pm: it was possible to book a passage on this flight but you had to return the same day or wait for a week!

Mr Khumalo, a large grizzled African, was the Senior Livestock Officer in charge of Ghanzi District, and very cross about it he was.

'This district should have a Veterinary Officer in charge, not an uneducated man like me. Every time I see Dr Falconer, I tell, please send me a veterinary officer and do you know what he say?'

'No,' I said. This was our first meeting; you do not joke with well-respected senior men on first acquaintance and Mr Khumalo was considered the best of them all.

'Dr Falconer say, these Boer farmers with your help can look after

302

themselves. I need to put vets where the farmers are not educated, to help them improve.'

Mr Khumalo might have been short of book learning, because he joined the service long before the Botswana Agricultural College was started, but he was not uneducated. He had native wit, and intelligence, an insatiable desire to learn, the ability to work hard: he had loyalty, integrity and perhaps the greatest gift of all, he knew his own limitations and when he needed to get help. I did not know this at the time, but I sort of guessed that this was a man of stature that Jack would treasure as the best of the best. More will be heard of Mr Khumalo and his tenacity. At the present he was telling me about his district.

He dealt with three groups of settled farms the most important of which were the settled ranches round the town and which extended 100 miles to the north and south. These had been settled by Boer farmers who trekked across the Kalahari to get away from intrusive Afrikaner government in the late nineteenth century. They were good solid farmers who were not receptive to new ideas, kept themselves to themselves and looked after their staff. To the south at Mamuno are a group of ranches owned by people of 'Cape Coloured' descent, probably from the same group that settled southern Botswana. The third group of settled ranches were owned by black Batswana and were way into the desert at Metsimanshu (Blackwater) and a long hard drive over deep sand. There are many cattle posts out in the desert but not as many as in the east. Many of the farm workers on all the farms were Bushmen and there were many different clans wandering across the Kalahari. Mr Khumalo was full of admiration for these people who could survive forever in a waterless world.

'They know where there is underground water, and if going on a long journey they bury ostrich eggs filled with water in the sand to supply the return. They know which plant has a big root filled with water and they know where to find the game. They are very clever people.

'I was wondering, Sir, if you would be kind enough to come with me this afternoon to a village where there are settled Bushmen and they have a problem of calves dying, but I have no more information?'

'I have no equipment with me but if you can supply me the post mortem kit and sample bottles and a case of drugs, we should make out.'

'I will prepare our usual field case, and thank you for agreeing to come. This is a big area without a single good road: several farmers have their own plane and can bring in help when it is required. The others have to depend upon me and my staff.'

Mr Khumalo then talked fondly about the Kalahari desert.

'It is not a real desert but I am concerned that it is becoming so. The grass can only support one beast for twenty hectares and so to make a living the farms need to be very big. Some of these Batswana farmers, they have too many animals and the mouths and their feet are destroying the vegetation, and I am afraid, Sir, that once it is gone we will not see it back and we will have desert like the Namib which can support next to nothing. The government is trying to stop this overgrazing, but people are greedy and do not think of their children.

'You would be amazed to see how the grass can grow after we have been blessed by rain. You can almost stand here and watch it grow. At the same time you can see the cattle getting fat. We had a bad drought that lasted for more than two years and during that time none of the Bushman ladies produced babies. Then the rain came, the grass grew and the Bushman ladies' bellies all grew full. It was a happy time Sir.'

We started talking about the disease problems in the area; it was the same story as the rest of Botswana, except that there was no rabies. But this worried Mr Khumalo, because there was a strange manifestation of the disease across the border. The disease had established itself in kudu; normally ruminants are 'dead end hosts' and do not spread the infection. In this part of Namibia this does not hold true. The kudu, almost uniquely among ruminants, have a habit of grooming each other and it is thought that this practice spreads the virus. The virus can be present in great quantities in the saliva and so the licking could introduce the virus through breaks in the skin. Infected kudu were known to enter human dwellings and attack people. Mr Khumalo was afraid they would cross into Ghanzi and bring the disease with them.

'But we are ready Sir; Missee Hobday when she was here set up the red box system.'

This was a wooden box painted scarlet with a lid that could be locked with a padlock. The padlocks in every veterinary office were identical and the laboratory had a key. Inside the box were two 2 lb Kilner jars, one half full of formalin and the other containing a solution of glycerine. The brain of the suspect animal was removed and divided longitudinally. One half was put into the formalin and the other into the glycerine which prevented bacterial growth during the journey, so that despite the time and the high temperatures the brain would arrive in Gaborone in reasonable condition. The sample in formalin was used for making histological sections in case we saw no Negri bodies. Buses, lorries or even private cars going to Gaborone were asked to deliver the locked box to the laboratory. No one ever failed to deliver the box: their child might be the next to be bitten,

After lunch we set off into the desert along a well-defined track. Mr Khumalo had a double cabin Toyota Hilux and so Alford and Azi sat in the back while Mr Khumalo's staff were in the open back (or 'the back back' as my children called it). The village was about an hour's drive but we did not get there, more is the pity, because the cattle were held a few miles nearer Ghanzi. There were several thin calves 'blowing a bit' and there was one that had died that morning. They were obviously suffering from a *Pasteurella* pneumonia. I opened the dead calf and carried out as complete a post mortem examination as I could with no proper protective equipment: sure enough both lungs showed severe pneumonia. There were no other lesions to be seen. Samples were collected to go to the laboratory and I suggested that in the meantime all the calves be treated with intra-muscular streptomycin, and this was done. Treatment for the next two days was left with the farmers. It appeared that these calves had all been moved on foot for twenty miles at one go and so transit fever was what it was.

By agreeing to visit the farm I had made a friend for life in Mr Khumalo, but what vet would have done otherwise? Besides I had had the best of the deal: I had met and talked to Bushmen under conditions where they were really pleased to see me! The deal became even better on the way back when we met a troupe of Bushmen out hunting. We stopped the car and through the interpreter found that they were after a kudu. One of the younger men approached the interpreter and through him asked if I wanted to purchase his hunting bag. I had seen tourist versions of these in the shops in Gaborone on sale for about Pula 75 (then about £30), but this was the genuine article: the bag made from springbok hide, with beads made from ostrich shell sewn on. There was a bow and a quiver of arrows made from a hollowed out branch and a box of the same material sealed with hide at both ends which contained the arrow heads; there were also the two well-used fire sticks.

'How much does he want for it?' I asked. After some discussion I got the reply.

'Two pula.'

'I cannot pay two pula,' I said. 'I will give him P40.'

The bushman shook his head when he heard my reply.

'No, he wants P2 because he wants to buy a packet of cigarettes.'

'Tell him if I give him P40 he can buy 20 packets of cigarettes.' This was the first and only time in my life that I have bargained to pay more. Here Mr Khumalo stepped in.

'You do not understand Sir, these people have no understanding of money and he does not appreciate that P40 will buy more, he is frightened that it will buy less and so not be enough. Give him P2 and take the bag; then you give him P20, that will be quite enough for him and he will probably spend all the money left from the cigarettes on drink.'

I had got a bargain and one Bushman was very happy – the essence of good business. Without anything more of interest we returned to Ghanzi. I said my goodbyes to Mr Khumalo, sure in the knowledge that we would meet again.

We had an early dinner in the hotel and an even earlier breakfast the next morning as Alford wanted to be on the road by 6.30 am so that we could get to Francistown by dark. We stopped for a drink and a sandwich in Riley's Hotel in Maun and it was just after dark that we pulled up outside the Grand Hotel. Alford had driven well: I offered to share the driving and on later safaris we did, but not this one: he was out to impress the boss.

We left at a much more respectable time the following morning and still made Gaborone before the lab closed. It had been a wonderful trip: I had learnt a great deal about the country, its people, agriculture, and even veterinary medicine. Jack had been right, in ten days I had learnt a great deal about Botswana, and I was now in a much better position to make a good job of running my first laboratory.

The transition from journeyman to master had been confirmed.

17

Getting to Grips with the Administration

'Detectives need good memories.'
Sir Arthur Conan Doyle, *The Sign of Four*

During the many hours in the Land Rover I had given great thought to making the laboratory function for the benefit of the country. What was needed was to ensure a new mindset – for the laboratory to become more dynamic, more responsive to the needs of the field officers, and for them to believe that they were a vital part of the disease control team. It was noticeable that the laboratory was held in low esteem by the Directorate – staff took no part in the daily radio conference – and yet it was capable of responding to a serious problem outside working hours with speed and accuracy. This was obvious from the way they had sorted out the rabies case from Selibe Pikwe, and over and above its overt function it was able to provide the hospital with human rabies vaccine. This was basically a good outfit that needed to be moulded into a team with a single objective – service.

The key to success was Stan. Soon after my return Stan suggested that I come round to his house after work for a beer or two and some supper. Stan's wife Hazel was working with the UN Commission for Refugees – what with the problems in Angola and Southern Rhodesia, not to mention South Africa itself, Botswana was a haven of tranquillity among the violence, and so there were refugee camps scattered over the north. Hazel was an administrator involved with several camps and that required her to travel on a regular basis. During her absences Stan was looked after by Joyce, an excellent cook/housekeeper, another lady of traditional build. Hazel was there that evening but apart from the meal I hardly saw her. She understood why I was there.

I thought it best to lay my cards on the table and tell Stan exactly what I wanted to do. I carefully pointed out that I wished to avoid making the same mistake that Mik Mares had made, of imposing a system from above on a group of people who had been working, as they thought, reasonably well together for years. I did not want them to feel that I knew all the answers and that their experience counted for nothing.

'What I want, Stan, is to install the system that works so well in British Veterinary Investigation Centres,' I explained, and I spelt out in basic terms what I would like to see happen. 'First and foremost, the professional staff are to take control of their work and cases. You carry out the post mortem examination then you are responsible for that case till the final report is sent. It will be the same with Ken and Mike. There is no need for the veterinary staff to be involved with the routine samples that come from Lobatse, Ken can write and send the report and if it requires a veterinary signature, then you or I can countersign. The work that Mike does in Nata can equally be reported by him. It is only when a veterinary opinion is required that the veterinary staff need to become involved.

'This will necessitate the installation of a duty officer system both for veterinary and technical staff. With only you and me this may well be a bit irksome but we have to show we mean business, and that starts at the top. I suspect that we may be able to recruit Jean Bradley when Mik goes, which will ease the load a bit, although the throughput of samples is not great.

'The submission form that you have, with a few tweaks, will do nicely until we can get a new one printed. Each field office will be issued with a book bearing unique numbers so we can always trace the origin if it is not clear from what is written on the sheet. The blue copy will remain in the book and they will send us the white (top) copy, together with the pink. After it has been registered here and given a species submission number, which will be written on both white and pink copies, Magdalene will put the white sheets in a loose leaf folder until the time comes for the report to be typed. Meanwhile the pink copy is used as the laboratory work sheet and all tests required and results will be written on the back. The initials of the duty vet will be put on the top right hand corner and hopefully he will write what is to be done on the back. The pink sheet and sample/s will be taken to the required laboratory for analysis.

'Once the system is underway all senior staff will meet in the bacteriology laboratory at nine am and the duty vet will take us through each case. In this way we will all know what is going on, without detracting from the authority of the person in charge. For recording purposes we will have "Species" reception books for cattle, small ruminants, avian (for poultry and all other birds), rabies (irrespective of the species), and miscellaneous – cats, dogs, horses, donkeys, wild animals and humans.

'The reason behind this is that the individual results will be analysed on a species basis so that we can make meaningful projections of what might happen based on what has happened.

'At the end of each month the senior staff will meet to produce the Monthly Report, which will be circulated to all veterinary offices, livestock offices, the Medical Department and, provided the Director agrees, to the Directors of Veterinary Services of all our neighbours. This report will tabulate our confirmed diagnoses and will carry reports of interesting cases by the officer concerned.'

And with that I drew breath.

'I have to hand it to you Roger,' Stan said, 'you certainly seem to have it all sorted out.'

'It's not surprising really. I have been waiting for this moment ever since I undertook that first field trip with Maryk Gitter in 1966, and realised that being a detective was what I really wanted to be. I have been trained by many people, including some who showed me how not to proceed. And that is why I so need your support.'

'You've got it bhoy.' With that he turned to me and shook my hand. 'Your ideas are just what we need to make this place hum. You will have not the slightest problem with any of the senior staff.'

'But look what happened to Mik's plan,' I said.

'Mik is a nice enough man but he is a bureaucrat with the mentality of a permanent secretary; you have a pedigree and your work is known. I know all about the fine work you did with CBPP in Kenya, and that vaccine you made at Muguga for us in Uganda worked a treat. Ken knows about your work on strep meningitis and avian TB in pigs and he is brimful of ideas of possible projects.'

I did not know that my fame had spread so far!

'Make yourself scarce in the morning,' he said, 'and I will have a chat with Ken and Mike. I might even bring Leonard in. By tomorrow afternoon you will be able to have your meeting.'

The following morning it was announced that Mik was being transferred to the Botswana Agricultural College. He had had a meeting with Jack and, according to Mik's version of events, Jack

309

had been very tactful and told Mik how valuable his contribution would be to the training of young Batswana. While reluctant to go, Mik could see how important it was that I had a fair chance to cock it all up.

I did not see Mik and was therefore unable to wish him well in his new job before I set off to the Botswana Vaccine Institute, in the middle of the industrial estate, where the foot and mouth vaccine was made. There I met Dr Jean Jacques Guinet, the director who was employed by the famous French pharmaceutical company Merieux who were the leading players in the BVI.

It was immediately obvious to me where Dr Guinet's loyalties lay. He was responsible for making the vaccine and testing it, but I had the responsibility for supervising the testing and I had to sign for every batch. This irked him somewhat and he felt that it rather clipped his wings, which was exactly what it was designed to do. He suggested that it was not necessary for me to do anything: he would take care of it all and I just had to sign. This was no way to endear himself to me, because I have always had a firm belief in the importance of professional integrity. And so I said to myself, if he can try and persuade me to behave incorrectly then there is every possibility he is prepared to behave incorrectly himself. But I kept my thoughts to myself. Some time later he was found to be diluting the vaccine after it had been tested, in order to increase the profits for the company and so increase his chances of promotion.

It was obvious that relations between the director of the Vaccine Institute and the laboratory were becoming strained. Luckily the manager of the BVI, Bill Shaw, had the ear of Jack Falconer and informed him where the real problems lay. Dr Guinet was recalled and a real diplomat was sent in his place. François Guilleman had obviously been told that he had to improve relations, and a normal healthy relationship was soon restored. François and his charming wife Christine were soon actively involved in Gaborone life and Christine became a piano pupil of Maxine's.

I looked into the module where they made the vaccine through one of the numerous windows. The module had been constructed in France, flown out and installed inside a custom-made building. I met Bill Shaw the manager, who was to become a close friend through our mutual love of the theatre. I also met several members of the technical staff including two young vets who were doing their 'military service' by working in an overseas French project.

I returned just before lunch to meet a beaming Stan, who said, 'I have arranged a meeting in your office at two thirty to discuss the future. I think it will be a good meeting.'

And so it was.

I put the plan of action to them just as I had to Stan the night before and there was a great positive response. I stressed to them the importance of personal commitment, and taking responsibility and 'ownership' of their work. Provided that their work was carried out, they were free to plan it as they wanted, I would not interfere. That did not mean that I was not interested, in fact quite the opposite, and I would always be there to give them support, help or back up if it was needed.

'It is vital that we get reports out quickly: when a PM is carried out then the veterinary office concerned should be phoned that day to let them know what we have seen. The same applies to all rabies cases. A written report on all samples *must* be sent within forty-eight hours even if it is only a holding or preliminary one.'

They approved of using the submission form as the worksheet and finally as the report form, as it would reduce the paperwork. They were not so keen on the idea of the work sheets being gathered up each evening and brought to reception, but came round to the idea that it would be easier to find them if they were all in one place.

The general view was that the system should be put in place as soon as possible and that it should be practical to start at the beginning of the following month (April 1981). It was agreed that all samples from a single animal should be given a single case number and all samples from the same outbreak should be given a single number: 200 blood samples from a herd with suspect brucellosis would certainly inflate the figures but would make year on year comparisons impossible to analyse.

'The success of our endeavours will be measured by the submissions: if we improve our services then the numbers will increase, of this I am certain. I saw this happen in Kenya and again in Argentina. The majority of the vets and livestock officers out there want to do a good job and they know that with our support they can improve their services to the farmer. If we give them the help they want, then they will use our services. Speed is essential, but accuracy is vital.'

I then broached what I thought might be a thorny topic – Saturday morning working. Animals do not stop dying because it is the weekend: what did they think of us opening from eight to midday on Saturdays? We would split into teams, and once we had three vets we could have three teams and take it turn-about. The staff would be compensated by receiving a half day off in lieu; people would be able to aggregate two of these (but no more than two) and have a whole day off, and so have a three-day weekend.

Surprisingly it was Leonard who spoke first. He thought that the junior staff would find this very useful: many of them had families a long way away and having a three-day weekend would give them more time to go and see their wives. Saturday working was on. That will make HQ sit up, I thought – it shows we mean business. The meeting came to a very satisfactory conclusion and we adjourned to the golf club, where Stan and Mike were members, for a couple of cans of Castle. The occasional drink together after work does wonders for the team spirit; it was such a pity the Africans did not join us.

Stan, Ken and I worked on the new submission form and we soon had one that was approved by all. Ken took over getting it printed and within a week we had them ready to send out, each set of three with its unique number. Ken also produced the letter that was to accompany the books to each office explaining how they were to be used. Three books were sent to each office and their numbers were carefully recorded so that when sheets came in incompletely filled in, as they almost certainly would, we could chase them up to complete the gaps.

Things were hotting up: the new submission books for each species were made ready, as were the ring binders in which to store the case papers once they were completed. The trays for the overnight storage of the case papers were set up in reception. People make fewer mistakes with small numbers than with large, and so at the start of each month the numbering would return to 1 – so the first rabies sample in April would be R1/4. It has always been my belief that the simplest systems work best.

Jean Bradley phoned to ask if she could come and see me: what a delight it was to have a telephone service that worked.

'When would you like to come? At the moment I am free most of the time. I hope that this will change.'

'Could I come this afternoon?' she asked tentatively.

'Of course, I will see you at two thirty if that is convenient for you.'

Promptly at two thirty Jean was in my office. 'I do not want you to

312

think that I am being foisted on you,' were her blunt opening words. 'I think that I have something to offer, not the least is my aptitude for work.'

Jean was a tall athletic woman who, although in her forties, still played in the Botswana squash team. She was also a keen golfer and sailor. She seemed competent and enthusiastic and we were here to teach people, and nobody said that they had to be black! While we were discussing matters, Magdalene popped her head round the door to say that Stan had phoned to say there was something interesting in the rabies room. Meeting over, Jean and I went to the rabies laboratory, a room dedicated to rabies in which no other work was carried out.

The brain of a goat from north of Nata had come in from the Francistown office; the smears had been prepared by the technique we had pioneered in Kabete and, as is always the case with goats, when the test is positive it is *really* positive. Goats with rabies produce so many Negri bodies that we kept the brains and used them for the control sample, which is always put up with field cases, to make sure that the test is working. It took just one glance down the microscope to see that the goat had died from rabies. In almost every neuron (nerve cell) there was a Negri body, that small, round, regular body that fluoresced brightly under the ultraviolet light – only some of them were huge, almost doubling the size of the cell.

There was no doubt about the diagnosis and it confirmed Tony Holmes's view that in the north, away from the towns, it was the jackal that was spreading the disease. Jack would not allow farmers to vaccinate their cattle (or other ruminant species) against rabies (there was now an efficient vaccine available), as he considered that cattle were a good indicator of the level of rabies among the jackals, which in turn indicated the population density of the jackals. As jackal numbers increased, as they did from time to time when there was plenty of food about, so too there was an increase in the number of animals infected with rabies. He would then suggest to the Game Department that it was time for a jackal cull, which was in due course carried out.

The next morning I went to see Jack to ask if Jean could be employed in the laboratory. I had not seen him since my return from the field visits, but he knew all that I had done, including my stay in Crocodile Camp. However, I was able to fill in some of the details and to say what an eye-opener it had been. I knew a great deal more

313

about the livestock industry than before and the information would be most useful in our developments. I explained about the changes that were to be made in the organisation of the laboratory.

'And do you think that the staff will go along with this?'

'Without a shadow of a doubt; they have been involved in the planning and their views have been taken into account. With your permission, I intend to open the laboratory on Saturday mornings. Don't worry, this will not cost you any money for overtime because they will get time off in lieu. They all seem very happy with this development. I need to recruit Jean Bradley to make my plans possible.'

'You have already indicated to the field staff that there will be an improvement in the service they receive and so it seems reasonable that we employ Jean. I'll just let you into a secret, there might be more staff coming your way if certain international discussions go as planned – but don't hold your breath, you know how long some negotiations can take. Just keep going the way you have started and we will see that new laboratory up!'

'I have yet another request: could I send a member of staff to HQ each day to take part in the radio conference?'

'Just arrange it with Eddie and he will make sure that you are included in the list.'

The new system in the laboratory got under way with almost no problems at all. As the work increased we initiated the role of Duty Technician: this was greatly resented, at first, by the junior staff as they could not see why they had to undertake administrative duties when they were 'scientists'. They objected to having to go to reception when samples arrived and do the booking in. 'This is a job for a clerk,' they said.

However, once they started doing the job they realised how interesting it could be taking down a history and having to decide whether or not to call the duty vet. They eventually agreed that it was more than just a job for a clerk.

At the start of the new system there was a massive surge in sample submissions. We all felt that this was the field staff testing us out and that the numbers would soon drop, but they did not. Getting the results out quickly was becoming a problem for Magdalene and so a new secretary was recruited. The morning meetings were going very well and were really appreciated by the staff, who sort of grew into them as they gained confidence in telling others what they were

314

doing. Jean was very reticent at first but the sympathetic hearing she received enabled her to flourish.

The first test was to come: the Monthly Meeting was about to take place. I had been through the books and tabulated the submissions and diagnoses, and although we had little to show for our efforts, it was a start. It was my practice to start the meeting with administrative and personnel problems so that any member of staff could get any complaint off their chest at the start and not let it fester as the meeting progressed. The surge in the work had taken everyone by surprise and so I asked Mike to go through the old diagnostic book for the March results so that I could produce a comparison to take to the director. More staff were required all round! We had not had a big intake of work on the Saturdays, but it was early days and people needed to get used to the idea that they could come to the laboratory on a Saturday.

There were no really exciting stories to tell: a few diagnoses of mastitis, a case of anaplasmosis in a bullock from Ghanzi, a couple of cases of erlichia infection in dogs (a nasty disease that often resulted in death), a couple of hens with Maryk's disease, and that was about it. Not a very stimulating report for readers of the first Monthly Report. But we were saved by a wonderful diagnosis, made through some good thinking by Stan.

We had received some well-roasted bones of a goat from the Central Kalahari. People had attended the wedding of a settled Bushman couple and had feasted on a goat that had been found dead: it was roasted to add to the celebrations. Within a few days four of the guests had died. The medical authorities suspected anthrax as the cause and the goat as the means. They collected what bones they could find and sent them to us. We split one thigh bone and set up cultures from the marrow. As was to be expected we isolated almost every bacterium known to man. We heated some marrow to kill all the vegetative forms of the bacteria and leave only the spores and that gave us masses of clostridia (the gangrene-causing bacteria) but no signs of *Bacillus anthracis*. Stan suggested that we try making a suspension of the bone marrow both before and after heat treatment and inject it into mice, as they are a wonderful means of filtering out the contaminating organisms. This was done and one by one the mice died of anthrax. We were able to isolate *Bacillus anthracis* from all tissues of the mice in pure culture, and then confirmed its identity. The medics were right; the goat and hence the people had died from anthrax.

That was great detective work and it made a wonderful story when written up in the Monthly Report. The really important information in such reports is the detailed figures given in the tables, but what makes people read them are the interesting anecdotes and stories of investigation that the reader might be able to use in the future.

Maxine and family delayed their arrival until the summer holidays, so that Guy could complete the academic year before going to join Richard at Orwell Park School in Suffolk. This time the house and garden were in good order and there was no soot and ash to contend with. There was also running water, both hot and cold, constant power and a telephone on which you could actually make calls. Maxine even had her piano somewhere between London and Durban.

When we were packing she asked if we could afford to bring her piano. We could, and this was the best joint decision we ever made: it changed her life. Before many weeks had passed she was in demand to accompany singers and instrumentalists and she met David Slater, 'Mr Music, Gaborone', a teacher at the Maru-a-Pula School, and the real driving force for music in the city. He ran the Gaborone Singers and the orchestra and conducted both. He was an English-speaking South African who deplored the Afrikaans government's racial policies and so came to live and work in Botswana. He was a great inspiration to Maxine and started her playing in public and teaching the piano. By the time we left Botswana she had a large number of pupils of all ages and nationalities, and had started studying for the Teaching Diploma of The Associated Board of the Royal Schools of Music. She remained in Botswana to take the examination after I left, which she passed with flying colours. With her children preparing to lead independent lives she needed something to fill the gap. Having devoted her life to her own children, she was now to devote her life to other people's children and to instil in them her great love for music, with all the happiness that brings.

She approved of the new three-piece suite and the Beetle – the Nissan would soon be with us and the Beetle gone, but it had served its purpose. Stan had already found us a housemaid, Dinah, of Bushman descent and a real treasure: she was less than 5 foot in height with the classic Bushman posterior, and she was always smiling, willing and hardworking, and the children loved the way she carried everything on her head, including a bottle of Branston Sauce. Maxine also approved of Dinah who remained with us throughout our time in Botswana. We knew that we would not always be in Botswana, and Dinah could not work for ever, and so we opened a savings account for her. Each month we paid in a pension contribution, so that she would have a small nest egg when we left.

Not only did Stan find Dinah, he also found Blue and Behra and a more unlikely couple of dogs you cannot imagine. Their former owner insisted that the dogs must not be separated and so they came together. Blue was short-haired with Labrador blood and the most intelligent dog we have ever owned: loving faithful and clever were her main characteristics. Behra by contrast was a pedigree keeshond (Belgian barge dog), a small husky, with a coat designed for northern climes; she was the dimmest, but the most beautiful, dog we have ever possessed.

The children rapidly adapted to their new environment and soon made friends. It was easier for Claire because she lived in Botswana the whole time, while the boys were going back to school in England. In fact Claire did the whole of her primary education in Botswana. There were two old established primary schools and a third had just been set up. Thornhill School was just over a quarter of a mile away. Claire was accepted for this school and she loved it and prospered there; it trained her well for her secondary education. We were delighted when she went into the third year and had Mrs Harwood for a teacher: she was known to be a real tartar but a brilliant teacher. A week after the start of term we received a call from her, asking us to go and see her. What had Claire been up to? We need not have worried, Mrs Harwood had decided that Claire was too able for the class and she wanted our permission to skip third year and go straight into fourth.

One great advantage of Maxine being a musician and my private passion being the theatre is that we know different groups of people, which results in us getting involved in each other's activities, so that we have a wider circle of friends and probably get involved in more things. Life in Botswana was never dull.

Farmers are always looking for a cheaper way of raising their animals, and those in Botswana were no exception. Concentrates are always expensive and again in Botswana this was even more true – because of the climate it was not possible to grow cereals or leguminous crops other than in a very restricted way. Consequently they all had to be imported over great distances from South Africa. So when

317

the boffins came up with the idea of feeding urea to cattle as a cheap source of non-protein nitrogen (which is much cheaper than protein nitrogen) the farmers jumped on the bandwagon, little realising the problems that urea can cause.

The urea works in the rumen (the first and large stomach, which is like a huge vat in which bacteria break down the food into fats and sugars so that the animal can absorb the nutrients): the bacteria there are capable of turning the urea into protein nitrogen, which is then available to the animal by the normal processes of digestion and absorption. For this to be successful and profitable it is essential that the animal gets enough carbohydrates in the food to provide energy for the bacteria to convert the urea. This requires considerable skill on the part of the farmer or he ends up in trouble. If not enough energy is fed or the animal has access to too much urea, then the micro-organisms in the rumen cannot cope and ammonia is produced which is absorbed through the wall of the rumen into the bloodstream. The liver converts the ammonia back to urea which is excreted by the kidney: the urea that was in the sack is now urea in the soil, having undertaken much animal energy use in the process. The problems do not end there, because if too much ammonia is absorbed into the blood, then urea and ammonia circulate in the blood, causing poisoning.

This happened to an old Boer farmer just outside Mahalapye. The farmer was convinced that he had a serious outbreak of rabies because his steers were bellowing, staggering and salivating. Senior Livestock Officer Mr Njui phoned and asked if we could rush up and sort out the problem as there were several dead animals and more were showing signs of rabies. It sounded serious enough to warrant an immediate visit.

Following the maxim of Sherlock Holmes that 'it is a culpable mistake to theorise before one has data', I normally prefer to examine a dead animal in the calm of the laboratory before taking off to the field as it gives you the opportunity to read round the possible causes. It is often said in the detective world that it's not what you know that matters, but knowing where to find the answers. I asked Leonard to come with me, and we took Geoffrey Mpeto with us in case there was heavy work to be done. Geoffrey was an extremely likeable young man who had a strange deformity in the last phalanges of his fingers which looked like mini table tennis bats: the last joint was round and almost double the width of the others. It

318

tended to make him a little cack-handed. However, what he lacked in dexterity he made up for in enthusiasm. We took with us a post mortem kit and several containers for samples and set off to the Mahalapye Veterinary Office, and directly from there with Mr Njui in his truck as guide to the farm which was about ten miles from the town on a fairly rough old track.

'Never rush in' has always been my motto and so we all sat in the farmer's kitchen drinking rooibos tea. After Mr Njui had introduced our team I set to asking questions. It did not take long to find out that urea was being used on the farm and access to it was not carefully restricted. Never rush in ... but even without seeing the animals I was fairly certain what we would find.

For me a classic diagnostic sign of urea poisoning is disturbance of the ground, indicating that the animal had been 'paddling' before it died. There were four dead animals which had been paddling. Unfortunately there were no real pathological lesions. The dead animals all showed signs of bloat with their left side abdomen as taut as a drum. We carried out a post mortem examination, with Leonard and I doing the cutting and chopping and Geoffrey the recording. Before we were half way through the work I asked Mr Njui if he would mind going to the office and bringing me a Drinkwater gag, a medium-sized stomach tube and a plastic funnel, and then I wanted him to go into the supermarket and buy a couple of gallons of vinegar. I saw his surprised look and said, 'It's OK, you can charge it to expenses!'

A bemused Mr Njui departed, thinking I had gone mad. By the time he returned we had finished the post mortem examination and washed up. There were five live animals in various stages of intoxication, including one that was lying down paddling its feet. I suggested to the farmer that he shoot that one. We put the stomach tube down the throat of the first beast and after releasing the bloat we poured down about fifteen litres of water and a couple of litres of vinegar. We did this to the other three, and I then tried to explain the chemistry of what was going on in the rumen of the animal, about the urea being converted into ammonia and absorbed. The water was to dilute the contents of the rumen and lower the temperature so that the micro-organisms worked more slowly, the vinegar was to combine with the ammonia to produce ammonium acetate and so reduce the pH (a measure of the acidity or in this case the alkalinity) of the rumen, which also slows the rate of ammonia production. I have little faith in this treatment because by the time the farmer sees that the animal is sick the damage has been done. However, it is always a good thing to do *something* – provided it is not actually harmful – because activity gives the farmer hope. I said that I thought it unlikely any animals would survive but, if there were survivors, then he should contact Mr Njui who would come and repeat the treatment the next day.

If the farmer wished to persevere with feeding urea it had to be done really carefully and only a weighed, determined quantity of urea should be fed. I told him that in my opinion urea should never be fed unless it is given mixed with some crushed or rolled maize. Under no circumstances should the animals have direct access to the urea.

It was now well past lunch time and so we adjourned to the Mahalapye Inn, where we were all able to get some food and a cold drink.

'You are a very bad man, Dr Windsor,' said Mr Njui, wagging a finger at me but with a twinkle in his eye. 'When you told me to buy vinegar you did not say what it was for and I could not ask. I thought you were pulling my foot, but I thought to myself, he said buy vinegar and so I buy vinegar. I see you are a clever man.'

'Not clever,' I said, 'but, well, knowledgeable and with a very good memory for diagnoses that I have seen before or read about. Although I am still learning about Botswana, I know quite a bit about nervous disease in animals, having been responsible for rabies diagnosis in Kenya. Remember the paddling Mr Njui; if you see cattle doing that and they have access to urea, you can bet your life that that is what the problem is.'

'I am not a gambling man, Dr Windsor, but I will remember your advice and I humbly thank you for coming to our aid so quickly.'

It was time to get on the road back to Gaborone. It had been a profitable visit and a most satisfactory one with another satisfied customer. We shook hands.

'I thank you all again for coming to our aid. Go well, young men; go well, Dr Windsor and go with God.'

There is nothing better than to sort out the problems on a farm, particularly when it is the first time that you make a clinical visit to the area. If you start with a success, then immediately (and usually permanently) the client or farmer trusts you and thereafter you can do no wrong! We were a happy party in the truck going home.

*

I attended several theatrical performances in the Moth Hall before plucking up courage to join the group. It was Mike, who was a backstage stalwart of Capital Players, who finally persuaded me to audition for a part in *An Inspector Calls*, one of J.B. Priestley's 'time plays'. I was lucky enough to land the part of Gerald, the son of the owner of the business where the young girl dies. Amateur dramatics is a time-consuming business but luckily I was concentrating on building up the laboratory services at the time and there was no requirement for me to go away from Gaborone. Rehearsals were always very hard work and went on from 7.30 to 10 pm when we adjourned to the bar for a drink and a discussion of the rehearsal.

Capital Players was a very friendly organisation which had been going since the capital of Botswana had been moved to Gaborone from Mafeking, but it had no black members. The older members had grown up with a colonial view of black people and suspected that they would not put in the hard work necessary to make a successful production: there was no antagonism, just an unwillingness to give them a chance.

The theatre was on the outskirts of Gaborone on the road to Molepolole and was in the grounds of the Masonic Lodge, from whom it was rented. As with most buildings in Botswana it was constructed from a mixture of white asbestos and cement, and walls and roof were made of the same material. It seated about 150 people with a raised area at the back. It was a classic proscenium arched theatre with adequate space backstage. The major problem was that it was not possible to fly scenery but Mike had overcome this problem by having a system where the flats were held in rails above and below: these flats could be wheeled on and off the stage and each one rotated. It was a very clever system which meant that we could stage musicals and plays that required changes of set. There were only two changing rooms, one for the men and one for the women, and no such luxuries as a shower. There was a good sized bar to one side of the auditorium which after its makeover was known as the Lem Morgan Bar and we instituted a 'door of honour' on which visiting professional artists signed their names. Many big cities would have been proud of the quality of some of the productions that were staged on the edge of the Kalahari Desert.

The British Council and the cultural organisations of other nations such as the Americans, French and Russians were very active in Gaborone. The London Shakespeare Company was almost an annual visitor to the city and they worked wonders with the Bard's plays with only five actors and no set. *Twelfth Night* was my introduction to Frank Barrie; he was the best Malvolio that I have ever seen. The British High Commissioner invariably gave a cocktail party when the Company was in town and Capital Players members made up the bulk of the party goers. It was at the *Twelfth Night* party that I met Frank. We had a long discussion about the play and his role, then he casually mentioned that he had written and performed his own one-man play *Macready* about the great Victorian actor and friend of Dickens. He had been asked by the British Council to bring *Macready* to Africa the following year. I was determined to get him to perform in Gaborone, not just for the adults but to stage a couple of performances for secondary schools in the town and do a workshop for Capital Players members.

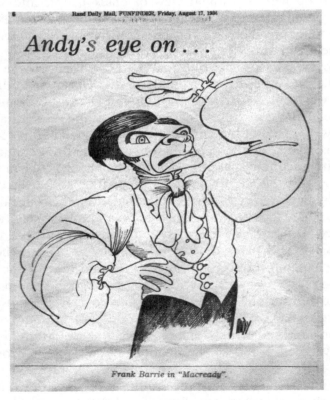

Rand Daily Mail, FUNFINDER, Friday, August 17, 1984

Andy's eye on . . .

Frank Barrie in "Macready".

Frank Barrie in his one-man play *Macready*, as seen by the theatre critic of the *Rand Daily Mail* which is sadly now defunct.

Dr Quett Masire, the President of Botswana, was a regular attender at all productions in the Moth Hall. There is the lovely story about his attendance just after his election as president, when he was very unsure of himself. His bodyguards were stationed round the theatre leaning against the walls. Unfortunately nobody had thought to warn them that in the middle of the second act there was a black-out. When the lights came back on, to a man the bodyguards all had their pistols at the ready! By the time I was working in Gaborone the president only had one bodyguard when he came to the theatre, one of the twins – Mr Churchill or Mr Smuts Setloboko.

After some discussion with the British Council it was agreed that *Macready* should come to Gaborone and that there would be two public performances, three performances for schools and a work-shop for members of Capital Players. All would be paid for by the Council. They were happy that Frank should stay with Maxine and me while he was performing in Gaborone and we later learnt that his wife Mary was accompanying him as his stage manager and tech-nician. Mary, Maxine, Frank and I hit it off from the moment that they arrived and we had a great deal of fun.

To enable all the schoolchildren to attend the performances the seats were removed from the theatre and replaced by beer crates and planks: in this way almost 1000 children were able to see the play. They were a wonderful audience, paying rapt attention to Frank's words and thrilled by his agility as he turned cartwheels on the stage. There is one part of the play when Macready's daughter dies of tuberculosis – only Frank used the Victorian word 'consumption'. This convulsed the audience: to the Motswana child consumption meant eating, and they all thought that the daughter had died from over-eating! Frank changed the line for subsequent performances.

The adult performances were sold out and the show was a great success. The workshop was seriously over-subscribed and so dear old Frank did two, much to the delight of the participants who learnt a great deal from this wonderful, professional actor. The whole trip was great and we even managed to show Frank and Mary some of the delightful countryside around Gaborone, including Livingstone's cave and the house where he lived and where some of his children are buried. We were sad to see them go. Maxine and I took them to the airport and saw them go through 'Immigration', but we did not wait until the plane took off. Big mistake.

I had a Capital Players council meeting and so was out when the phone rang. It was Frank's agent in Johannesburg wanting to know what had happened to him. Maxine explained that we had seen him off. The agent informed us that the plane had arrived and the Barries were not on it. What could have happened? It was a time of great unease in southern Africa – a meeting of the Southern African Development Community (an organisation set up by the frontline states to counteract apartheid in South Africa) had just come to an end and President Masire was due back in Gaborone that afternoon. We were concerned lest the Barries had been taken off the plane by SA intelligence officers when it had landed in Johannesburg.

Maxine informed Frank's agent that I would be seeing Lem Morgan, the Communications Officer from the British High Commission (and widely thought to be a member of MI6) that evening, and that I would phone him back at the end of the meeting. I explained to Lem what had happened and he immediately contacted his opposite number in Pretoria who told him that the plane had landed and that all the passengers had disembarked uneventfully. This information we duly relayed to Johannesburg and suggested that the agent should wait for Frank to contact him. He was greatly concerned as Frank was due to perform in Swaziland the next night.

Maxine and I spent a very troubled night, worried that our new friends were in the hands of the SA secret police. When the phone rang at 7 am there was a race to answer it. It was Frank. All our worries were misplaced and compounded by wrong information. Frank and Mary had boarded the plane, but it could not take off until the president's plane had landed and so it was dispatched to a far corner of the airstrip to wait for well over an hour. When their plane came to take off it had developed a puncture and by the time a new wheel had been obtained it was going to be too late for the DC4 to set off. So all the passengers were taken off the plane, given their luggage, put on a coach and taken to the Morning Star Motel, a grotty hotel at Tlokweng near the South African border. They had not phoned us, not wishing to bother us: little did they know what we had gone through the previous night.

I dressed and rushed out to the motel, picked them up and brought them back home for breakfast, which had to be hurried because they had to get back to the airport for their flight to Johannesburg. Frank phoned his agent and put him out of his misery explaining that they would be in Johannesburg in time for the Mbabane flight. Maxine and I took Frank and Mary to the airport and this time we waited until the plane had departed before we left the airport. As Frank was about to board the plane, he followed the lead of Pope John Paul II and knelt and kissed the ground before climbing the steps.

18

Increasing the Numbers

'An experience of women that extends over many nations
and three separate continents.'
Sir Arthur Conan Doyle, *The Sign of Four*

I was sitting at my desk when Magdalene knocked on the door.
'There is a Mr Sachania at the door who wishes to see you although
he has no appointment.'

'Please show him in, Magdalene.' I rose from my seat and walked
to greet him. 'Mr Sachania, it is a pleasure to meet you and what can
I do for you?'

'I have a problem, Dr Windsor, but before telling you about it,
please accept my apologies for making this unannounced visit, but I
was in the hospital . . .'

'Nothing serious I hope,' I interjected.

'No, no, nothing like that. I am working in the hospital. I am from
Mombasa, Kenya and I am an architect and the hospital is doing
some building. I did not know that there was a laboratory here and I
thought I would come in and speak to the man in charge about my
daughter.'

'Let me stop you right there,' I said. 'This is the veterinary
laboratory, the medical laboratory is next door.'

'No, my daughter is not sick, she is in fact quite well; she has just
returned from studying in Britain. She has just completed her BSc in
biochemistry from the University of Essex and she has come to live
here with her mother, brother and myself. She would like to work
with you.'

'Well,' I said, 'if your daughter wants a job here, then she herself
must come and see me. I will be very happy to talk to her and if we
can use her talents and skills then we will offer her a job.' I rose.
'Please ask my secretary to give your daughter an appointment
whenever it is convenient for her. Thank you for coming to see me.'

326

Mr Sachania made an appointment for his daughter to come the next morning and at the appointed hour Varshika arrived. She was tall and very slim with bobbed hair, enormous spectacles and an even more enormous grin which lit up the room; not conventionally beautiful but extremely attractive, bright and cheery. I guessed she was in her mid to late twenties. After she had sat down and we had exchanged pleasantries I asked her to tell me something about herself.

'I come from Mombasa in Kenya,' she said in a strong South London accent, 'but I went to school in Weybridge and then to the University of Essex where I studied for a degree in biochemistry and I want to be a biochemistry technician.'

I do not know what it was about her but she was so positive about herself and life that I thought she would be good member of the team. So I phoned Mike and asked if he could spare the time to join us.

'This is Varshika Sachania,' I said to Mike. 'And this is Mike Fortey our head of the Biochemistry Section,' I said to Varshika. 'Mike, this young lady has a degree in biochemistry from Essex and wants to be a lab technician.'

'Does she?' Mike said, and started, in a very friendly way, to put her through her paces. When she knew the answers she gave them in a positive manner, and when she didn't she said so. I was getting to like her more and more.

'We are a small laboratory and we cannot afford too many specialists because when one section is busy we all have to help out.'

'One of my courses was in microbiology and I really enjoyed the plating out and making the smears and of course you have to use biochemical tests to identify many of the organisms.'

She was rapidly talking herself into a job. But it was time for the coffee break, a ritual that I dared not touch. There was a table in the car park under the trees where coffee was taken. The HQ staff did not like it because the staff could be seen by passers-by taking coffee. I believe that Elizabeth Hobday had started this practice as a means of getting staff, who all worked in different labs and some in different buildings, to spend time together, with the same motive as my morning case meeting. When HQ staff complained, as they did regularly, that it showed us in a bad light to the public, my reply was always, 'But the public can see that for most of the time there is no one sitting at the table.' The practice continued until the new

327

laboratory was built, and HQ staff were never too opposed to refuse to join us. It was cool and there was often a breeze.

I invited Varshika to take coffee and meet some of the other staff and she joined us at the table. Varshika made a good impression on us all. When she left I told her that I would speak to the director and let her know his decision.

'Well what do you think?' I asked the others. They were unanimous that Varshika would be a great asset to the laboratory. The director agreed and Varshika was given a local contract. She was indeed a great asset and in my time in the laboratory she ran the Biochemistry, Food Hygiene, Microbiology and Rabies Sections and made a great success of them all, and learnt how to cut good histological sections.

The next addition to the ranks was Elspeth Benson, whose husband was employed on overseas terms by the Medical Laboratory. Both had worked in a hospital laboratory in Glasgow. Jim Benson had been introduced to us and he had spoken to Ken about the possibility of employment for Elspeth, a small wiry Glaswegian with much experience and a great deal of knowledge. She too was taken on, on a local contract, and proved a very meticulous and capable worker. Like many Glaswegians she did not suffer fools gladly, she had a sharp tongue and she was well able to make the junior staff squirm. On more than one occasion I had to point out to her that the best way to teach people was not to make them think they were idiots. She found it hard to understand that the Batswana had not had the same educational opportunities as she had, and that she would get more out of them by building their confidence rather than damaging it.

Subathra Sinnathamby came from Sri Lanka and had arrived with her father who, like Varshika's father, was an architect. She had studied biochemistry in Colombo and she phoned the laboratory and asked to see me. It was almost a repeat of the interview with Varshika, and Mike put her through her paces. While she seemed to have a good knowledge of biochemistry she had nothing like the self-confidence of Varshika and her university course seemed much more restricted. However, Mike needed more help as Mabatho was off to Britain to study. The team seemed happy with her and Jack gave her a contract. She proved to be a meticulous and conscientious worker, always friendly and willing to perform the tasks required, but her shyness prevented her from fully joining the team and she was unwilling to leave the 'safety' of the biochemistry lab. Working in the bush was not on, whereas Varshika loved seeing the country and was always willing to work out in the field.

Jack's negotiations with the international agencies finally bore fruit and one morning, out of the blue, he arrived at the laboratory, something he rarely did. With him was Mik Winnen: I could not believe my eyes; how had he got here? We had last met in Salta, Argentina, when we both worked for FAO. We sat down in my office and I asked after his wife Gemma. She was not with him but would be coming. He informed me that after he left Salta he had been taken onto the books of the Dutch Aid Agency as a fully fledged 'expert'. Because of his experience in the Argentina Project he had developed a taste for detective work and when offered the chance of coming to work with me again in Gaborone he had accepted.

'But why didn't you write and tell me you were coming? I could have helped ease your arrival.'

It transpired that after months of procrastination the Dutch government acted with great speed. Mik had been given two weeks to prepare to leave and that was the reason Gemma was not with him as she was sorting out things back in Holland. Jack stayed for coffee where Mik was introduced to all the staff and I felt that he was rather impressed at the level of discussion that went on round the table. We had been receiving reports and samples from the Tuli Block of abortions in cattle, which were beginning to give cause for concern. Various possible agents had been put forward to account for the problem but no satisfactory conclusion had been reached.

This seemed a good moment to approach Jack about visiting the Veterinary Research Institute in Onderstepoort. I had been wanting to do this for some time because the laboratory needed back-up. It was frightening to think that I, in the form of the laboratory, was Botswana's last line of defence. We required a link to a laboratory that had specialists in the different disciplines, to whom we could refer. We could always use the CVL in Weybridge, where I still had many friends and contacts, but importing pathological material into Britain required permits and special containers, and of course there was the inevitable delay caused by distance.

'Jack, how would you feel about my visiting Onderstepoort to see how they can help us? I appreciate the political problems of dealing with the apartheid state, but we definitely need a back-up laboratory

329

to sort us out when we get stuck and Onderstepoort is only two hundred and fifty miles away while Weybridge is nine thousand miles.'

'Diseases don't recognise country boundaries,' Jack replied. 'South Africa received its disastrous outbreak of Rinderpest from us 80 years ago, so successful disease control must know no boundaries either. Erasmus, their Director of Veterinary Services, is a good friend of mine and will be very pleased to see you. There will be no political fallout if you go.'

Having helped Mik to settle in, I felt the laboratory was now adequately staffed and the new systems were working well enough for me to take a few days off to go to South Africa. I phoned the director of Onderstepoort and received a very warm response. They would be delighted to see me at any time; when did I want to come? I thought that the following Monday would be fine if it was acceptable to him.

Dr Rudolf Bigalke proved as delightful a man in real life as he was on the phone. I had allowed four hours for the journey and had time to book into the Boulevard Hotel (recommended by regulars) and I arrived in good time. 'I have phoned my deputy Tom Naudë to ask him to join us,' Dr Bigalke said. 'You have some old friends and indeed a former member of your staff working here. Jane Walker, a lady of some distinction is she not? Then there is the virologist Attilio Pini who worked with you in Kabete – but they all worked with you in Kabete! How about Dr Ogonowski the Polish serologist? I have saved the best to last – your old lab tech Wally Ashford is here with Pini, trying to make foot and mouth vaccine. You may know others but these are the only ones I have tracked down.'

'You have certainly done your homework on me,' I replied. 'It will be lovely to see Jane again.'

Jane was a leading expert on the ticks of East Africa when I was working at Kabete and was always willing to give advice. Wally and I had a special relationship as he was my chief technician in Kabete and he was a delightful man.

'You will see Dr Pini and Mr Ashford tomorrow when you visit the Foot and Mouth Disease Vaccine Laboratory where Dr Pini is battling against the bonehead Afrikaaners on our board. Yes, I am an Afrikaans speaker and can use those terms, even if Dr Pini cannot. But he will tell you the story of how Botswana stole a march on its giant neighbour, and why we are buying our vaccine from you. I understand it is a very good vaccine. Ah Tom, come in. Tom, this is Dr Roger Windsor the Director of the Botswana National Laboratory.'

'Not quite,' I said hurriedly, 'nothing so grand.' (Little did I know that that would become my title before I left Botswana.) 'I am just the head of the Diagnostic Laboratory Service for Botswana who is here seeking help.'

'Help, we can offer; money might be a little more difficult.'

I explained my predicament as 'Mr Veterinary Medicine, Botswana'. I told them what we were trying to do with the laboratory and how we were trying to provide farmers with the service they needed. The numbers of staff and the expertise that we had was laid bare.

'Please tell us exactly what you want us to do for you and we will let you know if it is feasible.'

'First of all I would like you to act as a reference laboratory so that we can send you cultures we have isolated and to confirm our identifications. We do not at this time plan to carry out virus isolations as we have neither staff nor facilities for this work; we would like to send samples to you and, perhaps this is the most important, to allow your experts to come when we have problems, to undertake disease investigations on the spot. I have discussed this with my director and we will be happy to pay all the expenses of such visits. Basically what I need is a sympathetic ear at the end of a telephone – someone who wants to help.'

'Is that all you are asking for? It's yours! I thought you would be coming with a great shopping list of requests, that you would want reagents, sera ...'

'Botswana is not short of money: what the laboratory needs, I have the money to pay for. What we lack is bodies, and not dead animals (although we could do with more of them) but trained staff: we only have thirty vets for the whole country. I am the only specialist we have, and I am a specialist in general diagnosis!'

'I think that we have the basis for a really good relationship here,' Dr Bigalke said. 'As a general principle, if we can spare one of our disease specialists they will be given permission to come and assist you, and I would not dream of asking your department to pay: it will be our contribution to helping a neighbouring service; besides, the bureaucracy involved would cost more than we will save. If I may make a suggestion, when you are going round the departments, please discuss this matter. I think that you will find that they will be clambering over each other to come.'

The conversation then turned to clinical and diagnostic matters concerning various diseases, and how Botswana was getting on with foot and mouth disease control in the light of the political controversy over the fences. Finally, Dr Bigalke looked at his watch and exclaimed in horror, 'You have to be going. I took the liberty of arranging for you to meet my director. I thought it better to get him out of the way this afternoon, so that you can have two whole days in the Institute without having to rush back to Pretoria.'

I returned to Pretoria. I had been staggered by the reception that I had received from the director and his deputy. We had an ally who was prepared to help if we got stuck. Major government departments were all controlled by the Afrikaaner mafia – the Broederbond – and here were two leaders offering a black African country all the help they could. What a strange mixed-up place was South Africa!

Dr Erasmus was charm itself, wanting to know how his good friend Jack Falconer was and whether Drs Bradley and Stewart were in good health. I was able to inform him that Tom Stewart had retired and gone back to live in Scotland. He enquired after the health of the national beef herd and our control of foot and mouth disease, and like Dr Bigalke congratulated us on our vaccine against the disease.

'But we have Dr Pini working on the matter. Soon we will catch you up and you will decide to buy the superior South African Vaccine.' He was laughing as he said it, but from what I heard the next day, I reckoned South Africa would never catch up. He talked about the beef trade and how Botswana was a valuable supplier of beef to the black community: 'Your beef is very lean with little fat, which means it can be sold very cheaply to the natives.'

What he really wanted to talk about was the new veterinary college for black people at Venda. He was on the board of the college and most impressed with the facilities they offered.

'The problem we have is that secondary education for blacks is not up to that for the whites, and the college is determined that its degree is to be equal to that of the Onderstepoort Faculty.' That faculty was just across the road from the Veterinary Research Institute and shared many of their personnel. 'What we are having to do is to take in the brightest and train them up to the standard of the white entrants at Onderstepoort before we let them in; we cannot have two standards of degrees, one for the blacks and one for the whites.'

I thought to myself, then why have two veterinary schools within

332

fifty miles of each other, when one in Cape Town a thousand miles away might have been a good idea? But I said nothing, as this was the essence of the South African conundrum and the whole illogicality of the Afrikaaner position. How can you accept that some people are inferior and yet expect them to reach the same standard? The whole premise was untenable and indeed within a few years it had collapsed. At least Erasmus's heart was almost in the right place and he wanted *his* Africans to succeed. It was an interesting visit and again I was offered any help that his department could give. I told Dr Erasmus of the kindness of his colleagues at Onderstepoort, and said how grateful I was for their offers of assistance.

What was strange to me about the Boulevard Hotel was the complete absence of any black faces in reception, dining room, or bar. I caught sight of a black woman in the corridor – she was obviously a member of the cleaning staff. What a contrast with my final visit to the hotel some five years later, when there was hardly a white face to be seen and even the head waiter was black.

What a feast was put on for me by the staff of Onderstepoort. The programme was so arranged that I visited the departments Dr Bigalke thought I would find most useful, although I started with Jane Walker.

'Roger, how lovely to see you again after all these years.' She gave me a great bear hug. 'I hear that you have three children now, you must bring them to see me.' And indeed we did, on a return trip from Maxine's uncle's farm at Ixopo in the Drakensburg mountains. She had moved from Kabete to Onderstepoort because it was getting more and more difficult to work in Kenya. Since coming south she had worked with Gareth Jones (who had been DVO in Ghanzi) to produce *A Field Guide to the Ticks of Botswana*. Now close to retirement, she was dreading the long hours at home after the camaraderie of the Institute.

'But dear Rudolf has told me that I can keep my laboratory here for as long as I wish and he might even be able to find an assistant. Because of this rotten leg [she had had polio as a child] I do need someone to help me: Rudolf is such a lovely man.'

'He has already been most generous to me and promised me any help I need in Botswana.'

'If he has said he will do it, it will be done: he is that sort of a man.'

Jane gave me a tour of the Sir Arnold Theiler building with its wonderful photographs of the great rinderpest outbreak on the wall.

Theiler was the founder of the Institute and one of the leading parasitologists of those days. Jane and I talked of ticks and Kenya, until my minder was sent to move me on to Stan Herr's laboratory.

Stan was a short, curly-haired Russian Jew who had managed to escape from the country during the chaos that followed the Second World War, and now headed the Department of Breeding Diseases. After some general chat about reproductive diseases, I casually mentioned that I thought it a waste of time to undertake post mortem examinations on foetuses in the tropics.

'Excuse me saying so, but you are totally wrong, Dr Windsor. If you have adequate resources you can determine the cause of abortion in eighty percent of cases. The question to be asked is, do the results justify the costs? In many cases the answer is no.'

I told him about the abortion outbreak that we were seeing in the Tuli Block in Botswana.

'Are these farms close to the Limpopo River?' he asked.

'Yes. All the affected farms have some grazing along the river.'

'Already you can see the benefits of international cooperation! We are having a problem with leptospiral abortions on the other bank.'

'Would you be prepared to come and help us investigate it?'

'It would be a great pleasure for me as I have never visited Botswana. Rudolf has already told us that he wants us to cooperate.'

Stan was in fact the first Onderstepoort scientist to come and help us.

We were deep in conversation when my minder came to take me on to Dr Balthus Erasmus, the Head of Virology.

Balthus was a tall Afrikaaner with a long family history in South Africa. Again there was a very warm welcome. He was a most distinguished scientist, having made major advances in African horse sickness, bluetongue in sheep, malignant catarrh in cattle and various other less important diseases. He could not have been more helpful. He understood that it was not practical to have a virology unit in a small laboratory. He was also very keen to visit Botswana.

I was introduced to Dr Gavin Thomson, and realised that we had met before, but I could not place him until he told me where we had met, which was on Newmarket Racecourse during an evening meeting!

After lunch the next department to visit was the new Foot and Mouth Vaccine Laboratory, which had been built in the midst of some of South Africa's most productive dairy farms. For that I had

334

to take the car and my minder accompanied me to make sure that I did not get lost. It was great to see Wally again and he looked not a day older, but then he had been silver-haired when I knew him in Kabete. He had seen the writing on the wall in Kenya; his days there were numbered so he had written to Onderstepoort and been offered a job, first in bacteriology and then when Dr Pini had come he transferred to virology to work with him. The work making foot and mouth disease vaccine had been a nightmare.

'But I will let Attilio tell you all about that.'

We sat in Attilio's office and drank coffee. Attilio was a tall, greying Italian charmer who had made his name making a blue-tongue vaccine in Kenya. Like Wally he felt that there was no long-term future for him in Kenya, and his Peruvian wife did not want to live in Italy so they had moved south. Rudolf's predecessor had been in charge when the whole foot and mouth project was mooted. He was furious that Botswana was producing vaccine before South Africa, but everything he did was wrong. He had invited the same pharmaceutical company that had built the Botswana Vaccine Laboratory, Merieux, to come and view the possibility of setting up a vaccine unit in Onderstepoort. This they did and they gave the director a quotation to carry out the work. It was going to cost 5 million Rand, and Merieux would charge them a design and supervision fee of 3 million Rand. Apparently the Director was happy with the building costs but he was not going to pay 'those thieving Frenchmen' R3 million for something he could do himself.

Attilio was told that he was to take charge of the project, but the director continued to make all the decisions and it was he who decided to put the lab in the middle of rich farmland. Attilio had battled and battled over this one. Why had Botswana put their facility in the middle of an industrial area? Because if there was an escape of virus, there would be no cattle to infect – here if there was an escape the entire cattle population of the district could be wiped out. He got nowhere. Industry was having a real boom at the time and farmland was much cheaper than industrial land. He was told that 'if you build the building correctly there will be no escapes!'

'He was supposed to be a scientist!' Attilio fumed.

A firm of Pretoria architects was given the brief, and came up with what looked like a fine building which was duly erected and cost three million rand more than Merieux would have charged in total.

Attilio decided that all systems needed to be tested before a single vial of virus was opened. The animal testing facilities were on the ground floor. There was a marvellous chute to deliver concentrate feed to the animals with a double door system: the top door was opened and the required amount of food was dispensed. Then the top door was shut and the bottom door opened to dispense the food, after which the door was shut and it was then sterilised by steam before the top door could be opened again. It worked perfectly ... once. What the designers had ignored was that when concentrate food is mixed with steam it forms a sort of glue, which stuck the doors firmly shut. They would have to use the Botswana system of just feeding hay.

The designers had used stainless steel pipes, the welding of which was a nightmare. When Attilio realised there were fundamental flaws and the pipes had to be changed, the New York firm of welders had to return because no one in South Africa had the relevant skill. That added a further million rand to the bill. At that time the rand and the dollar were more or less at parity (two to the pound sterling).

The litany of disasters went on. They were now at Attilio's mercy because if they insisted that he make vaccine and there was an outbreak of the disease in the neighbourhood ... By now Rudolf Bigalke was the director, but it was too late; the building was up and it had to be made workable. Attilio was hopeful that in a couple of months they would make their first test batch of vaccine. A tour round the building showed a very impressive series of laboratories, it was just such a pity that the system did not work.

Wally was insistent that I come home and meet Joan, and we had a wonderful evening talking about the days in Kabete. Wally told me how delighted he was when Bob Roach had resigned as Head of Diagnosis.

'For such a common little man, he was a dreadful snob and he looked down on us technicians as second-class citizens. It was a great delight to work with someone who actually valued my services.' I had never noticed this facet of Bob's character myself.

My first port of call the following morning was to the Bacteriology Section and Dr Ogonowski. We had lived next door to him in Kabete but had seen little of him. Like Maryk Gitter he was a Pole, but the two had little else in common and were not friends even in Kenya. I then spent time with the mastitis team whose welcome became even warmer when they knew I was a disciple of Dougie

Wilson. He was revered in Onderstepoort for his pioneering work on the control of mastitis.

I had a different minder, who was much more chatty, and he took me to the vaccine unit which was very impressive with the huge range of vaccines that it produced. The isolation of South Africa because of its racial policies had had an incredible effect on their self-sufficiency; a similar effect was being seen in Southern Rhodesia as the international community was putting pressure on that country to make it into a proper democracy. The massive investment in the vaccine unit meant that the country was producing all the vaccines it needed for its livestock industry, foot and mouth disease being the sole exception.

The next stop was the Poultry Department where I met a tall, slim German who had come to South Africa as a child after the Second World War. Dr Henryk Huchzermeyer was an avian specialist whose main work was on the bacterial diseases of poultry. After discussing the major disease problems of the industry, he said to me, 'Would you mind if I invited my wife to join us as she is very keen to meet you and your programme does not include the Pig Department?'

'We have almost no pigs in Botswana but I would be delighted to meet her, and you never know when we might need a pig expert.'

He phoned and Dr Hildegarde joined us. We shook hands and almost her first words to me were, 'Are you *the* Dr Windsor?'

'I am Dr Windsor, but I do not know about *the* Dr Windsor.'

'Are you the man who did that wonderful work on avian tuberculosis in pigs? I have so wanted to meet you because I think that we have similar problems in this country.'

No more was said of poultry, as husband and wife embarked on a whole prearranged series of questions about TB. It was lucky for them that I was the relevant Dr Windsor.

After lunch instead of going to the Pathology Department my minder took me to the director's office.

'I am so sorry to disturb your schedule, Dr Windsor. I had planned to speak to you at the end of the afternoon to find out how you had got on with my colleagues, but I have been called to see the Minister and I am afraid politics have to take precedence over science.' Dr Bigalke was as gracious as ever.

'Thank you so much for your excellent organisation,' I said. 'I have had a fascinating, productive and valuable couple of days. Your staff have been most kind and helpful: I am sure that I have

337

disturbed their schedules and I am most grateful to you and to them all.'

'The gain has not been all on your side: I understand that we now have some members of staff who know a great deal more about avian tuberculosis.'

He certainly had a superb network of informers.

'It has been a great pleasure to meet you Dr Windsor. I thank you for coming and I know that this will be the start of a very productive relationship for our two laboratories. The more that we know of the disease situation in your country, the better able we will be to protect ourselves.'

We shook hands and I went off to pathology where I met Dr Kuis Coetzer, who seemed to be far too young to be head of the department. He was soon to have the additional role of Professor of Pathology in the Faculty at Onderstepoort. There was an incredible dynamism about him. He never seemed to hurry, but things got done. I like to think that I was instrumental in persuading him to rewrite that wonderful book by Dr Henning *A Handbook of the Diseases of Livestock in South Africa* – years out of print but still the very best book for a vet in the tropics. (Some years later Dr, by then Professor, Coetzer was the senior editor of *Infectious Diseases of Livestock, With Special Reference to Southern Africa* in two volumes and a wonderful and worthy successor to 'Henning'.) We had an interesting discussion of the role of diagnostic laboratories in the economics of animal disease.

'I asked Rudolf to send you to me after lunch, because it is at this time we have our pathology consultation among the professionals in the department. Please follow me.' We went into a small darkened room which contained a table on which stood a microscope with five sets of eye pieces and five empty chairs. He sat me on his right side and took the chair in front of the microscope itself. Other people filtered in and sat down. I had never seen a multiple-headed microscope before.

'This is the most important piece of equipment that any diagnostic laboratory can possess. You obviously do not have one: my advice is get one. Make it the first purchase you make when you get back. I was taught in the days when the teacher sat at the microscope and said, "At 11'oclock you will see the small blue dot," and you swapped places at the microscope. Do you remember?'

I certainly did remember – we were still doing it in Gaborone!

338

'Well this puts all that into the garbage can of history; if you look down the microscope, it will become clear. Instead of telling you where to look, I show you.'

He did something, and a pointer appeared and indicated the precise cells he was talking about. It was like magic. We had to get a couple of these, one for rabies and one for the bacteriology laboratory. We did, and this changed our teaching. Dr Coetzer was absolutely right and I kicked myself for never having come across this before. Had the rest of the trip been a waste of time (which, of course, it was not) then it would have been worth coming just for this. We spent a most enjoyable half an hour discussing various pathological microscope slides. It was with regret that I dragged myself away to go to what I thought was to be my last port of call.

Dr Farnie Kellerman was the last on my list; he ran the Department of Toxicology although his real interest was poisonous plants, on which he was a world authority. He considered that many people underestimate the importance of food plants as a cause of poisoning and he mentioned lupins, the seed of which, if fed to animals uncooked, can be very poisonous. Rape is a temperate crop which caused huge mortality. Some grasses under certain conditions can produce cyanide, and even our potato, if allowed to go green, can cause poisoning. In Botswana he thought that the two most important plants were gifblaar or *Dichapetulum cymosum*, and mogau, *Pavetta harbori*, both bushes that remain green when almost every other plant has shrivelled from the drought. The clinical picture with both was the same, namely sudden death, but the results were brought about by different mechanisms. With *Pavetta* the poison causes death of individual muscle fibres in the heart and when there is sufficient damage, then with sudden excitement the heart cannot cope and the animal drops dead. *Dichapetulum*, on the other hand, is an acute poison that has an immediate effect and the animal dies: in this case the body is usually found near water, because it is drinking water that promotes absorption of the poison.

Dr Kellerman and his colleagues had produced a series of beautiful coloured leaflets on individual plants and their effects. He sorted some out for me and he later wrote a superb book, *Plant Poisonings and Mycotoxicoses of Livestock in Southern Africa*.

We were interrupted by my minder coming in bearing a note. Dr Kellerman read it and said, 'I am afraid you are requested to go to the Faculty to meet the Dean. Before you go, you are expected at my

339

house for a couple of beers and a braai and there are one or two old friends coming.'

How could I refuse? He lived near the institute so he wrote out the address and directions and told me to go there direct from the Faculty, and I was off again, literally just across the road.

The Dean, Professor C. Hofmeyer, had heard that I was visiting and just wished to make my acquaintance.

'Next time you come I will give you a conducted tour of our impressive facilities. If you ever require any help that the Institute cannot provide please call me and we will try to assist you. And now we have a little surprise for you, one Rudolf did not know about. My secretary will take you to the Department of Equine Physiology. It has been a pleasure to meet you, and remember, if we can help, we will.'

'Thank you for your time. I hope we meet again.'

I was wondering what would happen next when we arrived at the Department of Equine Physiology and knocked on the door.

'Come in, Roger,' came the reply, and there was Sandy Littlejohn sitting behind a large desk. I had not seen Sandy since my final year at college. Sandy had been working for a doctorate in equine anaesthesia and earned some spare cash by showing the students how to administer anaesthetics and control anaesthesia in horses.

'What a pleasant surprise to learn that you were on the site!' Sandy said. 'I decided that I must see you. I phoned Rudolf but he had gone off to another of his interminable meetings. His secretary said that you would be with Farnie this afternoon, and I knew that the Dean wanted to see you and so he sent a note across, and here you are. You've filled out a bit since student days but what are you doing in these parts, I thought that you were in Kenya?'

'It is eight years since I left Kenya. I have been in Cambridge and Argentina since then, but why are you here?'

'Have you forgotten my story? I was born in Scotland but then came the war and I was sent to a branch of the family here, while brother Jimmy stayed in Scotland.' I knew his older brother Jimmy because he was Professor of Anthropology in the University of Edinburgh when I was a student. 'I completed my secondary schooling here, got a place in the Vet School here and never looked back. Equine surgery was in its infancy then; if you opened the abdomen of a horse there was a good chance it would die of shock. I thought that it was time to return to Scotland and at the same time do my doctorate, with a view to remaining in Scotland when I finished my thesis on electrolyte control in the horse during surgery. But I could not really adapt to the place, particularly the cold in the winter, and so when I finished I returned here – and here I stay.

'Do you remember that mad Rhodesian, Bob Schwanepol, who was doing his PhD on Rift Valley fever? He ran off and married the gorgeous librarian at the college? He is here now, and he's Mr Big. He is the Director of the South African Virus Research Institute that does all that work with the ebola and other haemorrhagic viruses: a vet as director of a medical institute! Next time you're in Johannesburg go and see him, because the inside of that place looks like one of those satellite stations up in space, as they all wander around in replicas of space suits with long tubes trailing out of 'em.'

We had a great old chat until he looked at his watch and said, 'Time to go to Farnie's house – his braais are legendary.'

It was indeed a wonderful braai, but it was more the companionship and camaraderie that made the evening. It was certainly a great end to my first visit to Onderstepoort; I was hoping that there would be further reasons to visit this vibrant and exciting laboratory. I was careful not to drink too many cans of Castle, knowing I had the long drive home in the morning.

On my return Maxine said, 'While you were away an old friend of yours called at the house: Monyi Gadek.'

'Never heard of him. '

'Oh yes you have and it is not a him, it's a her. When you last saw her she was called Brenda Mtui.'

'Brenda? From Muguga? What is she doing here and why the name change?'

'She is married to Joe Gadek, an American of Polish origin. He's a water systems engineer working here with the World Bank. Because she now has a European surname she decided to use her Chagga first name to show her Tanzanian origin. She wants to see you because she wants to work with you again in the lab.'

'She was stardust, and she could be a real role model for all the young Batswana trainees. She can point out that when she first worked with me she was in the same position as them and she is now in a senior position.' I used the same argument with Jack when I asked him to give her a contract.

She came to the laboratory the next day and gave me a great hug.

'What a delight,' were my first words to her. 'But what on earth are you doing in Botswana?' She had met Joe when he was working in Tanzania: she had finished her technical qualification before she married and since then she had lived in Washington and Ghana before coming to Botswana. I called Ken and asked him to join us. Monyi made a big impression and they did not want to hear about my trip to Onderstepoort. Eventually I was able to talk about the wonderful reception I had received at the Institute. They all had a good laugh at the foot and mouth saga: 'Typical pig-headed Boer' was the general consensus.

There was great interest in the multi-headed microscope. Everyone agreed we needed one for the Bacteriology Section for teaching purposes and one for the rabies laboratory for diagnostic purposes. It was often of life saving importance that we got the rabies diagnosis right and so all senior staff who were in the laboratory examined the smears before a final diagnosis was made. Ken was asked to look into the matter and we soon had a pair of double-headed microscopes. It was felt that two people at a time was adequate for our needs.

The whole team were delighted by the response I had received from the different sections. Mik thought that it would be a good idea to invite Stan Herr to come and look at the suspect leptospiral abortions in the Tuli Block.

'If we do that, we will need to get some guinea pigs for the isolation of leptospira,' he said. We had a small, experimental animal colony but it consisted only of mice which we bred and used for rabies diagnosis. Because of their use they were kept at one end of the rabies laboratory. If we were going to breed guinea pigs on a regular basis then we would need a proper house for the experimental animals.

Month on month we had shown an increase in the number of submissions of samples. Armed only with the figures for the first two months I went to see Jack to inform him of my visit to Onderstepoort and to request a local contract for Monyi. He was in good form that morning and told me that he had been in contact with Erasmus, the South African director, who told him that he had enjoyed my visit. Jack was delighted that I had made a good impression. I went through the visit department by department, pointing out what each had to offer us in terms of back-up and support. He did not know Rudolf Bigalke, who had only just replaced Zimmermann as director, and he had a good laugh at the foot and mouth vaccine story. I ended up by giving him the statistics of the submissions, telling him of the visit of Monyi and requesting a local contract for her.

'If we recruit her we will have a senior member of staff for all the different sections of the laboratory.'

I explained to Jack that it had taken only a few changes to get the laboratory working efficiently. 'We will also be able to put into action the next part of my plan for developing the services. I want to visit all the dairy farms in Botswana and undertake a mastitis survey on each and work out a control plan for them.'

This was not as grand as it sounds, because there were only a dozen dairies in the whole country and most of the milk was imported from South Africa.

'What is more ambitious is that we aim to visit each of the settled ranching areas and carry out a breeding disease survey. In each case we will need to send out a team of people to collect samples. We will have to take the laboratory out into the field – microscope, incubator, agar plates, and a generator to power them. Ken and Varshika have been working preparing a detailed list and will see how we can carry the equipment securely. Blood and faeces samples will be taken to give us some biochemical and parasitological information. As well as giving you valuable information on the health of the national herd, it will give the laboratory and the Department a high profile.'

'You have a knack of preparing a case so that I cannot turn you down,' Jack said. 'However, the results indicate that the reforms you have instigated are working and so yet again I am happy to give you what you want.'

Although it would be some years before the term was coined, we now had a 'rainbow coalition' in the senior staff of the laboratory, and I had recruited women from Asia, Africa and Europe. However, the staff had not finished growing: a few weeks later I was asked to go to HQ as Jack wanted to see me. Sitting in his office was a man of about my age with black curly hair and an open friendly face.

'Roger, I want you to meet Carl Berg, a veterinary surgeon who has been recruited by Norwegian Aid to help you in the laboratory. He arrived this morning and is staying at the Holiday Inn. Please help him to settle in and explain what it is you want him to do. I hope that you have no more requests for staff?'

'Not at the moment, Sir, but if the work continues to increase, you never know.'

343

In the car on the way back to the laboratory Carl told me something of himself. He was married with a daughter the same age as my son Richard. His wife was a very high-powered laboratory technician, and had been working in the breeding disease department of the Oslo Veterinary School. She had not been too pleased at having to resign from her post to come to Botswana, as she was very career minded. Carl was a very intense man, most friendly and pleasant but given to bouts of serious depression. He had worked in several countries, mostly on short-term contracts and Anne, his wife, had not gone with him. He wondered if the laboratory could employ her. I told him that I was not keen to employ a husband and wife team because when one went on holiday we lost two! However, I felt sure I could find her a job at the Botswana Vaccine Institute, or where she actually ended up, in the research laboratories at Sebele. He had some experience of laboratory work although it was mostly with fish, but he proved a reliable and dependable colleague, hard working and eager to fit in with the team.

Until the African staff returned from their overseas training courses our team was complete. Our number would remain stable but the number of submissions would continue to increase.

19

Diseases, Theatre, and Schools

'It seems ... to be one of those simple cases which are so extremely difficult.'
Sir Arthur Conan Doyle, *A Study in Scarlet*

Rabies was not a major problem in Botswana; we confirmed about seventy-five cases a year, about half of which were in dogs. The remainder were in a variety of animals, and of course humans, as we did the rabies diagnosis for the hospital and Medical Department. Perhaps the saddest human case that we had was a man who had been given a corneal transplant from a rabies victim (although, at the time, it was not realised what had been the cause of death) and he succumbed to the disease. In this case we were able to diagnose the disease from corneal smears made while the patient was alive and so were able to inform the doctors that he was suffering from rabies, so that they were able to ease his pain until he died. They were also able to inform his family that there was no hope of his recovery.

Another human case was of great importance to the country: a Bushman farm worker was sitting outside his house in western Botswana one night when a jackal walked into the yard and bit him on the face. He shooed the animal away and did nothing more. One week later he was unwell and his family took him to the Ghanzi hospital where the staff diagnosed encephalitis of unknown origin. Within a few days the man was dead. Mr Khumalo the senior livestock officer in charge of the Ghanzi Veterinary Office had heard of the case and went to the hospital and asked them to carry out a post mortem examination. The medical staff declined to carry out the examination on the grounds that the disease could not be rabies because the incubation period was too short: it certainly was much shorter than I had ever heard of. The man was duly buried. Mr Khumalo was not happy because he felt that this might be the first case of rabies ever recorded in Ghanzi. He went to the local magistrate and after a battle with the Medical Department that

345

lasted almost a week, the magistrate ordered that the body be exhumed and the brain removed for examination.

We received a Kilner Jar of goo in glycerine. It was impossible to determine which part of the brain was which, as it was almost completely liquefied. I do not know how many slides were made and examined, but in one Stan saw a single Negri body, standing out in the ultra violet light. We all saw it and agreed that this was a Negri body and not a piece of grot. The slide was sealed and preserved while we waited the results of the biological tests. The test mice all died but from bacterial infection and not rabies, and so we repeated the tests with more antibiotics. But it was no use, there was too much contamination.

We decided that this was too important to make a decision on a single Negri body. We sent the brain to Colin Cameron (an Afrikaaner) who was the South African expert on rabies in the Onderstepoort veterinary faculty, along with the slide: we had identified where on the slide the Negri body was to be seen. He was certain that what we had seen was enough to diagnose rabies, which we did, congratulating Mr Khumalo for his diligence and perseverance.

Our confidence was justified a few weeks later when we received a brain of a cow from the same farm in Ghanzi, and there was no doubt that this cow had rabies. A new minimum incubation period of seven days for rabies in humans had been confirmed. We watched as this new rabies epidemic slowly moved east across the Kalahari Desert towards Kanye as we confirmed the disease in jackals and cattle; the few field staff that we had in this part of Botswana were on the look-out for the disease.

A cat bit two children in Lobatse; the cat was found and killed, and the brain sent to us. It was positive for rabies without any shadow of doubt and the local veterinary officer discussed the case with the medical officer who rushed out to see the families of the bitten children. He found one easily and persuaded the mother to bring the child to the clinic for vaccination – not the 'seven-a-side' of yesteryear (the Pasteur Vaccine required fourteen daily injections given in two lines down the abdomen, the sites of the injections becoming more and more painful as the course went on) but five painless injections over three weeks. The family of the second child could not be found; the doctor was informed that the mother and child had gone home to Francistown but nobody knew where (or, at least, they were not telling). The child in Lobatse suffered no ill-effects, but a few weeks later another child was taken to the Francistown hospital where she died of rabies. We confirmed the sad diagnosis and were furious with the mother who, in fear, had run away.

Cat rabies gave us nightmares – it is not possible to vaccinate all cats as there are so many feral ones living in urban areas, surviving on what they can scavenge and small rodents. Cats do not generally suffer from rabies as they are agile enough to escape from most canine attackers. However, they do get bitten by mongooses, and if the mongoose is infected with rabies ... Normally the disease in cats dies with the cat, but occasionally the infection is transmitted to humans before the cat dies. The Lobatse outbreak ceased with the two children and there were no further cases.

I do not know how many cats lived under the Grand Hotel in Francistown (many buildings in Botswana are built on a platform two to three feet off the ground to prevent flooding during those rare flash floods), but there were more than 100. It was a nightmare when one of them became infected with rabies; so many animals living so close together made it inevitable that the infection would spread. The population of cats had to be eliminated. Using poison in a town presents serious risks of the poison being taken away and other animals being killed by accident. They had to be flushed out and shot, but again this is not a very pleasant activity and with the guests about it had to done at night and without too much noise. The cats were not completely eliminated but their numbers were substantially reduced and the outbreak died out.

In an earlier chapter I described a great success for the laboratory, when the wife of the manager of the Selibe Pikwe copper mine was walking in her garden and was attacked by a strange dog. Thanks to the rapid response of all concerned, by 5 pm the woman had had her first dose of rabies vaccine and all was well. It is such cases that make the reputation of a veterinary laboratory. Even when things go wrong, as they inevitably do, people will forgive a great deal if they know that everything possible has been done.

Plant poisonings were a regular problem, particularly in the dry season when the grass dries up and often the only green material available to the animals is poisonous. Perhaps the most dramatic outbreak of giblaar poisoning was in buffalo in the Okavango, and there was nothing that we could do. Alan Wellwood phoned one morning at the end of the dry season to say that he was going to

347

investigate suspicious deaths in buffalo, and were there any special samples that he should take. He mentioned that all the animals were found dead on the banks of a tributary of the Okavango and some were actually in the water. Bells rang. I remembered Farnie's comments about *Dichapetulum cymosum* poisoning, and how it is drinking water that enables the toxin to be absorbed and become effective. I told Alan the story about the plant and asked him to take unselected samples of the rumen contents of half a dozen of the buffalo, examine the hearts of a couple of the freshest and put some samples of heart muscle into formalin. I suggested that he should also examine the area where the buffalo were grazing to see if any of the plants were visible and I told him what to look for.

He phoned me at home that evening to say he was convinced that it was *Dichapetulum cymosum*: the whole area was covered with the plant and it was the only green thing to be seen. Large numbers of leaves were present in the rumen and he could find no lesions at all. The problem here is that there is nothing you can do, except pray for rain. The samples duly arrived from Maun but they added nothing more to the diagnosis.

There is a well-documented story concerning mogau poisoning. About seventy beasts were in the holding ground at Mahalapye station awaiting loading on the train for their journey to the Lobatse abattoir. When the train arrived it tooted its hooter and 18 animals dropped dead. At the time Botswana was experiencing one of its periodic droughts. Everything in the bush was shrivelling up and dying, or giving the appearance of dying.

We were in the middle of a drought and yet *Pavetta harborii* was still looking as green as it ever did, and reports were reaching us of animals dropping dead. I had a phone call from Mr Njui, saying that he had a suspected outbreak of mogau poisoning at the southern end of his district and could I possibly assist him once more. It was just over an hour's drive to the meeting place and I asked Emmanuel and Gift to come with me. We also had a very bright student, Kereng Masupu, at home for the holidays from Tuskagee Veterinary School (an old established black university in the States) and I suggested that he join us.

In no time we were on the road. Mr Njui was waiting for us at the cordon fence and led us to the cattle post. The post itself was completely devoid of life. The trees stood listlessly round the house, their leaves brown and lifeless. There were some healthy looking beasts standing aimlessly under the trees, worn down by the heat and drought, looking at the ground. Their faces seemed to say, 'Where has all the grass gone?' We got out of the car and Emmanuel slammed the door shut with a great bang. One of the steers dropped dead more or less at our feet. There could have been no better indication of the cause of death. Had I been a doubter of the train station story, I would have had a Damascene conversion.

We set about examining the beast which despite the drought was in fair condition. There was some fat and all the tissues appeared normal. I took the whole heart and put it directly into the cold box to examine back in the laboratory. When we opened the rumen the diagnosis was confirmed (although in this case the absence of the plant would not have ruled out the possibility that mogau was the cause because it is a chronic poison and the animal might have eaten and digested the leaves some time previously). We took samples of the rumen to show the staff. I was asked if the meat was fit to eat. When I said that it was, I was asked if I could put some meat in the cold box and Emmanuel and Gift negotiated with the farmer to purchase some choice cuts: not the fillets but the meat with fat on it.

Their transactions concluded and the meat safely in the cold box, we began to discuss with the farmer what he needed to do. It was a pretty thankless task cutting down mogau because it has budding underground roots (rather like ground elder in Britain). If you tried to dig it up you were certain to leave some part of the root in the ground, chemical treatment was prohibitively expensive and the only real hope was to cut it down to the ground and burn it, which is fine round the borehole but not so easy over an area of 200 square kilometres. The only solution was to sell some of his stock and use the money to buy hay for his animals until the grass started to grow again. It is amazing how difficult it is to persuade farmers to take this course of action. They could not understand that it was better to sell ten and save ninety rather than allow fifty to die. Like Mr Micawber they always expected that 'something would turn up'. With Mr Njui supporting my recommended course of action, there was some hope the farmer might follow it. Mr Njui was a definite Windsor supporter.

The next interesting case of poisoning occurred when Stan was the duty officer and a member of the Game Department drove into the car park with ten dead or dying vultures on the back of the truck. One look at the birds told Stan the cause of the problem: they had

349

been poisoned with strychnine. There is no mistaking the signs: all the muscles go into intense spasm and the animal or bird dies because it is unable to breathe. It is a foul poison.

The source of the poison was not hard to find: the vultures had been seen feeding on a dead cow on a settled farm near Mochudi. The farmer was fed up with the vultures making a nuisance of themselves, or at least they upset the farmer by doing what vultures do best, namely getting rid of dead bodies. The farmer had laced a carcase with strychnine. He was prosecuted for possessing strychnine, which was a controlled substance, and for using it with the intention of killing protected birds. He pleaded guilty, and so we did not have to give evidence, and he was fined a substantial sum. But to return to the vultures in the post mortem room: six were dead and four still living but in a sorry state. We attended first of all to the living and gave all four hefty doses of acetylpromazine. We did not carry anaesthetic-quality barbiturates, only the highly concentrated phenylbarbitone used for putting animals to sleep. We diluted this with sterile salt solution (saline) and small doses were injected under the skin until the birds relaxed (none of us felt confident enough to try and find a vein to give the anaesthetic intravenously).

With four sleeping vultures in the post mortem room we had a look at the dead ones, more from interest than to make a diagnosis. The only lesions seen were those associated with severe muscle spasm: the tissues were full of blood and there were splashes of haemorrhage on the surfaces of the muscles, heart and lungs. After the post mortem room had been cleaned, we shut the door and left the sleeping vultures in peace. At the end of the day we found that two of the four had died, but the following day the two remaining birds were showing signs of activity so we gave them a glucose saline drip under the skin and some vitamins into the muscle. By the end of day two there were real signs of activity, and when I opened the PM room door on the Saturday morning I was almost knocked over as the last two vultures charged to get out. They took off and flew away. A twenty percent success rate is not bad when treating strychnine poisoning!

I am not sure whether the next case was strictly a poisoning but cattle died from botulism toxin. It is not known why it should be, but there seems to be an affinity between *Clostridium botulinum* (now famous for the Botox beauty treatment) and dead tortoises. Perhaps the organism likes the taste of dead tortoise. In periods of severe drought, which are not uncommon in Botswana, tortoises die, probably from dehydration, and cattle eat them. In periods of severe drought cattle often suffer from mineral deficiencies, and in particular lack of phosphorus. For some reason the soils of southern Africa (as in South America) are particularly deficient in this element and as a consequence animals suffer from a depraved appetite, which is called 'pica', and they will eat anything: I have seen a cow chewing away on an old tin can. So it is not surprising that if they come across a dead tortoise they will chew it, ingest the botulinum toxin and die.

David Brown, the vet in Serowe, had an outbreak of this problem and he suspected that the cattle which were paralysed in their back legs were suffering from dumb rabies. He put one to sleep and removed the brain and sent it to us. It was not rabies. However when we examined histological sections of the hind brain (called the medulla oblongata) where the brain is becoming the spinal cord we saw strange lesions – big holes were present where they should not have been, indicating oedema of that part of the brain. This was Mik's case and going through the texts he found that botulism could cause these lesions in the brain. Stan remembered the story about tortoises, so David was asked to check and see if there were any dead tortoises about and if so to send one to us. He was also asked to take a blood sample from any new case. To our delight we isolated *Clostridium botulinum* from the tortoise and we demonstrated the toxin in the blood. To do this we injected the serum from the dead animal intravenously into three mice; serum from the animal was mixed with the antiserum to *Clostridium botulinum* and injected into three more. The untreated serum produced posterior paralysis and death in the mice, but the protected mice all survived.

The case was solved, the diagnosis had been made, but as Sherwin would say, 'We are not in the business of making diagnoses, but of solving problems.' It was possible to vaccinate against *Clostridium botulinum* but if the farmer loses three or four animals every ten years, this is not an economic solution. It is not like vaccinating against blackleg (a gangrenous condition) or tetanus, both of which are common in young cattle (and both caused by clostridia) if they are not vaccinated. Vaccination in this case was not the answer. The solution was that the farmer had to feed bone meal supplement to his animals to treat the pica and so stop the cattle eating anything they could find to alleviate their craving. This he did and no further cases

351

occurred. Perhaps no further cases would have occurred had he done nothing. That we shall never know, but it is as well to take the credit when there is any going.

Stan thought it was time I came up to Motopi to watch a vaccine trial. I did not have the time to spend a whole week in idleness but decided that I would fly up on the Friday with the plane that would be bringing the team back to Gaborone. It was the first time I had ever flown with a woman pilot – Wyn Wylie was to become a good friend. She was South African, about my age, short, slightly built with a mop of blonde hair, a cheerful grin and a ready wit and tongue. She worked as a commercial pilot for a private company for fun, not the money: her husband Loch had a huge road building company which was improving the Botswana roads.

It was a plane which could seat ten although there were only four of us on board – there would be more on the way back. Wyn was checking out her co-pilot to see whether or not he should be taken on by the company. He was not, although I could see nothing wrong with the way he flew the plane. Wyn explained that there had been one or two niggling little problems with the plane, but this was the first flight after a major overhaul and so all should be well. We saw some game as we flew over the Mgkadikadi Pans, and when we arrived at the grass landing strip outside the Motopi Security Unit we made a low-level pass to frighten the impala off the runway. When she was doing her landing drill Wyn realised that the landing gear was not coming down. The air was blue with her comments about the company that had serviced the plane: because one of the niggling faults had been that the contact for the landing gear was not always engaging.

'Don't worry,' she said, 'we can always wind it down, but the problem with that is that we have to fly back with it down, which will add at least half an hour to the journey. Would you please move round the plane, jumping on the floor?'

This we did, until somebody jumped on the right spot – down came the undercarriage, and her co-pilot made a perfect landing! Stan was there to greet us. Wyn made the plane safe and we all went off to the main building for a coffee before starting work. There were twelve animals to examine: three controls, three animals vaccinated a month previously with a full dose of the latest batch of BVI foot and mouth disease vaccine, three with a third of a dose of vaccine and three that had received a ninth of a dose of vaccine. These animals

352

had all been challenged on Monday by injection in the tongue with a fixed dose of virulent virus.

The animals were all shot in the order ninth, third, full dose and control, and tongues and feet were all carefully examined. In none of the vaccinated animals were there any lesions of foot and mouth disease in mouth or feet. The control animals all had the classic lesions of foot and mouth disease on the tongue, and in one the whole lining had died and was about to slough off. All animals had lesions in one or more feet. It was a very satisfactory trial: there was no need for statistics to see if this vaccine worked even when diluted. The abdomen and chest of each animal was opened and liberal quantities of diesel were poured in, to ensure that the staff buried the carcases rather than ate the meat, or even worse sold it in the village.

Throughout the week the animals had all been housed in a sort of covered yard to which entry was via a securely padlocked door. This stood in a field about fifty yards square which had a high fence to prevent the entry of game animals, and again a locked gate. Outside this paddock was another in which cattle susceptible to foot and mouth disease were grazed. This was to determine whether there had been any escape of virus. Round the whole 1800-hectare unit was a double fence: the inner fence was about eighteen feet high and the outer fence, which was about six feet from the inner, was about four feet high. The purpose of this double fencing was to prevent game animals jumping in; with a good run up some antelopes can scramble over an eighteen-foot fence, and the double fencing was to prevent the run up. The system at Motopi worked well; to my knowledge there has never been an escape of virus even to the sentinel cattle. The dry climate ensures that any small droplet of fluid evaporates quickly and so the virus is killed.

When we had completed the work, disinfected our clothes, showered, and had lunch (fresh fillets of tilapia of course), we returned to the plane with our colleagues, personal effects, and Stan's cold box of frozen tilapia: he had had a good week on the river. I have to admit that it was a pretty impressive setup, which seemed to work like clockwork. We had an uneventful flight back, and this time the contact was made and the undercarriage came down.

We were cleared by the control tower for landing and on our final approach for touchdown when Wyn noticed a larger plane coming up the runway to meet us! Landing was aborted, as we took to the skies to get out of the way of the plane taking off. Wyn was not amused and again the language was choice: what she called the staff in the control tower had to be heard to be believed. We landed without further mishap. I flew on many other occasions with Wyn and never again did anything untoward happen.

Perhaps the oddest problem we ever had to deal with was also associated with flying; it was the case of the sick aeroplane. This was a fairly new, small twin-engined Cessna which was regularly maintained. It developed an unhappy knack of one of the engines cutting out. The plane could fly on one engine, but was far better (and safer) on two. Sometimes the engine could be restarted; sometimes it would not start again until the plane was back down on the ground. Both engines were affected from time to time, although never both at the same time.

The owner thought that some contaminant had got into the tank and so he brought a sample from the tank for us to analyse, and it was just my luck to be on duty that day. There are millions of different chemicals about, so how was Mike to choose what to look for? An analysis of the spectrum of light caused by burning the fuel suggested that it was pure aviation fuel. Mike took it to Ken and asked him to make smears to see if there were any particles in the fuel. There were; long, thin, cotton-like threads. Ken asked me to have a look because he thought that they might be fungi: specific staining techniques for fungi were used, which suggested that there was a fungal infection in the fuel tanks. It was decided that fungal cultures should be set up and a pure growth of a fungus that we could not identify was isolated: identification of fungi is the work for a real expert.

Out came the books – there was no Internet or Google in those days, although computers were making their appearance in our laboratory. The books gave us nothing. We informed the owner that we thought that his tanks were suffering from a fungal infection and it was he that supplied the solution. He brought in an article from an aviation magazine which described our problem. In places where there is a high ambient temperature, water condensation inside the tanks occurs, and if the fungus is introduced during refuelling it is able to survive in the condensate: it is also capable of limited growth by breaking down the fuel. If the fungus is present in sufficient quantity then it can cause an obstruction in the fuel line and the engine is starved and so stops. Problem solved. The tanks and fuel lines would have to be thoroughly cleaned and disinfected with a suitable fungicide: this would then have to be removed from the tank by repeated rinsing and finally everything would have to be thoroughly dried before the tank could be filled again. The owner was so grateful that Ken got a free flight over the town.

Meanwhile problems in the Tuli Block were continuing unabated. Mik asked if we should bring in Stan Herr, so I phoned him and he was delighted to be invited. He drove up and spent the night with Maxine and me, then he and Mik set off in separate vehicles early the next morning bearing a great load of equipment. Russell Leadsom, the DVO, was unable to join them but Mik took a couple of staff from the laboratory and Alford was driving: he proved very useful as an extra pair of hands and was not afraid to handle the animals.

At Stan's request, the animals in the affected group had been kept short of water from the previous morning until the laboratory team arrived, when they were allowed free access. Each member of the team had a beaker, and when a cow passed urine the idea was to collect some of it in the beaker for injection into guinea pigs. Once the collections and injections were done, everyone adjourned to the farmhouse to take the history, and to discuss likely causes and what should be done. The reason for using guinea pigs to improve isolation is that Leptospira species that cause abortion are very labile and do not survive for long outside the animal body; they are also sometimes difficult to persuade to grow in culture media unless you have a big inoculum. Once a diagnosis had been made, then Mik would visit the farm again to advise on control measures. Stan Herr did not return to Gaborone but crossed the border into South Africa and went directly to Pretoria.

Leptospira species were demonstrated in the guinea-pigs and then isolated in culture media. Mik took the cultures to Onderstepoort, and there the identity was confirmed as *L. pomona*. Leptospiral infection is often associated with wildlife and water, and the farm concerned stretched down to the Limpopo river which is the border with South Africa. There are many species of wild animal associated with rivers. Wild animals, particularly rodents, are the common source of infection for domestic animals. The infection usually responds to treatment with the antibiotic streptocmycin, and today there is an efficient vaccine. The Tuli Block abortions were brought to a rapid stop and we had another happy client.

At first we did not receive many poultry specimens because there were no poultry farms in the country, and local hen keepers were not keen to bring their dead birds into the laboratory but preferred to eat

355

them. With increasing prosperity the demands for poultry meat grew and so, instead of breeding their own birds, the villagers started to buy day-old chicks produced commercially in South Africa – and with them they brought fowl typhoid and Marek's disease. The former is caused by a salmonella species and appears in the first weeks of life. Most frequently the infection is passed into the egg from the mother and it only takes one bird in a group of day-old chicks to be infected for the whole group to become diseased. Treatment with antibiotics can be successful but affected birds never do really well.

Some of the villagers became very successful producers of broiler chicks, which was a tribute to the Advisory Service who toured the villages showing farmers how to improve their management and so reduce the mortality and improve their profits. We saw some large outbreaks of Marek's disease where the farmer thought that he would save money by not vaccinating his day-old chicks, but lived to regret it because after spending much money feeding the birds, just as they were coming into lay they would start to die. If the farmer was lucky then some of the birds would start to die at eight to ten weeks and we always recommended that they slaughter the rest to eat before they all died. After one major loss we found that the farmers were more punctilious about their vaccinations.

Parasitic conditions were common to all species and were seen on a daily basis: it has always amazed me that in such hot, dry conditions, internal parasites should be a regular problem: how do the worm eggs and larvae survive desiccation? It seems that even in the driest of habitats there are micro-climates in which these tenacious creatures can stay alive. Mange mites are another creature that can survive under the harshest conditions; once aboard a fresh host they can burrow into the skin and get protection from the desiccation of the sun, although the psoroptes mite (which causes sheep scab) and chorioptes, which affects mainly cattle and horses, both live on the skin rather than in it and they feed on the debris as the outer layer of the skin is shed. It is important that the correct sample is sent for analysis: deep scrapings for sarcoptes (pigs) and demodex (cattle and dogs), and shallow scrapings for psoroptes and chorioptes.

It soon became obvious to the team that the field staff had not been taught how to sample and what samples to take, and so remedial action was necessary. The immediate action was to ask the staff teaching the Veterinary Assistant and Livestock Officer courses at the Botswana Agricultural College to allow us to arrange a couple of teaching sessions. This was agreed and became a regular feature of their courses. We next set about writing a manual, and another of our regular ad hoc committees was set up to produce what ended up as several small leaflets. It resulted in a marked improvement in the quality of the specimens coming in.

Sherwin's great dictum was 'you only see what you know', and we were concerned that the farmers and Veterinary Department staff might be missing problems that they had always lived with and had come to accept as normal. We decided that we would take the laboratory to the veterinary offices and out into the bush. This would serve an educational role as well as a promotional one. If the farmers could see the laboratory staff working on their farms it would encourage them to submit samples when they had a problem. We now had sufficient staff to spare some to work out in the field.

It was not all work, as there were concerts to go to, an occasional visit to Gaborone's only cinema and, of course, the theatre. My visit to Onderstepoort had given me pause for thought. I was appalled at the way the white South Africans treated their African compatriots and yet the Gaborone Players were doing exactly the same thing: not treating the Africans badly, but ignoring them. I gave thought to the matter and decided that the best thing to do was for me to direct a play that had a large number of Africans in the cast.

I was presented with a great opportunity when I found out that Alan Paton's book *Cry the Beloved Country* was the set book for the Cambridge School Certificate English examination. Christine Purves had been involved with a theatrical production of the book when she was a student in Oberlin, Ohio and she had a copy of the script, which had been written by a Japanese/American woman and first performed in St-Martin-in-the-Fields Church in London. It was a perfect opportunity to combine many different facets: it meant that we could stage the play for all the secondary school children in Botswana and bring them all to Gaborone to see a play. Many children had never been inside a theatre and did not know what a theatre was. How could they be expected to understand a play if they had never seen one?

Before saying a word to the Capital Players committee, I had a word with Chris Conyers, the Financial Director of Debswana (the Botswana mining company that was a joint venture between DeBeers,

357

Anglo-American and the Botswana government). Although he was a South African, Chris was very liberal and keen on education of African children: when they returned to live in Johannesburg his wife Sue set up and ran a multi-racial school. Chris agreed at once that Debswana would finance the transport and accommodation of the children coming to the play: some of them would take two days to get to Gaborone as they had to travel over 1000 miles! Discussions were held with the local secondary schools and they agreed to house and feed the pupils provided that they would be reimbursed their costs. The children would bring blankets and sleep on the floor.

Without the backing of a company such as Debswana such an undertaking would have been impossible as there were more than 2000 pupils to cater for. We would have to resort to the system we used for the schools' production of 'Macready' and remove the seats from the theatre, replacing them with beer crates and planks. Again the Kalahari Breweries came up trumps and provided us with everything we required. I had worked out that we would need to stage eight performances just to accommodate the schoolchildren. It was decided to run the play for two weeks, with performances for children from Monday to Thursday and performances for the paying public on Friday and Saturday. With the Gala Premiere, that meant a total of eleven performances over a two-week, three-weekend period. Capital Players normally put on only six performances even for a musical! I was now ready to go to the committee.

At the next committee meeting of the Players I waited until we got to 'Future Productions' on the agenda and dropped my bombshell. It had been meticulously planned in detail and only the date was lacking.

'You will never get the cast.'

'They will never learn their lines.'

'They will not turn up for rehearsals.'

'They will probably drop out half way through the rehearsals.'

The first criticism I could rebut, as I had spoken to several potential members of the cast and I had already found an actor to play the Rev. Stephen Khumalo: Hope Phillips a South African administrator in the Education Department, had been found for me by Jack Purves. Tshenolo Naledi from the University of Botswana, as the Black Narrator, and Adolph Hirschfeld, as the Rev. Mr Msimango, were found for me by a friend who was a senior civil servant in the president's office.

358

I carefully explained to the committee that this would be a wonderful opportunity for the Players to show the country that it was serious about involving the whole nation in theatre and so fulfil a major object of all amateur thespians, to get people involved. It was decided that Windsor could have his way, provided that I agreed not to bankrupt the group. The show was on the road with the premiere scheduled for July 1983. Auditions were held, arms were twisted, people were visited, old services were called in, and we had a cast. Rehearsals began and the African cast members dispelled the fears of the committee. They turned up for rehearsals, they learnt their lines and learnt them well before the European members of the cast, and above all they enjoyed themselves. They concentrated when they were working and recited lines to each other when they weren't.

I visited Radio Botswana to find incidental music for the play, but I wanted live music and so I played the recordings that I had selected to Hope and asked what we should do.

'Roger, there is no problem, we in the cast can sing this and you can record it.'

Hope selected the singers and we had an evening at home with Maxine supplying the sandwiches, Sprite and coffee and Hope controlling the singers.

'I will sing bass with Adolph and Edward; Tumanang and Tatho will sing tenor; John and Emmanuel, alto. Now let's try it.'

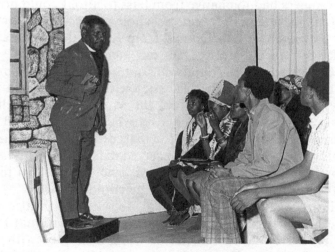

Hope Phillips as the Rev. Stephen Khumalo addressing his congregation in *Cry the Beloved Country*, directed by Roger Windsor.

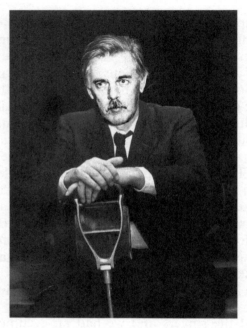

Bill Shaw as Jarvis, whose son is murdered by the son of the Rev. Khumalo in *Cry the Beloved Country*.

And they were away: if Hope thought that the balance was wrong, one of the singers had to change from bass to alto! I could not believe my ears. In one evening they had the whole musical score sorted. Reg Salisbury and Kinnear MacDonald from Radio Botswana agreed to record the tape for me and we had our incidental music.

When Christine Purves found out that we needed a drummer she told me that she had the perfect person for us, a twelve-year-old blind boy, Freddie Mogorosi, from the Mochudi Blind School. He sat on the side of the stage and played when necessary and without any prompting. He soon became the mascot for the show and when he took his curtain call he always received massive applause. I do not know what happened to him, but for a brief moment in his life he was a star and it did not matter that he could not see.

As with my veterinary management, so with my theatre management. We had people assigned to various organisational roles and these people were allowed to get on with their jobs with minimal interference from me. We needed the Gala Premiere to pay those schools' performance costs not covered by Debswana, and in an effort to ensure a sell-out it was decided that Alan Paton, the author of the book, should be invited. Surprisingly his number was in the South African telephone directory and so I called. His wife Anne answered the phone and I was not allowed to speak to the man himself; I told her the reason for my call and said that I would put the invitation in writing. I received a polite reply saying that he would consider the matter and let us know. We waited and waited for a confirmation until I could wait no longer, as we needed to know if he was coming so that we could publicise the fact. I phoned. Anne answered.

'Alan would love to come, but he is worried about the response he would get to the presence of a South African in an independent black republic.'

I assured her that he would be made very welcome, but she was not happy and so I told her that I would get an official answer from government sources: when I had that, I would call her again.

It just so happened that Maxine was playing in a concert that night, and I knew that the president would be in the audience. When Maxine plays I always sit in the front row so that she knows I am there. It happened that the president and his party were also in the front row, just across the gangway. At the interval I approached His Excellency and we talked about the play.

'Do not worry, Dr Windsor, the date of the premiere is in my diary and we will be there. It will be my birthday treat.'

That gave me the opportunity to explain my predicament.

'Dr Windsor, you can tell Dr Paton from me that all South Africans are welcome in my country and he in particular.'

That was all I needed: the following morning I was able to call Anne Paton and repeated to her what the president had said, word for word. The Patons were coming.

Everything was falling into place. Rodney Hodgson, under Mike's eye, had the sets organised and we even had the Gaborone Prison involved making some of the stage furniture. Els Velzoboer had the costumes in hand, including making the three Zulu women's outfits, the cassocks had all been borrowed from the Archbishop of Botswana and my loud check suit had been altered to fit the actor who was playing John Khumalo the flamboyant politician brother. The premiere was sold out and the Holiday Inn, who were providing the food and champagne for it, had erected their marquee behind the theatre.

Alan and Anne Paton used the opportunity of visiting Botswana

361

to have a few days' holiday in the Okovango Delta and they flew down from Maun on the Friday afternoon before the opening. The VIP lounge had been opened for them, and just before I went to the airport I received a message from the president's office that, if it was convenient, the president wished to meet Dr Paton at State House on Saturday 23 July at 10 am.

It was convenient. The Patons were delightful and Alan handled the assembled press corps with charm, tact and evident pleasure. I brought them to Tawana Close to our house where they were staying, for a well-earned cup of tea. Alan was thrilled at being invited to State House. There was a mini-drama when he found that he had forgotten to pack his black shoes: luckily John O'Brien who taught at Maru-A-Pula School and was a friend of Alan's son, had similar size feet, so Alan was able to visit His Excellency, and attend the premiere well shod. Just before ten the following morning I drove into the grounds of State House to introduce Alan to Churchill Sethloboko, the chief bodyguard, and the two went to the president's private office. I intended to wait in the car, but after a brief moment Churchill was back saying the president wanted me to join them and so I went in. The respect that each man had for the other was obvious: I did not say a word but sat and listened to the two wise men putting to rights the ills of Africa. It was a fascinating hour or so but we returned home to find that Alan was the centre of a political storm back home and our phone just rang and rang. Poor Alan had little opportunity to rest before the evening's entertainment.

Alan had been told that it was the president's birthday and had brought a signed first edition of *Cry the Beloved Country* as a present, neatly wrapped in gift paper. The champagne reception started the proceedings, at the end of which Alan made a short speech and wished Dr Masire a very happy birthday and the crowd sang the birthday song, after which the book was handed over. All wrapped presents had to be opened by the bodyguards in case they were booby trapped, but Dr Masire was thrilled with the book. The audience took their seats while I went and said a few words to the cast and handed them over to the stage manager. The lights went down and the show was on the road.

Having met the author, the cast were determined to do their best and a wonderful performance resulted, especially by Hope and the Black and White Narrators. There was scarcely a dry eye in the house as 'Nkosi Sikelel' iAfrika' drew the play to its close.

362

Maxine cooked the curry but Chris and Sue Conyers had arranged the lunch party for the Patons in their beautiful house and the whole 'Cry' team were invited. I said a few words of thanks to the Patons for coming, to the Conyers for their hospitality, and to the whole team for all their hard work. Alan replied, telling us that despite there having been two films made of his book, this was the finest interpretation that he had seen, that the acting was wonderful, and that he felt the scenes between Hope as the Rev. Khumalo and Bill Shaw as Jarvis were even more moving than he had written. He said that he was proud to be in Botswana and how impressed he had been by the local people and the women in particular; in South Africa no woman ever shook hands with him, but offered him a 'limp lettuce'. He and his wife had had a wonderful stay in their country and he hoped that one day South Africa would be as happy.

It was a marvellous conclusion to a wonderful weekend. Before they left to fly home, Alan gave Maxine and me a copy of the book he wrote on the death of his first wife, *Kontakion for You Departed*. Soon after his departure I received this charming letter, which I was able to share with the team, to their great delight.

PHONE 752120

P.O. BOX 278
HILLCREST
3650 NATAL

July 29th 1983

Dear Roger & Maxine

We returned home safely on Sunday night, after having spent four hours in the plane flying from Johannesburg to Durban and back again, because the plane couldn't land at Durban owing to bad weather. We finally got home at midnight, cold and wet!

We are writing to thank you for having us as your guests last weekend and for the splendid evening on Saturday, and the splendid luncheon on Sunday. We both felt that the atmosphere of Gaborone was very different from that here, and what I had to say about the handshakes of the Botswana women was nothing less than the truth. I must also thank you for arranging for me to meet the President.

I hope Botswana continues on its sensible and peaceful course. It certainly serves as an example to us, not to mention the other countries of Africa.

I shall leave Anne to add a postscript.

With affectionate wishes from us both

Yours

Alan Paton

Alan Paton

Thereafter, each time we travelled to Natal we visited their beautiful home in Hillcrest, and even after we left Botswana and went to live in Perú we kept in touch with Alan until his death in 1988.

The seats were cleared from the theatre and the planks installed for the first of our schools' performances: we started with a mixture of high schools from Gaborone and up country. The response from the audiences was fantastic: they laughed and they cried; they cheered and booed; and almost all went away with the idea that theatre could be fun as well as educational. The adult performances sold out and we were delighted with the number of Batswana who attended; for many it was the first time they had visited the MOTH Hall and I hoped that it would not be the last. The critics on the committee had been silenced – the show had been a success and made a profit, and the local actors had learnt their lines, come to rehearsals and performed with aplomb. During the run several of the actors came to me to say that they could not perform on such and such a day, but I was not to worry, because their friend so-and-so would do their part. It was amazing how many of the cast were interchangeable as they were word perfect in many of the parts. The changes went unnoticed.

Reg Salisbury phoned me to say that Radio Botswana wished to record the play to go out in three parts. Tim Holdcroft, who played Father Vincent, was unable to be present for the recording and so I had to read in his part. The last night of the play came to a close and we finished with a great party in the theatre. As always at the end of a successful run, I felt desolate when it was all over. However, it was time for me to return my attentions to my day job and begin the next phase in the development of the laboratory services.

20

Field Work and Small Animals

'It is a capital mistake to theorise before one has data.'
Sir Arthur Conan Doyle *A Scandal in Bohemia*

When any new venture was proposed, the first thing to be done was to hold a meeting to discuss what to do and how to do it. The idea of a national disease survey was thrashed out: this was an essential perquisite before the decision makers could make plans for developing the livestock industry in Botswana. Nick Buck from the Food and Agriculture Organisation's Agricultural Development Project at Sebele was asked to contribute his views as we did not wish to duplicate the efforts of his team.

It was decided that we should start with the dairy industry: there were two reasons for this. First there were only about a dozen dairy farms in the whole country, although some were fairly large with 100 or more cows. The second reason was that we could collect the samples on the farm but they would all be examined in the laboratory. We would therefore be able to cut our teeth before undertaking large-scale field work. Ken was asked to put together a set of sampling equipment that would be adequate for units of up to 100 cows. Even this was a large undertaking because it required at least 400 universal bottles, which are small wide-mouth containers that hold thirty millilitres of milk. Holders for four bottles – one for each quarter of the cow's udder – and racks for all the bottles were required. We also needed paper towels to clean each udder, methylated spirits to sterilise each teat end to prevent skin bacteria from contaminating the sample, and buckets of disinfectant to clean really dirty udders. Sheets for recording the animal numbers or names were needed. We soon found that it was not possible to number the bottles as we went along and so they were pre-numbered before we went out and each number was recorded alongside the name/number of the cow.

365

I am a great believer in starting with the simplest. By far the best-organised dairy farm in Botswana (if not the world, in my experience) was that of Robert and Elena White of Annandale Farm, Pitsane, who had a herd of about eighty Brown Swiss cows. The cows were milked in the morning and then the calves were put with their mothers for the day. In the evening the calves were taken away from their mothers and kept away overnight. The cows were milked by hand and each cow had an udder cloth with her name embroidered on it by Elana – woe betide any milker who used the wrong cloth. On arrival the milkers had to don boots, gowns, and hats, and then wash their hands in disinfectant before putting on disposable rubber gloves. This was a dairy herd that rarely experienced mastitis problems and so it was a good place to start.

Mik and I were to take the samples, and Ken and Monyi were to do the recording. We drove down to Lobatse after work with the equipment packed in the back of my Land Rover and we had booked into the Cumberland Hotel. We had an excellent dinner in the hotel restaurant and were in bed early as we had to drive the thirty miles to the farm in order to be there at 6 am. Apart from the problem with the numbering of the bottles everything went smoothly and there was no need to wash a single udder as they were all spotlessly clean. After we had taken the samples the cows were milked. By 8 am all the samples had been collected and we went into the farmhouse for an excellent breakfast. By 11 am the samples were being processed in the Bacteriology Section. All four samples from each cow were pooled and a California mastitis test (which indicates whether or not there is mastitis in that gland) was carried out. For this test the milk is mixed with an equal volume of a strong alkali solution; if there are cells present they coagulate and can be seen as clumps. Drops of the milk were then put onto various nutrient media and incubated to see if anything grew.

Ken decided that if we were to do this work properly an electronic counter was required which was much more specific than the California mastitis test. Our budget was adequate to purchase one and soon it was being tested in the laboratory, in time for our next mastitis investigation visit. This was to a small but much less well-organised dairy farm run by the Brigades, an organisation set up by an South African philanthropist Patrick van Rensburg, to teach agricultural trades to young Batswana. As there were only twenty cows to sample I went on my own and stayed the night with the young Blackbeards in Serowe. Roy, the elder son, was running the family cattle posts and looking after the trading business because his father had been appointed Minister of Works and Communications. Roy's wife Anne was Danish by origin, born in Kenya, reared in South America, educated at an English public school for girls, and studied at the Glasgow Veterinary School. Her father had been an agricultural adviser, hence the moves. Staying with the Blackbeards was always fun as Anne was a great cook and Roy had a fund of great stories about early days in Botswana and growing up in an almost totally black environment. His brother was the only white private in the Botswana Defence Force but soon rose to sergeant. On that night it was early to bed though, as we had an early start.

The farm was ready for us when we arrived; again the cows were milked by hand but with no individual cloths and only one bucket of water to clean the udders. They did not wash the udders unless they were really dirty. For that morning at least, and I hoped for ever, each udder was wiped with a fresh dry paper towel. The milkers did not wear protective clothing nor even wash their hands before commencing the milking. It is amazing what you can get away with in a dry climate! It has to be said that the whole parlour could have done with a good spring clean. But on this occasion I said nothing and just sampled the cows, while Anna did the recording. Despite the poor hygiene I was pleased with the apparent health of the udders and generally the cows were in good condition. I would return with the results, watch the milkers milking and discuss with the manager improvements to management and hygiene but there was a good basis for a successful dairy enterprise. I drove Anne home and after a cup of coffee and a bacon sandwich I was on the road to the laboratory, where I arrived in time for a late lunch.

To check on the bacteria in the milk sample, three different media were used: Edwards agar which is specific for streptococci, perhaps the most significant of the mastitis-producing bacteria; McConkey agar which is a wonderful medium for identifying the Gram Negative bacteria that indicate sloppy hygiene or, even worse, contamination of the milk by faeces; and the third medium used was the bacteriologists' catch-all, blood agar, on which the majority of bacteria will grow. The day after inoculation the plates are examined for bacterial growth and the findings obtained are compared with the results of the California Mastitis Test. If mastitis or sub-clinical mastitis (which is when the udder has problems but no obvious

367

clinical signs can be seen) is suspected then the bacteria isolated are identified and an anti-bacterial sensitivity test carried out. In this way a picture of the udder health of the herd is produced. If there were problems, then the farm was revisited and questions were asked about the management and feeding of the animals: the milking process was then watched and obvious defects in technique or husbandry were noted. The team then sat down with the owner or herd manager and discussed the defects and how they could be remedied.

We grew in confidence with every farm visited and we ventured further afield, including a visit to the only dairy herd in Maun: we flew up there with all our equipment because we could not afford the delay in testing the samples that a journey by road would entail. We felt a special interest in this farm as we had been involved in setting it up. The owner had been a big game hunter and on his retirement he bought a plot of land along the river in Maun with a view to setting up a dairy to provide Maun with fresh milk. We explained to him that with his limited area of land he would need to import all his forage 1500 miles from South Africa, which was going to make it very expensive: he therefore needed to set up his herd with small cows that produced high-quality milk. Our solution to this was that he should have a herd of Jersey cows which, being small, have a small appetite. They produce a low yield of milk, but with a high butter fat content (five percent is not unusual). A further advantage to Jersey cows was that they were said to possess some zebu genes and hence were more resistant to African diseases. From the milk he could remove some cream and make butter, and still sell milk with an adequate fat content. We advised that he should start with only ten cows and build up the numbers as his knowledge and confidence increased. The staff of the veterinary office in Maun were keen to help, as they wanted the venture to succeed. Within a few weeks of the dairy starting, the milk and cream was being sold to all the hotels in the town. We were delighted to see the way the farm was working when we came to take our samples. Our advice had been followed to the letter and this novice dairyman was producing a high-quality product, which was in great demand in the town.

Once our electronic counter had arrived we were able to think about offering our dairy farms a routine monthly check of the cell count in their milk. In a healthy udder the cells lining the milk-producing glands die and are shed into the milk. This is normal; however, if the animal is suffering from sub-clinical mastitis then white cells from the blood join the gland cells and the number can reach astronomical proportions. When the count reaches 2 million per ml then the milk in that quarter is pus rather than milk! When a cell counting scheme was introduced in Britain, a count of 500,000 cells per ml of milk was deemed acceptable: today that figure is very much lower. We decided that we would aim for 500,000 as our maximum. Without exception, all the dairy farmers in the country enrolled in the scheme and agreed to send us a sample every month. We supplied the farmers with universal bottles into which we put a measured amount of fixative to protect the cells during the transport: they were asked to fill the bottle with a sample from each churn produced at a single milking.

The VRI, Onderstepoort, agreed to supply us with milk of a known number of cells so that we could calibrate our machine, and offered us the opportunity to join their laboratory control scheme in which they sent us samples each month and we had to undertake a count and report to them: it was wonderful to feel that we had someone checking us. What was most interesting was that our counts were always the lowest of all; we tried to find out why this should be, but we never succeeded. It did not really matter because our results always ran in parallel to the South African laboratories. The great advantage of examining milk on a monthly basis is that it is possible to determine trends. One single result was not considered important, but the trend was what mattered. If we noticed a farm showing a month upon month increase in the count, then we would contact them to arrange a visit in an attempt to find out the problem and stop it progressing.

Having developed a system for collecting specimens in the field and bringing them back to the laboratory for examination, the next step was to take the laboratory out into the field and perform most of the work out in the bush. It was the opinion of the laboratory staff that most of the problems with disease were associated with nutrition, and Mike and his team were working with the FAO project to demonstrate the effects of supplementary feeding with minerals on the fertility of cattle. We were able to build on his experience of taking blood samples on a ranch out in the bush, far from Gaborone, and bringing them back to be analysed in the laboratory. Ken and Mike worked out what equipment and reagents would be required to undertake a breeding disease survey across the Kalahari. A tent would be equipped with the apparatus necessary to examine

369

sheath washing samples for trichomoniasis and vibriosis (two of the most significant venereal diseases of cattle), and to check placentas (afterbirth) and foetuses (should we come across any abortions), and fluid from swollen joints for brucellosis, an infection that causes abortion in cattle and undulant fever in man. Blood samples would be taken and the sera separated and stored for examination back in Gaborone. Rectal faeces would be collected and stored, for examination for worm eggs back at base.

Meals had to be planned and the food purchased, enough for up to two weeks out in the field. Much to her dismay I put Varshika in charge of the food, and as always she made a great success of the job. Ice had to be brought from the Lobatse abattoir to put in the deep freeze to ensure that we had cold beer for the evening session round the camp fire! Since the teams would be mixed it was essential that there be adequate ablution and sleeping arrangements. Sanitary arrangements were simple: you took the team spade and disappeared into the bush.

The district veterinary staff were asked to arrange a timetable with the local farmers; one farm to be examined in the morning and a second one in the afternoon. There was no shortage of farmers wanting us to examine their stock. A camp-site was established so that we did not have to keep moving the laboratory. During the morning the laboratory staff would examine the afternoon samples from the previous day, bearing in mind that the samples for venereal pathogens had to be examined within four hours of taking. Luckily I had been trained in the CVL in Weybridge on how to take sheath washings, and I had had some practice in Kenya and Argentina, but nothing had prepared me for doing 100 samples in a day.

Sampling is an art, working through a crush and not getting your arm broken. A halter is put on the bull, a rope is placed round the hind limb of the animal on the side you are working and the leg is lifted from the ground. A good man holds up the tail and your life depends upon him. You then crouch at the side of the crush – you cannot kneel because you might need to make a rapid exit – put your arms through the bars and snip off the hair at the end of the prepuce, while examining the state of the testicles, penis, skin and the aperture to the prepuce. A rubber tube is then inserted into the prepuce, and you then have to close the exit from the prepuce while an assistant pours 200 ml of sterile saline into a filter funnel inserted into the tube which then flows into the prepuce. If the animal is going to object, then this is the time when he gets very restless. The prepuce is then massaged vigorously for 100 strokes: the animal normally enjoys this part of the process and stands quietly. When the massage is complete the filter funnel is lowered and the milky fluid flows from the prepuce. This fluid is then transferred into a universal bottle and is ready for examination.

It sounds simple enough, and it is when the animal is quiet and peaceful. Not so when the bull is restless and unhappy and he can jump and kick: this is where the leg and tail men come into their own. The leg must be held tight so that the bull cannot kick and if the tail man applies enough pressure on the tail, it takes the bull's mind off kicking as he is worried about what is happening to his rear end. Occasionally you have to leap out of the way of a swinging foot – and that was how I ruined my left hip in Peru. Taking evasive action results in the loss of the sample and you have to start all over again. Another problem is if the bull decides to urinate during the massaging: this you can tell when the sample is returned to the funnel – instead of being a beautiful opalescent white, it is yellow. The work then has to be repeated. Once the prepucial sample is in the bottle, a blood sample is taken from the caudal vein in the raised tail and another person puts a hand encased in a rubber glove into the rectum and takes a sample of faeces. On removing his hand the glove is inverted and the opening tied, so the faeces are on the inside. The blood tube and the glove are numbered, the samples are put into the cool bag, and you move onto the next animal, having recorded the state of the genitalia and the condition of the animal. We decided not to examine the cows in a herd, working on the assumption that if the males were infected the females would also be infected. A bull covers many cows but a fertile cow will rarely be covered by more than one male. If all the males are free from venereal infection then it is certain that the cows will be clean.

The faeces were stored in the cold box at more or less 4° C, for examination back in Gaborone: it would have been possible to examine them in the field but the technique requires a lot of water, which can be at a premium in the Botswana bush, and the samples require a great deal of time to prepare and examine; these samples will also not deteriorate on storage provided that they are kept cool. It would also have been possible to examine the serum samples for antibodies to brucella in the bush, but once the serum has been separated from the clotted blood, the samples will keep well in cold

371

storage. However, examinations for the venereal pathogens have to be carried out on the spot.

The sheath washings are initially spun in a centrifuge to remove the debris and examined under the microscope, first using low power to see if there is movement, and if any is detected then a higher magnification is used to find the trichomonas: under the microscope these appear as little 'boats' being propelled from the rear by three 'oars', or flagella to give them their proper name. The presence of these micro-organisms is sufficient to make a diagnosis. At the same time, cultures for vibrio are set up. Although vibrio will grow on simple culture media, it will not grow in a normal atmosphere; it prefers to have increased carbon dioxide and decreased oxygen in the atmosphere. To avoid having to carry cylinders of nitrogen and carbon dioxide with us, Ken devised a cunning system: the medium was prepared and dispensed in universal bottles. Before we went out into the field, a needle was inserted through the cap of the bottle, and the air was sucked out with a pump and replaced by a mixture of nitrogen and carbon dioxide. To inoculate the medium, some of the sheath washing was taken up into a syringe, a needle was inserted through the cap of the bottle and half a millilitre of the liquid was injected into the medium. Speed was of the essence with this work, because the pathogens responsible for these venereal diseases do not live for long outside the body.

Organisation of the field work was straightforward; the farmers had assembled the bulls the night before and one by one they were put into the crush, to be released once they had been tested. It was a simple matter to collect animals together under Botswana conditions as on the majority of ranches or cattle posts there was only one water point to which the animals had to return on a regular basis. It was thought that the maximum time a cow could last without having to come in for water was three days. One farmer had trained his cattle in such a way that management of them was simple. At six o'clock in the morning the gates to the kraal were opened and the animals were allowed in. At 9 am the gates were shut and no more animals could enter: late-comers had to wait until the following day. The animals remained in the kraal throughout the day and were given supplementary food. At 4 pm the animals were allowed to leave by walking through the crush: animals requiring special attention could be separated and the required treatment given before the animal could leave. The animals came to associate the crush with food and water, and were not shy about entering. The temperaments of the cattle varied from farm to farm – on some the cattle, even the bulls, were quiet and calm, whereas on others as soon as they were handled a rodeo started. I believe that the manner in which they were handled was reflected in their behaviour. The work went more smoothly if the cattle were placid!

Organisation of the laboratory work was much more complicated: everything had to stop when preputial samples were received, as their examination was the top priority. There were sera to be removed from the bloods, cultures to be inoculated, subcultures to be made and agar plates to be examined. Smears had to be made from the cultures, stained and examined under the microscope. It was little wonder that we required more laboratory technicians in the team than vets.

We started the work in the Tuli Block which was only a few hours' drive from the laboratory and where there were farmers we knew. We were able to set up camp near the farmhouse where they had running water and proper lavatories and showers, which made living much easier. From the Tuli Block we progressed to the Molopo where we had a permanent invitation to visit from the manager of the Commonwealth Development Corporation ranch, Tony Clayton. This was a great place to visit as Tony's wife Barbara was a wonderful cook and she always entertained the team to a banquet. We had visited this ranch on one occasion just before a visit from Prince Charles who at the time was Chairman of the CDC: he had expressed a desire to take a horse out into the bush. The quietest horse on the ranch was selected and I was asked to make a 'test drive'. Although I can sit on a horse I am no horseman, but I was able to take 'William' through his paces without falling off. If I could stay on then the Prince of Wales would have no problems. The desire of Prince Charles to ride put the Botswana government in a tizzy – what would happen were he to fall off and break something? The problem was solved by having the Prince fly to the ranch and Dr Alfred Merryweather, the head of the Princess Marina Hospital, was instructed to fly in a separate plane that was so prepared that it could carry a stretcher, if necessary. The plane was filled with splints for almost every bone in the body! They had no need to worry; the Prince had an enjoyable ride out into the country and returned unharmed, and the splints and stretcher were flown back to Gaborone unused. I have always wondered why he called his elder son 'William'.

373

We were now ready for our first foray across the Kalahari Desert. We took the easy drive to Ghanzi, going first to Maun where we stopped for the night before driving to Ghanzi, and setting up the 'laboratory' in the grounds of the Veterinary Office, where Alford camped to look after the equipment. Ken, Varshika and I stayed in the Kalahari Arms Hotel, the nearest thing to a 'Western Saloon', with a hitching post outside to tie up your horse, and a pair of half doors that could swing open in either direction. None of the patrons was carrying a gun! A good comfortable room with an excellent if limited menu was on offer.

This was a trial run to see how the team would cope; only two nearby farms were tested and only a small number of bulls were examined. I worked on the bulls while Ken and Varshika examined the samples: trichomonas was identified on the first farm which made us very pleased with ourselves, so much so that we had a few cans of Castle with our evening meal and decided to go for a walk after dinner down past the store to the airstrip. I do not know what the locals thought of three expatriates strolling arm-in-arm back to the hotel and singing as they went.

Again we cheated – the three senior staff flew back with all the samples on the Barclay's Bank plane on the Wednesday afternoon, while the Land Rover returned with all the heavy equipment across the Kalahari. Little did we know what we were in for! On arrival at the airstrip for the 3 pm departure, the pilot informed us that he could not take off until the temperature had fallen below 40° C. It was summer and afternoon temperatures were often in the mid forties; that afternoon was no exception. An additional problem was that we had to take off by 4 pm in order to arrive at Gaborone before dark, as single-engine aeroplanes were not allowed to cross the desert at night. By 3.45 we were getting very concerned, but in the nick of time the temperature fell below the magic number and we piled into the small plane with me in the co-pilot's seat. We rolled down to the end of the runway where the pilot made his final checks and we trundled off. At the end of the runway was a small house, but our ascent was so slow I thought that we would remove the roof. However, we cleared it with several feet to spare and continued our agonising ascent. I could see why he could not take off with the temperature over forty degrees because the air is so much less buoyant the hotter it gets.

We seemed to crawl up to 6000 feet (only 1500 feet above the ground) where the air was much cooler and we were then able to rise

374

rapidly to our cruising altitude. Problems over! Not so. As we approached Gaborone we hit an electric storm and the plane was thrown around like a cork bobbing in the ocean. I thought I was scared: the pilot was terrified and I could smell the sweat on him; what made matters worse was that President Masire was returning from Maputo after a conference of the Southern African Development Community, the 'frontline states' in the battle against apartheid, and as was always the case when the president was using the airport, it was closed to other users (see the story of the Barries in Chapter 17). The pilot decided to take us to Mochudi where the air was calmer and we pottered around until given permission to land. As we were killing time, an impassioned voice came over the airwaves asking for permission to land: it was denied. Then we heard the pilot say, 'I am making my first flight since passing my test this morning in Johannesburg and I can scarcely control the plane. I intend to land without your permission.' Which he did. What happened to the man I do not know, but in his position I would have done the same thing. We landed safely even if we were all a little green. I am not sure that it wouldn't have been more comfortable in the Land Rover.

We now felt ready to undertake a full-scale team exercise. Stan decided that he would rather hold the fort in Gaborone while the team were sleeping under canvas. He would reserve his field work for the foot and mouth disease vaccine trials in Motopi, where he could sleep in a proper bed and get in some fishing in the quiet periods. It was our policy to try and give all the staff an opportunity to take part in the field work and it certainly helped to build good relationships within the laboratory. To start with I led the team, with either Ken or Varshika leading the technical team, but I later relinquished my position so that the other vets could have a go.

The first large-scale exercise was an all-male affair. We managed to examine ten herds in the five days on the Ghanzi ranches and all went very smoothly. On this occasion we drove in two Land Rovers with Mik to assist me, and Leonard and Emmanuel working with Ken. We drove straight across the Kalahari, stopping at Kang to fill up with petrol and to camp for the night. Kang is about the only settlement on the road after Orapa until you get to Ghanzi. It has an amazing store in the centre of the desert run by an Afrikaans couple who managed to survive about ten years in the place and, having made their money, sold up to another Afrikaner and moved back to

South Africa. They stocked almost everything, including spares for many makes of vehicles together with a great variety of food. When we arrived there was a sunburnt European sitting under the shade of a thorn tree while he worked on some part of his Land Rover. We asked him what the problem was and could we help. With a shake of his head he replied that there was nothing we could do as the gearbox had packed up and he was waiting the arrival of a new one from Johannesburg. I asked him what he was doing in the Kalahari and he replied that he was making a film for Anglia Television about the bushmen. His was a solo effort because he thought that he would have a better relationship with them if he were alone.

'But how do you communicate with them?' I asked.

'I was born in Ghanzi and spent most of my childhood playing with bushmen children.'

'Then you must speak Bushman,' I said.

'I speak /Gwi [the '/' stands for the click that is the main sound to western ears of the bushman tongue] pretty well and I have a smattering of ...' and he rattled off a whole series of click sounds which I could not catch. He had been working with them for several months and luckily had been near Kang when his gearbox stopped functioning.

'When do you expect the gearbox to arrive?' I asked.

'I have been here for about a week and so it should be with me in a couple more days and it will take me a couple of days to put it all back together again. Time does not bother me, remember I was born in this country. It costs very little to live out in the bush and I am happy just to be back in the land of my birth, to mix with people I have known all my life and just to sit under a thorn-bush and let the world go by.'

We left him to his repairs and set off to find a campsite for the night. We washed while Alford and Jaapi set about preparing dinner. We did not bother about tents as it was only for one night, and we would sleep round the fire. I remembered, with some trepidation, Eddie's story about camping with some bushmen staff near Kang. He was disturbed in the night by a scream from one of the bushmen, who had awoken to find a lion looking at him: bushmen usually sleep under an old animal skin (in this case a bovine). The lion was terrified by the scream, leapt backwards and took off into the bush. The next morning when they examined the tracks they found that the lion had jumped backwards seventeen feet!

As it was our first night out we had steaks cooked over the open fire: meat never tasted better. We were up at 6 am and on the road by eight, and no western eye could have discerned that we had camped in the clearing. With Alford at the wheel the journey to the Ghanzi ranches was uneventful. We drove to the central ranch and there we set up camp upwind of the cattle crush. The whole trip was very successful and completely without incident and so a major visit to the area was planned taking in all three settled areas of Ghanzi.

The colonial racial policies were still manifest, as at Independence the Ghanzi ranches were all owned by white settlers, in the greater part by Boer farmers who, in the late nineteenth century, unable to stand the regulations imposed by their own government in the Orange Free State and Transvaal, had trekked their way across the Kalahari Desert to the good grazing lands of Ghanzi. The British masters of the Bechuanaland Protectorate had allowed them to settle and fence their farms. 'Cape Coloured' people from Cape Province had also migrated across the desert and were allowed to fence their farms at Mamuno, a much less hospitable land than the Ghanzi ranches. Black farmers who wished to have ranches in the area got the worst terrain of all at Metzimanchu (Setswana for 'black water'). I never established whether it referred to the fever of that name, although mosquitoes were uncommon outside the Okavango region, or whether it was the colour of the water that could be pumped from below the surface of the desert.

Although the grazing was good on the ranches, the road to the area was the worst in Botswana, deep, deep sand, where it was possible to get stuck, even in low ratio four-wheel drive. We did, frequently, and had to dig ourselves out on several occasions. Nick Buck of the FAO project had asked us to include Metzimanchu in our testing programme as they had a team stationed on the ranches to help the farmers develop their husbandry and feeding. We decided to do one long trip with a fortnight in the bush, going first to Metzimanchu, then to Mamuno and arriving in Ghanzi on the Tuesday night so that the samples collected and the cultures made could be flown back to Gaborone on the Wednesday afternoon Barclays Bank plane. I decided that we needed three Land Rovers for the journey because the road from Kang to Metzimanchu often only had one vehicle a week passing along it. This was in the days before mobile telephones and at the time the laboratory did not

377

possess a mobile radio. We would be on our own and should disasters befall then we had to have a lifeline back to civilization.

With a large team in three vehicles we decided that we could examine four farms a day, provided that each pair of ranches were not too far apart. Some of the ranches in Botswana were huge, 20,000 acres or more. The CDC Ranch in the Molopo was seventy miles long by fifty wide and it could be many miles between the centres of two neighbouring ranches. Despite the quality of some of the pastures, the land in Ghanzi could only carry one animal to about forty acres, a far cry from the European average of one cow to the acre. We had to carry extra fuel because there was no guarantee of petrol on those ranches between Kang and Ghanzi and low ratio four-wheel drive just drinks it up.

Varshika was again in charge of the feeding and because this team was large we decided to take two days on the journey to Metzimanchu: we drove from Gaborone to Tshane via Lobatse and Jwaneng and camped at the police station in Tshane for our first night. At Kang we left the 'main' Ghanzi track and turned south onto the very wild track to Metzimanchu, which is among the most beautiful areas of bush in the country. Almost immediately we saw a lone male greater kudu with his magnificent curly horns. Instead of running away when we stopped, he turned and looked directly at us as if to say, 'Yes, I am a splendid specimen, and I know it.' This area seemed to be teeming with game animals and we saw herds of impala and springbok, jackals and meerkats. I travelled with Varshika and Selahuru, and the latter was an excellent game spotter, which might have been the reason we saw so much game on this journey.

The journey from Kang to Metzimanchu is about 150 kilometres but it took us almost eight hours to drive because of the deep sandy roads. We saw a dead Land Rover on the roadside with a tree growing through it. Despite the land being flat with very few hills, the countryside in Botswana is never boring as the vegetation keeps changing and there is always the chance of seeing some wild animals. Apart from getting stuck and digging ourselves out, it was a delightful journey and all three Land Rovers made it safely to our destination. We set up camp in the Department of Agriculture Office compound and we were soon enjoying our first beer of the evening. Again Varshika was in charge of the food. It was obvious that her motto was 'simplicity, variety and flavour' and she brought with her several large bags of herbs.

When we started work the next morning it was clear that these farmers had far less money to invest in their farms than the Boer farmers at Ghanzi. However, it was Veterinary Department policy to build crushes around the country and so there was a decent crush in which to take our preputial samples. Diteko and Mik with their team went off to examine a couple of herds during the day and Carl and I set about our herds. The third Land Rover was used for ferrying the samples back to the laboratory established at base camp.

The most noticeable feature of the animals we tested was that they were of much lower quality of breeding compared to those that we had become accustomed to testing, and the quality of handling was very poor. It was obvious that, despite the best efforts of the agricultural advisers, the staff were not used to handling their animals on a regular basis and as a consequence were not very good at the job. It was very lucky that we had lab staff to show them how to do it. Because they were not handled on a regular basis the animals objected to being restrained and we had a bit of a pantomime with several samples being lost as a result. However, the farmers had many fewer bulls and so we were able to complete our allotted tasks.

There was now a Veterinary Officer in Ghanzi called Dr Oistroczech – known affectionately by all staff as Dr Ostrich Egg – but Mr Khumalo was still the driving force in the office and he insisted that whenever we worked on a ranch in his area a member of the Ghanzi staff should assist. This was good for us because they knew the terrain and the farm workers and it meant that we had an extra pair of trained hands to do the job which was invaluable in Metzimanchu. The district staff were happy to be involved because to a man (there were no women then) they were keen to learn and be of value to their community. Working with the laboratory team taught them new skills which they would later be able to use in their routine work. One of the most valuable outcomes to our field work was the team building that resulted, not just within the laboratory staff but between the lab and field workers. This had an additional spin-off in that, because the field staff now knew who was looking at the samples they sent, they began to trust us, which resulted in even more samples coming into the laboratory. This had been one of my justifications for the expenses of the field work.

After two days we set off from Metzimanchu to Mamuno and the ranches owned by the Cape Coloured people. They too suffered from a shortage of capital to bring their ranches up to an acceptable modern standard, but as at Metzimanchu the farmers were keen to improve their skills and the quality of their herds. We received a warm welcome and on arrival we were presented with a freshly killed goat, so we had fresh meat that night. We applied the same system as before, only it was Carl and I and the team who had to travel. Again we had a good crush at which to work and enthusiastic people to assist us. On these fenced farms, in contrast to the cattle posts, the farmers actually lived on the farm and this meant that we could discuss disease control with them.

On our journey from Mamuno to Ghanzi there were again many game animals to be seen and in particular there seemed to be greater kudu everywhere. We arrived in Ghanzi on the Tuesday evening and all the samples for Gaborone were packed and ready to go off on the plane. Three days were spent on the southern Ghanzi ranches and twelve more herds were examined. The senior staff even managed a trip to the Kalahari Arms Hotel one night for dinner and it was a delight to sit at a proper table with a tablecloth and napkins, and to have a glass of wine with our meal. Soon we were back in Gaborone having been on the road for almost two weeks.

I had been asked by President Masire to examine his herd, and since he owned nine ranches in Ghanzi this was work for a single trip. He wanted us to examine his animals in early July, but we made it a principle that we would only examine the herds if the owner was present and so it had to be at a time when he would be in Ghanzi. There was a sound reason for this, because if the owner was not present the staff could get up to all sorts of mischief; it was also essential that the owner be present if important decisions had to be made. President Masire asked if we could start work without him and for him to join us later as he had to host a garden party at State House; to this we readily agreed. When we looked at the dates, the president was due to fly to Ghanzi to join us on the day my sons were arriving from England for their summer holidays. I asked if it would be possible for him to bring Richard and Guy on the plane with him and he told me, 'Dr Windsor it will be a great honour to bring your sons to Ghanzi.'

The boys did not know of this arrangement and I am sure that they would not have agreed to it, had they been asked! They had travelled from school to Heathrow Airport and then an overnight flight to Johannesburg, followed immediately by a one-hour flight to Gaborone where they were expecting a five-minute drive home, a shower and a rest. Instead they were met by Maxine with an overnight bag for each of them and put on yet another plane to cross the Kalahari. Mrs Gladys Masire was kind to them during the flight, giving them fizzy drinks and sandwiches.

There was great demand to be in the team working on the president's ranch and the team was selected from the volunteers on the basis of length of service, so that there could be no complaints. As we had a mixed team we took the long route through Maun, which meant that we did not need to set up camp on the journey and as the ranches were north of the town we had less distance to travel. On arrival the farm manager showed us where the work was to be done and there we set up camp.

The following morning we set to work as there were more than 100 bulls to be tested. Luckily it was winter and so the day temperature did not get much above 35° C. but it was still hot work. In order to be comfortable I wore a minimum of clothes: Kenyan safari boots, no socks, a pair of shorts and a bush hat. Once my back had become accustomed to the African sun I preferred to work without a shirt which only got sweaty and clammy. After an early breakfast we were at work by 8 am; as there was only one crush Mik and I took it in turns to take the samples. We decided to stop for the day when we received the radio message that the president had left Gaborone. The plane should have left at 2 pm but finally left at 3 pm, by which time the team were exhausted. They returned to camp for a bush shower, some lunch and a rest for the remainder of the day, until dinner was served.

State House Ghanzi had its own airstrip which was only a couple of miles from where we were working and so I washed as best I could from a bucket of cold water, put on a clean shirt and set off to meet the president and my sons. When I arrived at the strip it was awash with brass: the Provincial Commissioner with all the lesser commissioners were lined up, together with the commander of the local barracks of the Botswana Defence Force, dignitaries of the various churches, the local mayor and many town councillors, all in their Sunday best; at the bottom of the line was Windsor in his shorts and bush hat. The plane, which was a twin engine military plane with a huge door at the rear to enable Land Rovers and trucks to drive in, lumbered down the airstrip, came to a halt and then taxied to the assembled throng and stopped. The door of the plane opened and a set of steps descended. The first person to appear in the doorway was the president himself; his eyes travelled down the waiting line until they got to me. He then gave a gasp of horror, put a hand to his mouth and said, 'Doctor Windsor! I have forgotten to bring your sons!'

He had obviously been working on this joke on the flight from Gaborone as, with that, Mrs Masire appeared together with Richard and Guy. Ignoring protocol the president and his wife came to me first and presented me with the boys: his personal affairs completed, he then returned to duty and greeted the dignitaries one by one in order of importance. Ceremony over, he again came to me and asked if the boys could stay with him and his family in State House, Ghanzi. I was happy for them to do so as it meant that they would have a proper bed to sleep in and I suggested that, as we were having a dinner in their honour that night, I should bring them to State House once they had eaten.

With that the assembly broke up; the president and his entourage with some of the dignitaries went to State House, the remainder to their various offices or homes, and the boys and I went off to the camp. There I learnt all about their doings during the term, and was told in no uncertain terms what they thought of me for dragging them away from home before they had even been home. This was during a very short period when the boys were at the same school. Richard was four years older than Guy and about to leave his prep school to go to Oundle School – they were never again at school together, as Guy chose to join his younger sister at Oakham, but that is another story. I think that by the end of the safari they had enjoyed themselves and were able to tell their school friends that they had stayed in State House with the President of Botswana. That night grilled steak, potatoes in their jackets, tomatoes and tinned peas was the five-star menu, washed down by the boys with 'Mellow Yellow', their favourite disgusting canned fizzy drink from South Africa. As soon as dinner was over I drove them to State House, knocked on the door and was amazed when it was opened by Dr Masire himself.

The following morning we were hard at work when the president joined us with Guy in tow. While Mik was taking the sample I explained what we were doing and why, how it might be of benefit to him with increased fertility and productivity, and how we were trying to build up a national picture of diseases round the country. The president spent the remainder of the morning with us, and we invited him and his wife and family to join us in camp for dinner that evening. He accepted on behalf of himself but said that his family was not keen on bush life and preferred the comforts of home.

We had delightful evening round the campfire, with the junior staff eventually plucking up courage to speak to their president and finding that at heart he was a simple cattleman like themselves. At the same time the president endeared himself to them by treating them as equals: he really was a lovely man and very different from many African presidents. We had finished with the sampling that afternoon and so all that remained was to tidy up the laboratory work, break camp and depart. When he heard that we were leaving, Dr Masire invited the whole team to lunch the following day, to help us on our way.

Guy had distinguished himself that morning: he had woken long before Richard and went into the kitchen to find the president at breakfast and was invited to join him. To his horror Guy found out that it was grilled liver on the menu, which was a dish he could not abide. To his credit he managed to eat it all and even gave the impression of enjoyment. He was definitely born to be a diplomat.

Lunch the next day was presided over by Mrs Masire and again the junior staff were staggered to be treated as equals by such exalted people. The president explained that there had not been time to slaughter a bullock, which was the normal way of treating important guests, and he hoped that we would forgive him for only serving goat. The meat had been barbecued to perfection and so the team were not only thrilled to be lunching with their president, but thoroughly enjoyed the taste of the food. I had to make a little speech of thanks on behalf of the team, the boys said their own 'thank yous' to the Masires for their hospitality and we set off for Maun.

There had been one black spot during our stay: the farm manager took me aside and asked for my help. He informed me that there had been a spate of 'lion attacks', mostly on one ranch. He did not believe this story but did not know how he could prove that it was not just the staff killing an animal to eat. Strangely it was always a prime bullock, ready for slaughter, and never an old cow that was killed. I thought to myself, how would Holmes approach this? I came to the conclusion that there was only one way he could go about stopping this killing without casting aspersions on the staff – he had to instruct the staff that when an animal was 'killed by a lion', before cutting it up to be eaten he had to be informed of the death. He would then visit the farm with some trackers and once the dogs had had a look and sniff round the animal then they could cut it up and distribute it among the workers on that farm for consumption. This instruction was issued and I heard later that the 'lion attacks' had come to a sudden halt.

There were two beneficiaries from this work: one was the farmer himself, as he was sent a report detailing such problems as he had, together with a list of recommendations; on some ranches follow-up visits were made to develop disease control programmes for the individual farmer. The other was the nation, which also benefited because the Veterinary Department could make plans for development based on a knowledge of the disease status of the national herd rather than on guesswork.

One of our principal findings was that brucellosis was widespread but at a very low level, and as such needed no national input other than that the farmers be recommended to vaccinate their calves between four and eight months of age with the S19 Vaccine. Vibriosis was present and undoubtedly played its part in lowering fertility, but the major problem which was present on almost all the Ghanzi ranches was trichomoniasis. The really interesting finding was that it was not present in any of the cattle in Metzimanchu or Mamuno. Why was this? The question was discussed by us all and the conclusion was that the unaffected ranches were owned by poor people who could not afford to purchase expensive bulls in South Africa but bought and sold among themselves: genetically the bulls were inferior but they were more fecund because they were free from venereal diseases.

However the major disease problem on all the ranches was deficiency of phosphorous in the diet. The soils of the southern African plains (as in the eastern parts of the South American continent) are notoriously deficient in this element, and deficiency is the major cause of infertility in cattle, as was shown by the work of Mike Fortey and the FAO team. For years the Department had been trying to persuade Batswana farmers to supplement the diet of their animals with bone meal, which is rich in phosphorous. The Botswana Meat Commission gave preference in the sale of bone meal to the farmers who supplied the cattle, but many farmers would not believe that it would be of benefit to their cattle and thought it was 'just a trick' so that the BMC could sell its waste product. There was one Ghanzi rancher of British descent who had such severe problems with phosphorous deficiency that his cows were not just infertile but dying. He told me that he could not afford to buy the bone meal. I told him that he could not afford *not* to feed the stuff, and I recommended that he should sell a few of his animals and with the money purchase bone meal for the remainder. Sacrifice a few for the good of the others. He did not take our advice, the animals continued to die, he became bankrupt and had to sell the ranch.

Over the years we carried out surveys on goat diseases, village poultry mortality, and even a survey on donkey mortality. In this way we slowly built up a picture of the national herd and flock health. Where there were problems we would revisit the farm and try to resolve them. Costs were rising and prices were remaining static and so it became more difficult for a farmer to make a reasonable living in Botswana. Consequently the laboratory had an even more important role in helping the farmers to reduce their losses.

Eddie and Jean decided that it was time to move on, and as Dr Diteko had returned from the States having completed her Master's degree there was no reason to seek a replacement, although the swap was not to the benefit of the laboratory. Jack asked me if I would join him in his small animal practice: with a growing family a little extra cash was not to be turned down and I readily agreed. The work was fun and brought me into contact with many senior members of the Botswana establishment. Lady Khama and her family were regular attenders at the surgery. Lady Ruth brought her Maltese terriers, Jackie and Ian brought their Alsatians and the twins brought a great variety of different animals – many, I thought, that they had found in the street. President Masire brought his dogs and waited in the queue, refusing to accept preferential treatment: what other African president would take his own dog to the vets, let alone wait his turn in the waiting room? He really was a delightful man. Festus Mogae, the permanent secretary in the Treasury, and later to replace Dr Masire as president, was a regular attender at the surgery. Archie Mokwe, then the minister for Foreign Affairs also brought his own pets: sometimes he sent his beautiful daughter, who spoke perfect English which was not surprising since she attended an English university.

We saw a wide range of animals, dogs, cats, chickens, budgerigars, snakes, tortoises and terrapins; we even had a human patient! Two Asian men were the last to be seen one evening and when they came

385

in, the first one said, 'My friend Sanjit has been bitten by a dog and we are worried that he might develop rabies. Sanjit, show Dr Windsor where you were bitten.'

Before I could stop him, Sanjit had dropped his trousers, pulled his under-shorts to one side and showed me the wound.

'I cannot tell from looking at the wound whether the dog had rabies or not,' I said. 'You must try to find the owner of the dog and ask the local veterinary officer to examine it. In the meantime you should clean the wound gently with a disinfectant and put a healing cream on it. But I should not worry, there is no rabies in Gaborone.' They went on their way in a cheerful frame of mind and I heard nothing further.

One of the really great deficiencies in our clinical services was the lack of an X-ray machine. With increasing traffic, the number of road accidents was growing at an alarming rate. We reduced and set the fractures as best we could, but the only means of immobilising a limb was to put it in plaster. That is until I met Lech Bazulczuk, a Polish bass singer, whose day job was as an orthopaedic surgeon in the hospital. I asked him to come and show us how to pin and plate broken bones. This he duly did, and there was a marked improvement in the quality of the repair work.

'I could show you much better how to do these things if you came to the operating theatre in the hospital,' he suggested. As a result, when he had an operation that he thought might be of interest, a message would come from the hospital, and if I were free I would cross to the operating theatre, gown and scrub up and join the team. A further bonus for us was that pins, plates and screws were only used once, and we were presented with items removed from patients. Surgical quality stainless steel items are very expensive. The quality of our work improved greatly.

When Jack retired I had to decide whether or not to continue the practice as it would mean converting the garage to provide a surgery. It was the opportunity to make an extra bedroom so that Guy and Richard did not have to share. The changes were made, the practice moved to Tawana Close and Alford became my assistant. After a few months I had a phone call from Larry Patterson, who had been a veterinary officer in Botswana but had moved to South Africa.

'Roger, I am thinking of setting up a practice in Gaborone, what do you think of the idea? I do not want to tread on your toes and so if you are opposed I will drop the idea.'

'By no means,' I said. 'I think it is a great idea; pet owners deserve a better service than can be provided by a laboratory vet in his spare time. If you don't mind I would like to continue with my surgeries, at least until I have recouped the costs of converting my garage.'

'I would want you to continue,' said Larry. 'If I cannot compete with a part time vet working only at the end of the day, I would not deserve to succeed.'

Larry opened his surgery in November 1984, in the centre of the town and within a fortnight, my private work had doubled! It was unbelievable. Larry was very busy and already it was obvious that his practice would be a success, and my work load had increased. There had obviously been an unfilled need. Larry was able to provide the facilities that I was lacking, an X-ray machine and closed circuit anaesthetic machine among others, and we sent our cases to him for examination and/or treatment. The laboratory received a large increase in samples from pet animals.

When Larry went on holiday, instead of getting a locum he asked if he could put up a notice telling clients to bring their animals to me. The first day was utterly amazing. I arrived home at 4.45 pm to start the surgery at 5 pm and I could not believe my eyes – the queue of patients stretched from the garage/surgery down to the gate and out into the street. We saw the last patient at 9 pm that evening and I was completely shattered. For the two weeks that Larry was away, I was run off my feet. The work was exhausting but the rewards were huge; in that two weeks I made more money than working in the laboratory (including my overseas aid top up) for three months. I told Larry that the next time he went on holiday he had to employ a locum, or I would need an early grave.

21

The 'Rainbow Coalition' and the Sign of Four

'There has never been anything like it before, nor will be again.'
Sir Arthur Conan Doyle, *The Sign of Four*

When I joined the laboratory there was only one African veterinary surgeon on its staff – Ignatius Nzinge, who was currently studying in Britain at the London School of Hygiene and Tropical Medicine. The general consensus was that he was a most able young man who, with experience, would make an excellent Head of Laboratory. The powers that be decided that this should not come to pass and on his return from the UK, having distinguished himself in microbiology, within a few weeks of starting work in the laboratory he was moved to the abattoir to understudy the expatriate in charge of meat hygiene. Why is it that bureaucracies never take into account the wishes of their staff members?

When I was promoted to Veterinary Investigation Officer, I was blackmailed into working in the State Veterinary Service Head-quarters with the threat that if I did not do this, I would never run a veterinary investigation centre. I loathed the work which seemed to me not about helping farmers, but more about telling them what to do; coercion rather than persuasion. It also happened to Noah Wekesa in Kenya, who was working as District Veterinary Officer in Kisumu when he was informed that he was to be promoted to Regional Veterinary Officer and would work with papers rather than cattle. It did not work with him, because within a few weeks he had resigned from government and set up in private practice, and it did not work with Ignatius, as he was keen to work with live animals rather than meat. He eventually left and set up his practice in Lobatse, and finally moved his practice to Gaborone. He was probably the most able Head of the Service that the laboratory never had.

Dr Tsholofelo Diteko studied veterinary medicine in Tuskegee University, a well-respected college for black Americans in the United States of America, but returned to Georgia to study for a master's degree in poultry science. When she had completed her studies she came back to Botswana and was sent to the laboratory to replace Ignatius (not a fair swap) with the intention of taking over from me. She was a tall, rather ungainly woman, with a mouth of teeth and unmarried with a young son. She had a rather moody disposition and she was not in good health. We suspected that she had contracted some infection during her second stay in the USA, as she was often suffering from glandular problems which entailed trips to the hospital both in Gaborone and South Africa. She seemed to prefer working in her room rather than partaking of laboratory activities, although when on duty she performed her work adequately. I could not persuade her of the importance of being part of the team, to which she replied that when she led the team they would do as they were told. I was never able to make her see that the role of the good boss was to lead and not to direct. I feared for the future of the laboratory under her direction.

I feared even more when the Mad Matz returned from northern Nigeria. Dr Matz Mosenyane had studied veterinary medicine in Maiduguri in Northern Nigeria, one of the many new, understaffed and underfinanced veterinary schools in that country. He returned as the messiah, the man who would lead his country into the animal health uplands. In short he knew it all: he was a Motswana born and bred: 'I have cattle in my blood.' My secret view was that he had water, or possibly something stronger, on the brain. His first posting was to Serowe, and I wondered if that was a deliberate move to put him in the hot seat, it being the spiritual heart of Botswana. He certainly charged off in all directions – we kept receiving reports of diseases in donkeys and goats, and long verbose dispatchess indicating that the laboratory was not doing its job. He suggested to Jack that he should come to Gaborone and take over from me until it was time for Jack to retire, when he would naturally take over. Pity poor Martin Mannathoko, who had been understudying Jack with great diligence and no little success for several years and came with some gravitas.

'Mannathoko is not a Motswana, he is a Kalanga, what do they know of cattle?' was Matz's scathing comment.

Unfortunately, Matz became a close friend of Diteko, as she was

389

known by most of the staff. It was widely suspected that they were more than good friends. Whether or not she became his mistress, he certainly had a serious and deleterious effect upon her behaviour towards all the staff and the expatriate staff in particular, especially the non-Europeans. Varshika, Monyi and Subathra were often the targets of her ire. Monyi suffered particularly at her hands because although they were both Africans, tall and slim, there the similarities ended – Monyi was graceful and gracious, warm and friendly, and consistently wanted to help and get things done.

The third member of the senior local staff was Mabatho Makobi, who was a very able and hard-working member of the biochemistry team. Mabatho had a degree in chemistry from a Nigerian university and a natural aptitude for the work of the biochemistry section, so much so that we are able to obtain for her a placement for a year in the Biochemistry Department of the Central Veterinary Laboratory in Weybridge, England. She was destined to head our biochemistry section. I do not know what happened in England, but she returned with a baby on her back and a massive chip on her shoulder. She became a close confidante of Diteko and constantly tried to undermine the harmony and working relationships we had so carefully built up. Our 'rainbow coalition' was developing a dark side.

During my tenure at the laboratory we had a very bright young Motswana student, Kereng Masupu, working with us while on vacation from the Tuskegee University Veterinary College. He was very able, but unwilling to learn from expatriate vets who could know nothing about animal disease in his country. He also felt that the world owed him a living and could not understand that when he qualified he would have to work under 'White Domination' as he put it. He returned as a graduate veterinary surgeon and was sent to work in the laboratory but not really part of it, as he was to be Botswana's first veterinary epidemiologist based in the laboratory. Secretly I thought of him as a veterinary *epidermiologist*, as he got under my skin! Had he been sent to me with instructions from on high that he was there to learn, I am certain that the lab staff could have made him a really fine field worker.

I met Masupu, as he was called by all, a decade later when I was sent to Botswana by the Food and Agriculture Organisation to assist in the control of contagious bovine pleuro-pneumonia which had entered the country from the newly independent Namibia. His incompetence cost his country dear, at least 100 million pula. Among his wrong decisions was the siting of the camp about twenty miles from Shakawe, along an unmade sand track. It took the staff at least an hour to get to the main road before they could start work, and even with a four wheel drive vehicle it was possible to get bogged down and have to dig yourself out. All water had to be delivered by tanker, until they built a twenty-mile water pipeline, as there were about 100 men based there and they all had to bring in their food. There was no mains electricity, only a small generator that kept breaking down. There was no telephone and no camp comforts at all. After a week living in a tent under very primitive conditions I decided to move out into the Shakawe Fishing Lodge, a mile off the main road along a well-maintained track: there I had a comfortable bed, a decent light by which to write up my notes in the evening, good food and cold beer. It would have been a simpler task to establish his base camp at Shakawe, on the main tarmac road, where there was a well-equipped veterinary office with telephone and radio, powered by mains electricity; where there were shops, cafés and bars. But that was the reason for putting the camp in the bush – he did not want the team to get drunk in the bars of Shakawe. Instead they got drunk in the camp where there were no police to stop the fights.

For many years Botswana had had a policy of building long permanent fences to stop the movement of cattle and so contain foot and mouth disease to the north of the country: they had worked brilliantly, despite upsetting the open-toed sandal brigade. Masupu decided that they would use fences in the control of pleuro-pneumonia. He did not realise that the fences designed to stop foot and mouth disease were in place when the outbreaks started. His main, very sound, intention was to stop the disease moving south into the rich cattle country of Ngamiland, but there were other good ways of stopping the movement of animals and preventing the spread of disease. In all, he built three fences in succession, diverting men, money and resources from disease control, and before each was completed the disease had already crossed it. As in earlier years he was impervious to advice. Instead of slaughtering the disease the moment it appeared he kept the animals alive, so allowing them to spread the infection, all the time hoping to receive authority to move them to the Maun abattoir and so save money. Authorisation never came and all the time the disease was moving on. It was such a waste; so much talent that could have been of real benefit to his country. He made up the four who wanted the expatriates out.

391

And then Matz hit the headlines. He was very friendly with a Kenyan surgeon in the Princess Marina Hospital. They regularly drank, or more accurately, got drunk together in the bar of the Holiday Inn. On one particular Saturday evening they got very drunk and started boasting about the women they had slept with; the Kenyan, to top the argument, stated that he had slept with Matz's wife. This precipitated a punch-up and they were ejected from the hotel.

On the Monday morning Matz was in the office of Kevin Cullinan, Head of the Criminal Investigation Department of the Botswana Police, demanding that the Kenyan be deported. Kevin the Irishman was a master diplomat and said to Matz, 'On what grounds do you think we should deport him?'

'For fighting in public,' came Matz's reply.

'Those would only be grounds for deportation if the police had been involved and he had been found guilty of a serious offence.'

'Well then what about carrying out abortions? That must be a deportable offence.' Carrying out abortions was a criminal offence in those days.

'I do not think that he has been prosecuted for that,' came Kevin's reply. 'But why, if you have the evidence, do you not report him to the police? Just go down to the police station in the village and lay a complaint.'

But Matz did not do that. Instead he wrote a letter to the local newspaper, alleging that the surgeon in question had been carrying out illegal abortions. I suspect that he must have had a friend in the paper or they would never have published such a potentially libellous article. The fat was in the fire: the surgeon sued for libel and Matz then had to prove his case in court.

He did not have much of a case and the public were eager to hear what he would say to the High Court in Lobatse, because surely he would not dare to lie to the court. He did worse: he put his wife into the witness box to fabricate a story that the surgeon had aborted her baby. The lawyer for the surgeon tore her testimony to shreds and the whole case collapsed. Substantial damages were awarded to the surgeon who left court without a stain on his character.

In most countries this would have finished Matz as a candidate for a senior civil service post, but not in Botswana, which was so short of trained people that it needed everyone, even the nutcases. When Jack retired, Dr Mannathoko was appointed Director of Veterinary

Services, but only for a couple of years before he was made chairman of the Botswana Meat Commission, the company responsible for the abattoirs and the export of all beef and beef products. And so Matz became Director of Veterinary Services and, as I was not prepared to work under him, I left the country at the end of my contract.

As director, Matz represented his country at meetings of the International Organisation for Epizootic Diseases, whose head-quarters were in Paris. I was at a meeting of the Society for Tropical Veterinary Medicine in Puerto Rico where I delivered a paper on the economics of veterinary laboratories with reference to Britain, Botswana and Peru. A delightful Trinidadian came up to me and introduced himself to me, telling me that he was the Director of Veterinary Services. He asked if I had been in Botswana when Dr Mosenyane was Director. I said yes and that he was the reason I left the country. I was given a tirade on this dreadful man: his behaviour at the meetings was fine in the mornings but he used to overindulge himself at lunch time and would then interject rude comments during the afternoon sessions, causing much embarrassment to his black colleagues. One day the Director of Veterinary Services for Trinidad could stand it no more and before the afternoon session began, he and a group of fellow black directors took Matz aside and told him he was a disgrace to the black community, that his behaviour was appalling and that if he did not shut up they would get up a motion to ban him from all future meetings. The Mad Matz said not another word throughout the remainder of the meeting.

I do not know whether or not his behaviour in Paris was the final straw that caused his dismissal, but when I revisited the country many years later for the pleuro-pneumonia outbreak, I had a meeting with President Masire in his office in State House. The first thing he said to me when he came into his office where I was waiting was, 'And how are Richard and Guy?' His next remark was, 'You will be delighted to learn that we have sacked Dr Mosenyane and sent him to teach at the Botswana Agricultural College.'

I did not think he would make a very good role model for his students, but did not say so. I was also a little surprised to find that he was still alive, for he was very promiscuous, and Dr Diteko had by then died from AIDS.

I was saddened to hear of Diteko's death, she was not a bad woman and could have been a good scientist; she had the misfortune to fall under Matz's spell and so learned to think that the only criterion necessary to run the laboratory was to be a Motswana. She did not want the post for what she could do for Botswana, or even for enriching herself. She wanted 'power without responsibility', the prerogative of the harlot throughout the ages.

Thanks to her malignant misrule, the laboratory had to be re-colonised. A team of Ghanaians were brought in, the same people who had visited the laboratory for the African Development Bank; they quickly returned the laboratory to what it had been. The export of meat to Europe was worth so much to the country that the laboratory services had to be maintained at a very high level.

In addition to the senior staff, the laboratory was blessed by a team of excellent young and not so young junior staff. Following the African tradition, the elders will be described first, and the doyen of them all was Mr P. Mpetholang, I never really knew what his job was but he was the marshal who organised the junior staff. He was small and grey-haired with big spectacles and a perpetual smile. He was never flustered or upset and was unfailingly polite and courteous. He treated all men alike and he had the happy knack of getting his staff to work for him. He was greatly respected by all and the expatriate staff held him in high esteem. Many, including me, had a great fondness for him as he had all the virtues of a good man: he was dependable, reliable, honest and truthful. Another of his endearing features was his ability to take the mickey out of the senior staff, particularly the expatriates, without ever crossing the line.

He and Jaape Khatola were great pals; the latter was not really a Motswana but a South African 'coloured', and Jaape could cook. No team left the laboratory for a prolonged field visit without Alford the driver and Jaape the cook. He was the master of the three-legged or black pot and out in the bush he could turn out the most delicious home baked bread, a good cooked breakfast and a warming nutritious stew with potatoes baked in the ashes, for the cold winter evenings. When we set out for the day's work, little old Jaape, small and wizened and looking much older than his years, would tidy the camp, wash the clothes, get in the firewood and get everything ready for the evening meal. He would then sit in a camp chair and I think that he emptied his mind and went into a sort of trance. Like pressing the remote control, at the sound of the returning vehicle he would spring into action. The fire would be restored to life and water heated for us to wash.

After a field shower and clean clothes, the team would sit round

the fire with their first beer of the evening and discuss the successes
and failures of the day. There were always cold beers because when a
field trip was planned, Alford would bring large blocks of ice from
the abattoir. These would be stored in the minus 70° C freezer until
required and taken to the field in a large polystyrene foot and mouth
vaccine box. The beer was put in for an hour or so before use, and
cold beer would be available for about ten days. Neither Alford nor
Jaape were drinkers but a cold Fanta or Coke was never refused. A
tot of whisky added to the evening Nescafé was a sure recipe for a
good night's sleep. Alford and Jaape between them were adept at
putting up and taking down the tents and returning the campsite to
bush; the rubbish was burnt and buried.

There is no doubt that conditions for the field team were luxurious
but we worked hard, often for long hours, in temperatures that could
be over 40° C. It was Jack's view that you could not expect a man or
woman to slog it out in the heat all day and then come back to camp
and set to and cook dinner. Alford and Jaape were worth their
weight in gold. Alford was also very good at handling animals and
when I took over Jack and Eddie's small animal practice, Alford
came to assist me with the surgeries: he soon made himself indis-
pensible. When Larry Patterson set up in Gaborone, he asked me if I
could spare Alford to join him. As this was a permanent full time
position I was happy for Alford to leave me.

Another senior member of the junior staff was David Keatimilwe,
short and rotund and always with a smile on his face. David was a
laboratory bench worker who had not the basic education to enable
us to get him further training, and as he said, 'I am too old to go
back to school.'

But he was dependable, reliable and once he had been taught a
task he would carry it out perfectly every time. He spent his time in
the Meat Hygiene Section 'plating out' cultures (taking a small
amount of sample and putting it onto plates of nutrient media to
ascertain if there were bacteria present) from the samples received
from the abattoir. He could be quite aggressive if he thought that he
was not receiving the proper treatment from his bosses and although
not a 'union man' he knew his rights. I respected him for it and we
developed a very warm relationship, such that when I visited the
laboratory many years later he gave me a ten pula note to keep as a
memento of Botswana: It is in my wallet to this day.

We were blessed with some beautiful young ladies who had brains as well as looks. Doris Kupe was the pick of the bunch, extremely attractive, very clever and hard working. She also studied at the Central Veterinary Laboratory in Weybridge but returned to us better trained, better informed and totally enchanted with her stay in England. Despite all Mabatho's blandishments she remained a member of the team until she was enticed away by a private company working in the Mkhadikhadi Pans who wanted her to run their simple laboratory. They paid her twice what the government did and so it was small wonder that she went: she went with our blessing. I was never one of those people who felt that as the government had paid for staff training they should stay through thick and thin. My view was that so long as they remained in the country and worked at what they had been trained to do, then they remained an asset to the country. Doris was such a one: sadly she had a boyfriend who was two-timing her with half the women in the village and he gave her AIDS. And so a beautiful, intelligent and educated young woman died.

Batswana men expected their wives to be faithful while themselves carrying on as they wished, and Thuli Lela who was another beautiful bright young thing also suffered. We sent her off to Swaziland to study on their laboratory technicians course, where she performed exceptionally well. When she returned, things were not well at home as her husband had been two-timing her while she had been away, and was continuing after her return. One morning she came to my office with red eyes. I sat her down and asked her to tell me what was wrong, and that opened the flood gates. There was a knock at the door and Mr Reuben, the storekeeper, barged in. I asked him politely to leave.

'But Dr Windsor I just want you ...'

I cut him off with, 'Mr Reuben can you not see that Mrs Thuli and I are having a private conversation and that she is rather upset. Please leave.'

'But Dr Windsor I just want ...'

'GET OUT,' I shouted, and he left. I rarely raised my voice with the staff, but on this occasion I did so, not for me but for Thuli. Mr Reuben reported me for racialist behaviour but his complaint was not upheld.

I was able to try and comfort Thuli and make her understand that the laboratory was with her and we would help her in any way we could. She was popular with the staff and within a few days they brought her back to her usual cheerful disposition.

Thuli's colleague was Martha Phiri from Lesotho, who had studied with her in Swaziland, where she met and married a Motswana. Martha was almost the opposite of Thuli; she was large and slow, and although very intelligent and able she gave the appearance of being rather dozy. The two were close friends, I suspect from the experience of being travellers in a foreign land. Both worked in the Food Hygiene Section, examining samples from the abattoir.

It was winter, and the mornings were quite cold: it was not unusual for me to arrive at the laboratory to find a line of junior staff leaning against the wall of the reception, which caught the first rays of the sun and so warmed up quickly. I referred to them as lizards, sitting on the wall to imbibe its warmth; they laughed and continued with the practice so long as the mornings were cold. One early morning Martha had a beakerful of alcohol which she was heating over the Bunsen flame with no asbestos mat under the beaker as protection for the glass. Of course it broke and the burning alcohol ran all over the bench and down on to her lab coat, and she went up in flames. Luckily, Godfrey Ndlovu was in the laboratory, saw what had happened, pushed her to the floor and rolled on top of her, so extinguishing the flames. His prompt action probably saved Martha from serious burns and scars. Thereafter she looked more favourably on Godfrey, who was a hard task master and stickler for getting the work done properly.

Godfrey was small, intense and had a great sense of right and wrong. He knew that he was good and yet at the same time knew his limitations. We considered that he was the man to head up the Food Hygiene Section and he did not let us down. He was sent to the Grimsby College of Food Technology where he studied for the Higher National Diploma and performed spectacularly well. I visited the college when he was a student there, to be informed that he was the star student of the year and easily outperformed all his British colleagues. I took Godfrey out to lunch in a local pub where we discussed his studies and his future. I asked if he would care to go to veterinary college with a view to joining the veterinary staff; we were always on the outlook for potential vets. Godfrey declined. His reason was that he felt that he would make a good leader in the Food Hygiene Laboratory but that he would always feel uncomfortable trying to go beyond his capabilities. Godfrey passed 'with honours', as top of the class and returned to work in the Food Hygiene Section where he and Varshika made a very good team; each having great faith in the ability of the other.

We were receiving great numbers of tins of corned beef and numerous large catering packs of tinned tongues which were being dished out to members of the section after the work had been completed. Ken thought this most unfair and a system of 'selling' the tins was started. Members of staff were invited to buy tins of corned beef for about 10 thebe (5p) a tin and a tin of three complete tongues was sold for a pula (about 50p). My children became sick of corned beef hash and tongue salad. The money raised was put into the 'staff party fund' and used to pay for food and drink at staff parties. The staff accepted this change as all thought that it was fair and in the end everyone would benefit from the money raised. Blood and bone meals were also sold to the staff although only the senior staff purchased them as fertilisers for their gardens.

Lee Masilomanthe was a tall, thin young man and the son of the headmaster of Thamaga Secondary School. He was friendly, outgoing and very capable. But he was my one real training disaster. I had heard of a laboratory training course in Norwich, where I had started my career in the Veterinary Investigation Service. Lee would be able to do his practical work in my old laboratory, where there were still many friendly faces and people who would care for his development and welfare. All started well and reports came back from Norwich that Lee had settled in, making good progress and enjoying himself. Imperceptibly things began to change, and one of the vets in the Norwich Centre wrote to me and said that Lee had started not turning up for classes and was behaving strangely. This preceded a complete mental breakdown. By English standards Norwich is a small city but it is much larger than Gaborone, with more bustle, more activity and traffic, and of course there were few black people. Lee became more and more isolated and yet unable to tell his troubles to the staff in the centre. He had to be sent home and it was a shadow of the young man we had sent to England who returned. I am not sure that he ever made a complete recovery and he certainly never worked at the laboratory again. He was not dismissed, he just left.

He was sent to Johannesburg for psychiatric investigation and treatment and I spent a great deal of time with his father trying to plan what we should do. I felt guilty about his breakdown, feeling that we should have noted something in his make-up that might have made us think twice about subjecting him to the strains of living in Britain, but he was so bright, cheerful and outgoing. Of all the people that I have been responsible for sending overseas, he was the only one who cracked under the strain. Staff management is part of the responsibility of running a laboratory and a vital task it is; being the boss, a teacher, a leader, a social worker and sometimes a banker is what makes the job worthwhile.

There were so many bright young people: there was Korapetse Magama who was always looking for a man but she was so choosy that no one ever measured up to her high expectations and she remained unmarried. She was the snappiest dresser in the laboratory and wore the shortest skirts and with her large bust, many of the young Africans (and not a few of the older Europeans) lusted after her, but she was having none of them. As far as I know she is single to this day and remains free from the dreaded AIDS.

Botswana has a serious AIDS problem which is not entirely of its own making. Heavy trucks from South Africa, Namibia and Angola pass through Botswana on their way to Zimbabwe and the copper belt in Zambia. There is a body of opinion that believes that AIDS was brought back to Africa by black West Indian prostitutes who followed Castro's Cuban Army into Angola when they were helping the communist government defeat the insurgents. Whatever the truth, the young people of Botswana paid a heavy price for this lorry transport. The drivers were away from home for long periods and there were always local girls at all the truck stops who would provide for their needs for a small fee. Monogamy is not the norm among Batswana men and they soon spread the virus far and wide.

We had a second Magama on the staff and she was known to all as Mamma. Only a little older than the others, she was married and a mother and she tended to mother all the young bachelors on the staff. She was kind and gentle, small and quiet, and just got on with her work in the bacteriology laboratory. She seemed older than her years but that was probably because she was more mature: families bring responsibilities. Because of her family commitments she was not keen to travel abroad for training, but we pointed out that if she did not then all the young people who had been trained would return and she would have to work under them! We found her a place on the training course that I had set up in Kenya fifteen or more years before, so that she was not too far from home should she need to

399

make a rapid return. The two Magamas worked together and, despite their differences in outlook, they were good colleagues and made a good team.

The junior staff – the ones who cleaned the laboratories and offices and did the washing up and made the media, tidied up and cleaned in the post mortem room – were mostly a jolly crew. Some would remain cleaners throughout their careers; others would join a training scheme and progress. In the washing up and preparation room there were Dorcas and Joyce; Dorcas was big, old, fat and slow whereas Joyce was young, small, slim and bright, and they were both totally dependable. Their work was always done on time and to a very high standard. Ken and Mike had drilled into them the importance of their work; how vital it was that bottles were properly rinsed after washing and that short cuts were not to be taken. Too often shoddy work is not the fault of the one who does it, but of the manager who has failed to lay down the rules and the guidelines. Dorcas and Joyce took a real pride in what they did and were always seeking to improve. They cherished every complimentary word they received.

There was a bunch of young men who were training to be laboratory technicians. Most had studied to be veterinary assistants on the course at the Botswana Agricultural College and had been sent to the laboratory on graduation. Geoffrey, of the funny fingers, Gift, Linchwe (the nephew of the Chief of the Bakgatla people), Robert Mackenzie, Sam Norris (both true Batswana), and Sehularo did not achieve the same high standards as Dorcas and Joyce but then Stan was not such a stickler for performance as Ken and Mike. Did it really matter if there was still some clotted blood on the post mortem room wall? Or if the knives were not of cutting quality? We could always sharpen them ourselves. They were young and enthusiastic and willing to learn, if somewhat slapdash in their approach to the work. There was something different about Sehularo: a spark that stood him apart from other young trainees, and so he was quickly moved into the bacteriology section where Ken and later Varshika could keep an eye on him and set him on the technician path.

The administrative team are an essential part of any laboratory and to start with we only had Magdalene Ngwanang (Mma Ramotswe!). She was a tower of strength, meeting the clients, booking in the samples, typing the reports, filing the case papers, answering the telephone and directing the calls, and generally keeping the laboratory running smoothly and efficiently. To take the strain off her, a rota of the junior technical staff was established, whose function was to screen all clients coming in, and calling the duty vet when necessary, entering the specimens in the diagnosis books and delivering the samples to the correct section. Despite this, Magdalene was soon over-run with work and so an assistant was employed, straight from the Botswana Secretarial College. Unlike Mma Makutsi in *The Number 1 Ladies' Detective Agency* Scholastica Mabeo had not gained ninety-seven percent in the final examination, but she was keen, enthusiastic and willing to learn. She was small, bright and attractive. Unfortunately she wore very low cut blouses without a bra, which meant that her large breasts were frequently on display, which was a great attraction to the young men and a great distraction to me when I was giving her dictation!

The store-keeper Reuben was a mature man, who had been brought up in the civil service and was stickler for routine and rules. He kept his store neat and tidy, and with Ken's guidance became proficient with storing and issuing all the chemicals, media and equipment. He was full of his own importance and treated the junior staff with disdain, and so he thought that I should deal with his requirements before those of Thuli. I prefer people who can deal with junior staff in the same way that they treat their bosses. After the altercation in my office Mr Reuben was moved to head office and replaced by Victoria Dikhudu, a young and very polite young lady who learnt quickly under Ken's tutelage.

All in all it was a happy team who pulled together for the good of their country and they also enjoyed themselves. We had a real rainbow coalition – Batswana, British, Dutch, Kenyan, Lesothan, Norwegian, Rhodesian, South African, Sri Lankan, and Tanzanian, and the relationships were warm and friendly. The laboratory in Botswana had never before had such a mixture of people. It has always been my belief that a good joke and a hearty laugh makes the serious work easier to perform and that people perform better in a happy and relaxed atmosphere. And I wanted the staff to take responsibility for their own work, so that they could be proud of their own achievements.

It was this happy band that Matz, Diteko, Mbatho and Masupu set out to destroy.

One of the shortcomings of Botswana was a lack of trained personnel; in a country of only a million people it is difficult to fill all the

401

management and professional posts. It is also impossible to staff a veterinary school in a country with only thirty veterinary surgeons, never mind the costs of running such an institute. With fewer than a dozen hospitals and only one veterinary laboratory, it is not economic to set up an institute to train laboratory technicians.

With the lack of basic training of most of our staff it was not possible to find training places for them overseas and so the first essential was to persuade the Botswana Technical College to set up such a course for laboratory technicians that would give them adequate qualifications to gain entry into further training outside southern Africa. The college was very keen to assist, provided that we would do some of the teaching, and Ken, Mike and Varshika readily agreed to help. So we had started on the road to providing the laboratory with a cadre of well-trained laboratory staff. With their qualification from the BTC our students could gain admission to training courses in Britain or the USA. In my view one of the major functions of an expatriate worker is to teach the local staff, and work himself out of a job by training them to replace the foreigners. The laboratory needed people to work in bacteriology, biochemistry, food hygiene, haematology, histo-pathology, parasitology, toxicology and rabies; and Botswana needed a supply of enthusiastic, well trained veterinary surgeons.

It was not the job of the laboratory to identify good candidates to study to become veterinary surgeons, but the country had a desperate need to replace the expatriates in the department. Many graduates of the Livestock Officer Training Course at the Botswana Agricultural College spent a month or so in the laboratory before they were posted to their districts and it was easy to identify the good ones. Three of those who passed through the laboratory as well as our own Sehularo eventually went on to veterinary schools round Britain. Sehularo was sent to the Polytechnic of East London (now the University of East London) and as with Godfrey, so with Sehularo. When I visited the college during his studentship, I was informed by his teachers that he should be studying for a veterinary degree. This was duly organised and Sehularo successfully completed the veterinary degree in my old college in Edinburgh.

It was the job of the laboratory, and indeed of all aid projects and possibly all academic institutes, to train their staff: it is also important that the needs of the department are matched to the ability of the staff and so it is important to select the correct courses for individual members of staff. Although we wished to end up with a laboratory staffed by high-quality veterinary surgeons and laboratory technicians, it was essential that the correct course be selected for the student. We have seen what happened when Lee was sent into an environment where he was out of his depth. In order to determine the needs of the individual person, all the junior technical staff were issued with a 'Technical Manual' showing what techniques they were required to master in each different section of the laboratory. Once the staff member was proficient in a technique the head of the section would sign that technique in the manual, indicating the level of attainment. Every four months these junior staff members rotated round the different sections and in two years each was expected to know all the basic techniques of the laboratory to the extent that they could perform the test unsupervised. These manuals were used to determine the training needs of the staff members.

Over the six years that I was in Botswana many different training institutes were used for our staff. These included:

The Botswana Agricultural College
The Botswana Technical College
The Botswana National Health Institute
The Botswana Secretarial College (we did not forget our administrators!)
University of Botswana
University of Swaziland
Nairobi Technical Training Institute
Central Veterinary Laboratory, Weybridge, England
Brooklands Technical College, England
North East Surrey College of Technology, England
Grimsby Technical College, England
The College of Food Technology, Norwich, England
North East London University, Stratford East, England
University of Edinburgh, Royal (Dick) School of Veterinary Studies
University of Liverpool Veterinary School
University of Iowa, at Ames, USA
University of Georgia, at Athens, USA.

Not only were our staff trained in many different institutes in three different continents, but the senior staff of the laboratory were also heavily involved in training students in other institutes and disciplines. The laboratory was regularly visited by parties of students from schools, colleges, universities and places of work, to see what we were doing in the battle to control animal disease. It was this happy industrious team that the 'Gang of Four' set out to destroy.

22

Windsor's Castle

'It has long been an axiom of mine that the little things are
infinitely the most important.'
Sir Arthur Conan Doyle, *A Study in Scarlet*

The second major shortcoming of the laboratory was the lack of
laboratory space: with the increasing workload, and more people
working, there was a pressing need for, among other things, proper
accommodation for laboratory animals, where they could be kept
and bred under the optimum conditions. We could no longer make
do and mend. There had been plans for a new building since the
laboratory had been moved from Mafeking to its temporary
accommodation in the asbestos sheds that comprised the government buildings. Each new laboratory head had designed his own
ideas and some had even been given to architects but none had gone
further, as Jack had not been happy with the performance of the
laboratory. In any case, a new laboratory would take several years to
accomplish and we needed space now!

I persuaded Jack that a couple of Portacabins would solve our
immediate problems and we set to, designing a modern animal
house. In one half there would be breeding and rearing facilities for
mice and guinea pigs; in the centre were food storage and cage
washing facilities; and there would be a much smaller section to
accommodate experimental animals. The second Portacabin was to
be used as a media kitchen in which media and reagents could be
prepared and sterilised.

The Portacabins were designed to our specifications and were
soon in place, reducing the size of the car park. We decided, for
security reasons, that the mice being used for the diagnosis of rabies
would continue to be housed in the rabies laboratory. At the same
time we set up a trial to see whether or not we needed to use mice
for all rabies diagnoses. After two years the results showed that in

405

all cases where the brains were adjudged positive in the smears it was not necessary to use mice to confirm the diagnosis and so the practice was discontinued. The old animal house was divided in two and one room was used for Elspeth to undertake the serology tests that were needed. The second was used to house laminar flow cabinets which enabled us to have greater control over sterility when examining products and other samples from the Lobatse abattoir.

The stimulus for developing the idea of the new laboratory came from an unexpected quarter. The Botswana Vaccine Institute had grown out of its cramped facilities and so a custom-built unit, capable of being used to make other vaccines, was built. For the official opening by President Quett Masire, the owner of the Merieux Institute, Dr Charles Merieux, came to Botswana, and addressed the audience after President Masire had formally opened the building. After the reception that followed, Jack brought Dr Merieux to the laboratory to show him what we were up to: it was almost unheard of for Jack to bring distinguished visitors to see us: we were definitely going up in the world.

After a discussion of the work that the laboratory was doing, a look at our monthly reports, and a tour of the laboratory, Dr Merieux turned to Jack and said, 'I do not know how they can do so much good work in such terrible facilities!' He had been particularly impressed with Ken's explanation of the work from the abattoir and Mike and Varshika's description of the sample from the field trial, together with the work from around the districts. He also expressed his view that our facilities for working with rabies were much too primitive and that he was amazed we had not lost any of our staff to the disease.

Following that visit, Jack gave us the go-ahead to look into the building of a new laboratory: a meeting of the senior staff decided that we would use the design of the man who had preceded Mik Mares. This had progressed as far as an architect's drawing. We asked Ian Cuthbert, who had produced the plan, to come and talk to us. It had been decided on high that the new laboratory would be built at Sebele, on the campus of the Agricultural College and the centre of agricultural research in Botswana. It is my preference to put veterinary diagnostic laboratories in the middle of towns or cities, where there are good communications, road, rail, and postal, and where there is little risk of farm animals being infected by the escape of pathogens. Sebele was on the edge of Gaborone and within a few years the city was likely to surround the campus.

Ian explained his concept in great detail, from the orientation of the buildings to make the most of the sun's warmth at different times of year to the fine details of our work flow within the site. He held our attention for a long time, and then the questions started, first a trickle and then a torrent. The first thing that he wanted us to do was draw up a list of all the tasks that the laboratory carried out and produce a massive diagram of how these tasks involved the different sections; in that way he could produce a plan of the most efficient layout for the laboratories. Numerous committees were set up, each with responsibility for designing a particular laboratory, the service areas, the offices and outbuildings: almost every member of staff was on at least one committee as it was important for the whole team to believe that they had had a part in designing their new home. It was a mammoth job, but we had a spectacularly successful outcome. Our aim, and their task, was to build a new laboratory that would serve Botswana until the end of the century.

As the design progressed, the laboratory was inundated with visits from structural engineers, mechanical engineers, and laboratory equipment suppliers. In addition to the new laboratory buildings we were to purchase new equipment to put in them and so a further committee was established to look at our needs. It was the dawn of the computer era and so the laboratories had to be provided with computer circuits so that they could be run on a network. It was time-consuming and the routine work still had to be done. Staff members stayed on after closing time to work on the new laboratory, it was all done with good will and was great fun.

The quantity surveyors looked at the finished plans and the equipment lists, and it all came to a grand total of five million dollars: four for the building and one for the equipment. Headquarters staff had been involved all the way and were as keen to see the building go up as we were. How was the government of Botswana going to finance the project? From being one of the poorest nations in Africa, the diamonds and the beef had made the country prosper, and the dynamic leadership of Sir Seretse Khama had prevented the African disease of corruption from taking hold; after his untimely death his work was carried forward by Dr Quett Masire, but in those days $5 million was a lot of money to spend on a laboratory when the country needed roads and schools and clinics. An approach was

407

made to the African Development Bank, in Abidjan, Ivory Coast, and the Botswana government was invited to send a delegation to present our case. With a team from the Ministry of Finance I flew to Abidjan and while I did the rounds of the agricultural and veterinary advisers the money men talked to the financiers.

After finishing at the bank on the first full day, I went for a walk in the city: the old part was very French with wide boulevards lined with trees but it was the new part that really attracted me. I am not normally a fan of modern architecture but there was real style to the new buildings and they complemented the environment perfectly. I persuaded one of my Motswana colleagues to join me for dinner and we took a taxi to the coast. There were numerous beach cafés where they grilled freshly caught fish and shellfish, and for a few dollars we had a feast.

On the final day of our time in Abidjan there was an open meeting of all interested parties, at the conclusion of which we were told that the Development Bank was interested in supporting us and would send a team to Gaborone to investigate the project on the ground.

A few weeks later we were visited by a delegation of Ghanaian veterinarians from the bank, led by Dr Emanuel Adom. We all thoroughly enjoyed the visit and towards the end of their stay I was taken aside by one of the bank team, Dr William Amanfu, who said to me, 'Roger, this is a really great project and the bank will definitely be supporting the work; however, your government should not ask for a commercial loan, they should apply for a Nigerian Trust Fund Grant, which has better terms.'

The government took this advice and within a few weeks we heard that the Trust Fund Loan had been approved.

We decided to break up the equipment lists into 'packages' of related items to give the small Botswana companies a chance to enter the bidding. The African Development Bank ruled that all purchases had to be put out to international tender. The tenders for the construction and the equipment were advertised in the international press. We received two bids from Botswana to put up the building – one from an international company based in Gaborone and one from a small African building company – and four bids from South Africa. Although we wanted to give the contract to the small local company we were certain that they would not have the financial strength to complete the contract; the international company made a very competitive offer and was selected as our preferred candidate.

Once we had completed our assessment of all the bids we sent our evaluation to head office, where they checked our arguments and our figures before passing it on to the Ministry of Finance: our team had done their work well and it was all accepted by the bosses. The African Development Bank was informed that we had completed our evaluation which was sent to them, and in due course we received an invitation to visit Abidjan to obtain their approval and consent to proceed. We returned with the loan agreed and authority to proceed.

There was great excitement among the staff as the building went up: Wade Adams who had won the contract were extremely efficient and had as their clerk of works Alan Rice, who was an absolute tartar; any sloppy work had to be replaced and on one occasion a whole section of the exterior wall had to be demolished and rebuilt. As a result of his efforts we received a superbly constructed building that has withstood the test of time; I cannot remember there being a single construction defect. The ground around the building was landscaped and trees planted, even the car park trees to shade the cars from the Botswana sun were in place and beginning to grow. When I revisited the laboratory twenty years after it was built, it certainly passed Ian's criterion that it should look good without a great deal of maintenance. The trees had grown, which gave it an air of permanence. Not only was Alan a great clerk of works but he doubled as a professional footballer and played for the Mochudi Centre Chiefs and is the only white man to have played for the Botswana National Team – The Zebras.

The equipment started to arrive. It was a massive task to unpack it all and to check that the items had not been damaged, and then to catalogue and install it all. Ken had left Botswana and Varshika replaced him in charge of the Bacteriology Section. Alan Whiteland, a friend and colleague from my Kenya days, had been recruited from Vietnam to be the Chief Technical Officer for the laboratory.

Alan and his team did a wonderful job of bringing order to the chaos and getting the laboratories ready for working on the day of the change-over. I had written a letter to President Masire asking if we could call the new laboratory the 'Botswana National Veterinary Laboratory' as presidential authority was required to use the word 'National' in the title of an organisation. To our delight, permission was given. Finally the day came when we turned out the lights in the hospital shacks and moved into our custom-built new and beautiful home. It was the start of a new era.

However, I had learnt by then that my time in the National Laboratory was to be short as Dr Mosenyane did not want my contract to be renewed. He had by now been appointed Director to replace Martin Mannathoko, who had moved to the Botswana Meat Commission, and Matz wanted Diteko to run the laboratory. It took away a difficult decision from me because, much as I wanted to stay to make sure the new laboratory worked well, I was certain I could not work for a man like Mosenyane.

I telephoned the president and asked him to come on an unofficial visit to the laboratory so that I could show him what we had achieved. He thought it better that it be a private visit after working hours, so he came alone with bodyguard Churchill and I showed him all round the laboratory, explaining the role of each of the different sections before we adjourned to my office.

The first thing he said to me was, 'Dr Windsor, I am very sorry that we shall be losing your services as you have done so much for my country, and this building will be a testament to what you have achieved. However, I dare not go against the policy of the government, which is to employ Batswana in the top positions throughout government services. I have no time for Dr Mosenyane, particularly when I compare him to Dr Jack Faulkner who dedicated almost his whole working life to my country: every decision he took was taken to improve the lives of Batswana. However, we have to use such material as we have.'

'I did not invite you here to ask you to keep me in my job, Sir,' I replied. 'I do not think that I could work with a man like Mosenyane who, in the mistaken belief that he knows everything, is unwilling to listen to any other professional and whose decisions are coloured by the nationality of the person offering such advice. Sir, I asked you to come here because I wanted you to see what we have achieved. Our team is a wonderful example of people working together.'

I pointed out to the president our rainbow coalition of Batswana, British, Dutch, Kenyan, Lesothan, Norwegian, Rhodesian, South African, Sri Lankan, and Tanzanian as I wanted him to know that it was possible to weld together a very happy team of disparate peoples if all were working to achieve the same thing. I felt that this was what was needed throughout his country: a country too small to produce all its own civil servants, bureaucrats, scientists, doctors, lawyers and vets, which for years to come would need to recruit staff from overseas. For this to be successful it was essential that the government select Batswana leaders of the right calibre. The later collapse of the laboratory services, and the 'recolonisation' by Ghanaians, proved the value of my words.

We had a delightful chat about his country and the importance of the veterinary department to livestock health. He ended by saying, 'Thank you Dr Windsor for all your services to my country; I hope that we shall see you in Botswana again in the future. I wish you well, wherever you go, and if you should return to Botswana, if only for a short time, I would be most grateful if you would come and see me, to tell me of your doings.' On that happy note we parted, I escorted him to his car and we shook hands. I believe that he understood my vision.

My contract ended just before the end of the children's school term: Maxine had to stay in the country as she was taking her music teaching examination in October. We decided that the children should have a summer holiday in Botswana and I would go home, look for work and then return to Botswana. Two friends had agreed to lend us their houses while they were away on leave. When Alan Whiteland arrived in Botswana to take up his post of Chief Laboratory Technician in the Laboratory, it had been agreed that he could move into our house when we left.

There seemed to be no shortage of overseas posts on the market at the time and so I was not too concerned about finding another job. I made a visit to Onderstepoort to say goodbye to all those people who had been so kind to me, and I was sitting with Farnie Kellerman in his office when the telephone rang. Farnie answered and with a surprised look on his face said, 'It's for you.'

The call was from Tony Irvin, the Veterinary Adviser to the Overseas Department Administration (now the Department for International Development) in London. He had phoned Gaborone and they had told him where I was. He wanted to know whether I would be interested in a job setting up a new laboratory in Arequipa, Peru. I had no idea where Arequipa was, but I had three children at boarding school in England – I was definitely interested in the job. I agreed to go up to see him when I was back in England. Farnie found an atlas and we saw that Arequipa was a city in southern Peru, up in the Andes and close to the Chilean and Bolivian borders: it sounded very interesting.

Back in Gaborone, the next call was from Australia; would I be interested in doing a consultancy for the World Bank lasting ten days in Addis Ababa, Ethiopia? I could easily fit that in on my way home and it would help to pay the children's fares to and from Africa. There was also the possibility that it might lead to a long-term contract. I gave them the dates of my availability, and a contract and a ticket soon arrived in the post. While I was in Onderstepoort I was told that the new veterinary school in Lusaka was still recruiting staff. I mentioned that I could be very interested in a job in Zambia and it was suggested that I should write to Professor Robert Lee, an Irish parasitologist who was dean of this developing veterinary school.

The last weeks in Gaborone were a round of parties, intertwined with handing over the control of the laboratory to Diteko and trying to persuade her that she should trust the staff to do their work, and lead by example and not by diktat. I could see the team so lovingly and carefully built over almost six years being destroyed in a few months. For me the greatest joy would have been to see the new National Veterinary Laboratory going from strength to strength. In fact after its initial collapse and 'recolonisation' the laboratory was handed back to Batswana and when I visited the laboratory again in 2004 it was in excellent health, so much so that a new wing was under construction.

It was sad to say goodbye to Capital Players, where I had spent such happy times, and the yacht club where we had passed such delightful moments sailing in the tranquillity of the Gaborone Dam. I did not say farewell to our many friends, as I would be back with the children and we would save that for when we finally left.

I flew to Nairobi on my way to Addis and spent a couple of days visiting friends. My job in Addis was to design and equip a veterinary laboratory service for the whole country. I was most surprised to be met at the airport by Dr Lindsay Tyler. He and his wife and family had been taken hostage in Ethiopia by the Eritrean Liberation Front while he was vaccinating cattle against rinderpest, and they had spent almost two years living in the bush while waiting to be freed. I was amazed that he had the courage to return to the country of his capture. He told me that although conditions were hard during their captivity, he had never felt threatened by his captors. Food was dire and not in sufficient quantity but they shared the same food as the freedom fighters. His wife had taught their young children to read during their captivity – the only book they had was Williams' *A Field Guide to the Birds of East Africa*.

412

Lindsay took good care of me and I had fun revisiting my old haunts at Debra Zeit and meeting former colleagues and friends. Ethiopia was still in the grips of the communists – the centre of Addis Ababa was full of portraits of Marx and Lenin and was not the happy city I had known a decade earlier.

My journey home was eventful because my flight to Rome was overbooked and so I was put on a flight to Athens with a hotel overnight and an early flight to Rome the next morning, and of course my luggage did not arrive with me. During my stay in Rome I was asked if I wished to be director of the Ethiopian Veterinary Livestock Project, and of course I said yes. My luggage caught up with me and I arrived in England in good spirits, hopeful that I would find a job.

My short time in England was spent visiting family and friends, and trying to find new employment: there was some urgency required, because the school fees for three children at boarding school was more than £7500 a term. In no time the Windsor family were on the plane back to Botswana. The first house that we stayed in was that of some Dutch friends, the Remmenzwaals, and their children Nils and Flora, both of whom were pupils of Maxine. The great attraction of the house to the children was an Apple Mac computer, a rarity in those days. They had great fun, playing computer games other than Pacman and tennis for the first time. But it was the second house that they really enjoyed, that of Al-Noor Manji the current boyfriend and later husband of Varshika. This was their ideal house, full of stainless steel and leather furniture, a dining table with a glass top, and a swimming pool.

All this time I was working on a thesis for a doctorate at Onderstepoort on the Control of Contagious Bovine Pleuro-Pneumonia in Africa. Time ran out. I had not finished the thesis and there was no time in my future jobs to complete the task. It remains unfinished to this day.

I had heard from the dean that the Chair in Pathology at the Veterinary School in Lusaka was available and that he would be very interested to interview me. I phoned him and explained that I could not get to the school, but I was taking the children home via Lusaka where we changed planes. He agreed to come to the airport and carry out the interview in the departure lounge!

We had a hectic few nights partying and saying goodbye to many friends. Maxine had to remain in Gaborone for another month to take her teaching diploma. Then the children and I flew to Johannesburg and on to Lusaka where we had to wait for the Air Zambia flight to London. Professor Lee was in the departure lounge waiting for me; how he got through immigration I do not know, but you could do these things in Africa before the terrorists took over the airports. We adjourned to a corner with a beer – he talked about what he wanted from his head of pathology, and I told him what I could offer in terms of teaching and research, and suggested that detectives make the best pathologists. I was offered the job on the spot. Prof Lee undertook to do all the organisation with the Zambian government. Now all I had to do was convince the Overseas Development Administration that they should support me in Zambia.

I arrived home excited at the prospect of being able to call myself Professor. But a couple of days later I had a telephone call from Prof Lee.

'Roger, we have a problem. You will probably know that the SADC meeting had just ended in Lusaka and that the plane of President Samora Machel of Mozambique was shot down on his way home from the meeting: the plane was crossing South African territory when it was shot down. As a mark of respect President Kaunda has decreed that the Zambian government will make no new appointments for three months. You will be appointed, but can you wait that long?'

I was not at all sure that I could.

Maxine returned from Botswana, flushed with her success in the music teaching diploma: her efforts and our separation had all been worthwhile. We discussed the situation: at a pinch we could pay the fees for the children for a term, but that was all. We visited the schools and explained our position to the head teachers: all agreed that they would do all they could to keep our children at their schools, as all three were performing well in the academic sphere.

Was it to be Ethiopia, Zambia or Peru? We decided that we would take the first job that offered a written contract ... My life as a veterinary detective was about to take another exciting and challenging turn; who knew where it would lead us?

Index

The names of farmers are not included, as many have been changed to protect the innocent/guilty.

415